Pediatric S K I L L S
for Occupational
Therapy Assistants

Pediatric SKILLS

for Occupational Therapy Assistants

EDITED BY
JEAN W. SOLOMON, MHS, OTR/L, BCP

Program Coordinator and Instructor
Occupational Therapy Assistant Program
Trident Technical College
Charleston, South Carolina

Illustrations by John M. Waddill and Graphic World, Inc.

WITH 20 CONTRIBUTORS

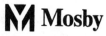 **Mosby**

A *Harcourt Health Sciences Company*
St. Louis   Philadelphia   London   Sydney   Toronto

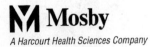

A Harcourt Health Sciences Company

Editor-in-Chief: John Schrefer
Editors: Martha Sasser, Kellie White
Senior Developmental Editor: Amy Christopher
Associate Developmental Editor: Leslie Mosby
Project Manager: Linda McKinley
Project Specialist: Cathy Comer
Designer: Renée Duenow
Cover photos: © PhotoDisc, Inc.

Mosby, Inc.
A Harcourt Health Sciences Company
11830 Westline Industrial Drive
St. Louis, Missouri 63146

Printed in the United States of America

Library of Congress Cataloging-in-Publication Data

Pediatric skills for occupational therapy assistants / edited by Jean
    W. Solomon ; illustrations by John M. Waddill and Graphic World ;
    with 20 contributors.
        p.   cm.
    Includes bibliographical references and index.
    ISBN 0-323-00092-4
    1. Occupational therapy for children.   2. Occupational therapy
assistants.   I. Solomon, Jean W.
    [DNLM: 1. Occupational Therapy—Child.   2. Child Development.
3. Pediatrics.   WS 368 P3713 1999]
RJ53.025P435   1999
615.8′515′083—dc21
DNLM/DLC
                                                                    99-40705

    01   02   03   TG/MVY   9   8   7   6   5   4   3   2

Contributors

KAREN S. CLAYTON, PhD, OTR/L
Program Director,
Institute of Occupational Therapy,
University of St. Augustine for Health Sciences,
St. Augustine, Florida

GLORIA GRAHAM, MA
Adjunct Professor,
Occupational Therapy Department,
New York University;
LaGuardia Community College,
New York, New York

LISE M.W. JONES, MA, OTR, SIPT
Certified Occupational and Physical Therapy
    Supervisor,
League Treatment Center,
Brooklyn, New York;
Private Practice,
Occupational Therapy Coordinator,
The Reece School,
Manhattan, New York

PAULA KRAMER, PhD, OTR, FAOTA
Professor and Chair,
Department of Occupational Therapy,
Kean University,
Union, New Jersey

KATHLEEN LOGAN-BAUER, MA, OTR
Senior Therapist,
Occupational Therapy Department,
St. Mary's Hospital for Children,
Bayside, New York

DIANNE KOONTZ LOWMAN, EdD
Assistant Professor and Director of Academic
    Performance,
Department of Occupational Therapy,
Virginia Commonwealth University,
Richmond, Virginia

PEGGY ZAKS MACHOVER, MA (Psychology)
Consultant,
Life Span Development,
Long Island, New York

CINDY TIMMS MATHENA, MS, OTR/L
Instructor,
Institute of Occupational Therapy,
University of St. Augustine for Health Sciences,
St. Augustine, Florida

PAULA MCCREEDY, MEd, OTL
Clinical Assistant Professor and Academic Fieldwork
    Coordinator,
Occupational Therapy Department,
New York University,
New York, New York

PAULA MURRILL, BA, AS, COTA
Private Contractor,
Charleston, South Carolina

DONNA NEWMAN, BS, AAS, COTA
Instructor,
Westwood College (Formerly Denver Institute
    of Technology),
Denver, Colorado

DAWN B. OAKLEY, MS, OTR/L

Senior Pediatric Therapist,
Early Intervention Case Management Supervisor,
Occupational Therapy Department,
St. Mary's Hospital for Children,
Bayside, New York

JANE CLIFFORD O'BRIEN, MSOT, OTR/L, BCP

Assistant Professor,
Department of Rehabilitation Sciences,
Medical University of South Carolina,
College of Health Professions,
Occupational Therapy Educational Program,
Charleston, South Carolina

GRETCHEN EVANS PARKER, BS, OTR/L

Palmetto-Richland Hospital,
Pediatric Rehabilitative Services,
Columbia, South Carolina;
Ride to Walk Therapeutic Horse Back Riding,
Granite Bay, California

ANGELA M. PERALTA, AS, COTA

Toddler and Infant Programs for Special Education
     (TIPSE),
Staten Island, New York;
Adjunct Instructor,
Touro College,
New York, New York

SHARON KALSCHEUER SUCHOMEL, OTR

Positioning and Mobility Specialist,
Morton Medical,
Neenah, Wisconsin

SUSAN STOCKMASTER, MHS, OTR/L

Charleston, South Carolina

JOYCE A. WANDEL, MS, OTR/L

Director,
Occupational Therapy Assistant Program,
Wright College,
Chicago, Illinois

PAMELA J. WINTON, PhD, MA, BA

Research Investigator and Director,
Research-to-Practice Strand,
National Center for Early Development and Learning,
Frank Porter Graham Child Development Center.
University of North Carolina—Chapel Hill,
Chapel Hill, North Carolina

ROBERT E. WINTON, MD, BA

Clinical Associate,
Psychiatry and Behavioral Science,
Duke University;
Medical Director,
Behavioral Health Services,
Durham Regional Hospital,
Durham, North Carolina

Reviewers

MARY BETH BROCK, MHS, OTR/L
Coordinator of Occupational Therapy Services,
Medical University of South Carolina,
Institute of Psychiatry,
Charleston, South Carolina

ANITA BUNDY, ScD, OTR, FAOTA
Professor,
Occupational Therapy Department,
Colorado State University,
Fort Collins, Colorado

JOANN CLICK, OTR
Occupational Therapy Department Head,
Adaptive Equipment Director,
Occupational Therapy Director,
Grand Junction Regional Center,
Grand Junction, Colorado

MARY BETH EARLY, MS, OTR/L
Professor,
Occupational Therapy Assistant Program,
Department of Natural and Applied Sciences,
LaGuardia Community College,
City University of New York,
Long Island City, New York

CLAUDIA LEONARD, OTR/L
Fieldwork Coordinator and Instructor,
Occupational Therapy Assistant Program,
Western New Mexico University,
Silver City, New Mexico

PAULA MURRILL, BA, AS, COTA
Private Contractor,
Charleston, South Carolina

JANE CLIFFORD O'BRIEN, MSOT, OTR/L, BCP
Assistant Professor,
Department of Rehabilitation Sciences,
Medical University of South Carolina,
College of Health Professions,
Occupational Therapy Educational Program,
Charleston, South Carolina

GRETCHEN EVANS PARKER, BS, OTR/L
Palmetto-Richland Hospital,
Pediatric Rehabilitative Services,
Columbia, South Carolina;
Ride to Walk Therapeutic Horse Back Riding,
Granite Bay, California

JEAN A. PATZ, MS, OTR
Adjunct Professor,
Occupational Therapy Department,
Towson University,
Towson, Maryland

PATRICIA P. SCHAEFER, MHS, OTR/L, BCP
Dorchester School District Two,
Summerville, North Carolina

SUSAN STOCKMASTER, MHS, OTR/L
Charleston, South Carolina

LINDA M. YORK, BS, OTR/L
Lourdes College,
Occupational Therapy Assistant Department,
Sylvania, Ohio

To my family and dearest friends:
I thank you for your love and encouragement,
which gave me the serenity to write this book.

JWS

Foreword

The task of presenting a complex and challenging subject to beginners is seldom easy, and yet Jeannie Solomon and her contributors have accomplished just that. In clear and direct language, *Pediatric Skills for Occupational Therapy Assistants* introduces a specialized practice area that many occupational therapy practitioners and educators have hitherto found daunting. Because it requires detailed knowledge of normal and abnormal development, clinical conditions, family systems, educational and health care systems, and therapeutic use of self, the practice of occupational therapy with children can be difficult both to teach and to learn. Educating the occupational therapy assistant (OTA) student in the subject has been a particular challenge because texts tend to be written for students in professional-level programs or for professional-level practitioners. *Pediatric Skills for Occupational Therapy Assistants* thus fills a recognized need. It facilitates the teaching and learning of a complex subject and provides inspiring, practical advice for students and entry-level clinicians. Further, it is a valuable resource for supervisors in pediatric settings because it clarifies the relationship between the professional and technical levels of practice. The text also recognizes and encourages the development of intermediate and advanced clinical skills by the certified occupational therapy assistant (COTA).

Of particular value in this text is the interweaving of performance context throughout. Case vignettes are drawn from many cultures and many socioeconomic and familial situations, with clinical solutions appropriate for each situation. The context of treatment receives the attention it deserves. In Part One the contributors explore the various systems that provide occupational therapy interventions for children. Placing the concept of *family*

prominently and early in the text prompts the reader to always collaborate with the family. In addition, detailing and clarifying the demands and constraints of the educational and medical systems alerts the reader to the ways practice differs in schools, institutions, the home, and the community.

The chapters on normal development (Part Two), pediatric conditions (Part Three), and the occupational therapy process (Part Four) provide essential information and theoretical foundations without overwhelming the reader with difficult terminology or unnecessary scientific detail. By clarifying ways in which the professional and technical levels of practice are different and complementary, the contributors define appropriate levels of responsibility for the COTA at beginning, intermediate, and advanced stages. Practical suggestions for establishing service competency and managing requests for inappropriate services are provided in Chapter 1 and reinforced by examples throughout the text.

The design and style of the book are highly accessible. The chapters focus on practical themes and are written in practical terms, emphasizing clinical techniques and solutions to commonly occurring problems. Important information is highlighted in boxes and is therefore easily located. "Clinical Pearls" focus on helpful hints for clinical practice; throughout the chapters, contributors list specific suggestions for handling techniques and sequencing activities within a treatment session. Frequent, engaging case vignettes illustrate key concepts. In addition, numerous helpful and attractive photographs and illustrations portray appropriate procedures, positions, devices, equipment, and other resources. Many chapters also include resource lists for further investigation of a topic.

Of particular importance is the respect shown for children as clients and collaborators in treatment. Regardless of the severity of the disability or communication impairment, the authors consistently elicit and address the child's goals and perceptions. The reader cannot fail to get this message. By adopting the child-centered (and family-centered) perspective modeled in this text, the OTA student and COTA are empowered to create effective and gratifying clinical partnerships with children and their families. Thus in many respects the publication of *Pediatric Skills for Occupational Therapy Assistants* is a milestone event for the profession and OTA education.

MARY BETH EARLY, MS, OTR/L
Professor, Occupational Therapy Assistant Program
Department of Natural and Applied Sciences
LaGuardia Community College
City University of New York
Long Island, New York

Foreword

As the field of occupational therapy begins the new millennium, the occupational therapy student and practitioner are endowed with the ability to access theoretical, clinical, and research information from several sources such as books, journal articles, conference proceedings, computers, and the Internet. The maturity of the occupational therapy profession has evolved to include a sizable number of textbooks that have been published to address the various aspects of education, research, and practice. Books for teaching focus on various theoretical foundations that guide practice. They provide occupational therapy students and entry-level graduates with essential assessment and intervention skills that are founded on tested approaches and frames of references. The texts provide interrelated sets of data that form the foundation for occupation concepts and theories. Moreover, the treatises include methods by which research investigations on occupation are conducted. In many instances, these same references also provide relevant information for clinicians beyond entry-level practice.

Another part of the information-explosion phenomenon is the increase in the number of newsletters and refereed journals for health professionals and the health service consumers themselves. Adding to this phenomenon is the increase in number of occupational therapy practitioners who are finally publishing their thoughts and research studies for occupational therapy and other professionals or health service consumers. The profession is beginning to recognize that such journalistic and scientific papers double their exposure when using publications read not only by their occupational therapy colleagues but also by members of other disciplines. The readership then takes on a wider base, comprising educators and health practitioners. On the other hand, evidence exists that

other professionals are writing about the profession, or about the approaches used by occupational therapy practitioners. The interdisciplinary exposure is also evident through scientific papers presented during interdisciplinary and intradisciplinary conferences. Thus the profession that promotes health through human occupation is recognized.

The use of personal computer databases or those of libraries located at institutions of higher learning have facilitated quick access to information. Before computer technology, searching the literature was long and tedious. Because of the new technologies, reviews of primary and secondary literature are done in front of the computer monitor. Therefore the search is much less tedious, and results are obtained much more quickly. As needed, the researcher or student can access full-text versions of research articles through various database collections. Information is also easily accessed through the Internet. Additionally, the databases are available through many universities and colleges that allow limited access to individuals who are not students.

However, this information-explosion era has created a dilemma: finding a way to condense massive amounts of information into the essential facts needed for entry-level practitioners or into a specific reference for students, practitioners, educators, and researchers. *Pediatric Skills for the Occupational Therapy Assistant* provides a resolution for this dilemma. By responding to her needs as an educator, a clinician, and a researcher, Jeannie Solomon has condensed all of the necessary information into one volume for the occupational therapy practitioner. Although the intent of the text is for use in the education of occupational therapy assistants (OTAs), it includes information that goes beyond that initial purpose. It is an excellent reference for occupational therapists who need information on collaborating with an OTA student or practitioner, it is an excellent resource for student learning activities, and it has appropriate information and structured activities that the practitioner can use for collaborating with OTAs and supervising both technical and professional levels I and II fieldwork students.

This textbook is a volume of useful information that drew material from primary and secondary literature sources and then supported that information with its authors' experience in academic teaching, curriculum development, practice, and research. The textbook contributors comprise a national representation of occupational therapy practitioners and related professionals from technical and professional programs, pediatric clinics, research institutions, and other related disciplines. The contributors all have the credentials and experience in teaching, designing, and implementing entry-level education programs for both occupational therapy and OTA educational programs. Clinical practitioners are also adequately represented and provide both scholarly and practical knowledge. In addition, an appropriate mix of theoretical and practical information in pediatric physical and psychosocial dysfunction is presented. From infancy to adolescence, issues associated with clients of all ages encountered in the pediatric clinic are addressed. The text maintains a balance between performance component and occupational performance information within the contexts of human performance as specified by the latest edition of AOTA's "Uniform Terminology for Occupational Therapy Practice." The need for collaboration with the family and an interdisciplinary team is emphasized, and the text highlights the core values, attitudes, and tenets that guide the practice of occupational therapy with total integrity.

Awareness of learning styles and adult learning issues are evident in the consistent formats of the chapters and sections. Each chapter provides concrete and conceptual information, followed by suggestions for learning activities and ways to measure learning. A logical sequence of information gathering, testing, feedback, and more testing is used, which facilitates learning in a safe environment. The approach used philosophically echoes that of John Dewey's but more importantly reflects the basic tenets of occupational therapy.

This scholarly text embodies the response by the author and her contributors to a need for a comprehensive textbook for educating OTAs. *Pediatric Skills for Occupational Therapy Assistants* goes beyond simply responding to that need—it is a salute to collaboration. It is wisdom passed on to a new generation of occupational therapy practitioners who will carry the profession into the new millennium.

RICARDO C. CARRASCO, PhD, OTR/L, FAOTA
Chairman, FiestaJoy Foundation, Inc.
The Foundation for Investigations, Education, and Support in Therapeutic Activities, Inc.

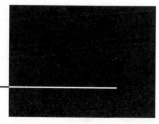

Preface

This book has been written for the occupational therapy assistant (OTA) student and the certified occupational therapy assistant (COTA) working in the pediatric practice arena. The language is consistent with the third edition of AOTA's "Uniform Terminology for Occupational Therapy Practice." The emphasis is on concrete, practical information that may readily be used by OTA students and COTAs who are working with children and adolescents. Because a wealth of information already exists regarding theory, frames of reference and practice models, these content areas are discussed on a limited basis. When possible, the text differentiates between the roles of the COTA and the registered occupational therapist (OTR). The term *occupational therapy practitioner* generally refers to OTRs and COTAs and is used during discussions of procedures that can be performed by either professional.

All of the chapters contain the following elements: a chapter outline, key terms, chapter objectives, a chapter summary, review questions, and suggested activities. The chapter outlines provide the reader with information on the specific topics that are discussed in each chapter. The key terms list contains important words appearing in the chapter that the author would like to emphasize for readers before they begin the chapter. The key terms are listed in the order in which they appear in the chapter. The chapter objectives concisely outline the material the reader will learn after studying a specific chapter. Each chapter has a summary that reemphasizes the key points of the chapter. Review questions included at the end of each chapter will help the reader synthesize the information presented. Suggested activities, which are also included at the end of each chapter, are activities that are to be performed by individuals or small groups of students.

Performing the suggested activities should help reinforce the information learned in the chapter.

Boxes, case studies, vignettes, tables, and figures have been used to reiterate, exemplify, or illustrate specific points. "Clinical Pearls," which are words of wisdom based on the clinical expertise of the chapter author, are also included. The clinical pearls contain helpful hints or reminders that have been consistently useful for pediatric occupational therapy practitioners. Appendixes are included at the end of several chapters of the book.

The book is divided into four parts. The first part of the book is an overall framework for the book. Chapter 1 presents information concerning recommended pediatric curriculum content, selected practice models, and COTA supervision and service competency. The next three chapters of the book present information regarding the systems in which a pediatric occupational therapy practitioner may work. These systems are the family system, medical system, and educational system.

The next part of the book discusses normal, or typical, development using AOTA's "Uniform Terminology for Occupational Therapy Practice" as a guide. Chapter 5 presents an overview of the periods and principles of normal development and also discusses the occupational performance contexts. The next two chapters present information on normal development in the occupational performance components and areas.

The third part of the book presents information on specific pediatric disorders that a pediatric occupational therapy practitioner may encounter. The first two chapters discuss single diagnoses, cerebral palsy, and mental retardation. Case studies are included at the end of these two chapters to help the reader apply the presented information. The following two chapters discuss various pediatric disorders that an occupational therapy practitioner may encounter while working with children who have special needs. Chapter 10 presents common psychosocial disorders found in children and adolescents. Chapter 11 presents information on other pediatric disorders not previously discussed. Chapter 11 is organized according to the systems that are affected by the disorder. Both Chapters 10 and 11 use vignettes to exemplify the content.

The final section of the book consists of five chapters containing specific program planning and intervention information. Chapter 12 provides the reader with an overview of the occupational therapy process from referral to discontinuation of services. Chapter 13 presents information on the occupational performance model and intervention strategies for daily living and work and productive activities. Vignettes are used throughout Chapter 13 to clarify the content. Chapter 14 focuses on play and playfulness. Chapter 15 discusses the neurophysiological, neurodevelopmental, and sensory regulatory approaches as they relate to pediatric occupational therapy intervention. The discussion of assistive technology is found in Chapter 16, and the final chapter of the book focuses on handling and positioning as it relates to pediatrics.

This book has evolved from many years of teaching pediatric skills to OTA students. The contributing authors and I have spent countless hours writing the text. My goal is to provide students with a pediatric textbook that will fill the void in OTA literature. I have contributed to and developed all chapters with the assistance of the contributors, who are primarily occupational therapy practitioners. I acknowledge the wisdom and skill of the contributors.

JEAN W. SOLOMON

Acknowledgments

I have been told that writing a book is a lonely process. I have learned that it takes a village to write a book and can at times be quite a solitary process. I would like to acknowledge and thank Mary Beth Early for her encouragement and assistance throughout this process. Several years ago Mary Beth convinced me that I could write a pediatric textbook. She helped me with the prospectus and has reviewed many chapters. She graciously consented to writing a foreword for the book. She has also encouraged me during my doubtful moments over the past several years.

I am privileged to have worked with the many talented people who have authored or coauthored many of the chapters. The knowledge and skills of the contributing authors amaze me. I would like to recognize and thank Jane O'Brien, Paula Murrill, Gretchen Parker, and Susan Stockmaster for helping me pull the final pieces together at the latest possible time. In addition to writing entire chapters or portions of chapters, these friends and colleagues have collectively spent numerous hours reviewing other chapters. Their feedback and comments have been invaluable.

I would like to thank the occupational therapy practitioners who reviewed specific chapters in preparation for the final draft of the manuscript. I would like to recognize Jean Lewis Patz for her contributions during the review process. I found the feedback and comments provided to me by all of the reviewers to be invaluable. I greatly appreciate the reviewers' participation in this project.

I would like to thank a dear friend for her help photographing subjects that have been used in various chapters or as models from which illustrations have been drawn. I would like to thank John Waddill, a close friend, for his illustrations. I would also like to thank Bill Colrus and Graphic World for the illustrations that they provided. I am very impressed with the artistic style presented in the pictures and illustrations.

I appreciate the hard work of the Mosby editorial staff—Martha Sasser, Amy Christopher, Chris Lange O'Brien, Leslie Mosby, and Cathy Comer. I am especially thankful for having had the pleasure to work with Amy. She has been most helpful throughout this entire process.

I thank my sisters, Amy and Tish; my dearest friends, Mary Ellen, Faye, and Neva; and other family members for their patience, support, and understanding while I was writing the manuscript. I would also like to thank my sister's sister-in-law, Jan Waring, for typing portions of the manuscript.

In closing, I would like to thank the occupational therapy assistant students whom I have had the pleasure to teach. You and the children with whom I have worked have been the motivating force that has allowed me to write this book.

JEAN W. SOLOMON

Contents

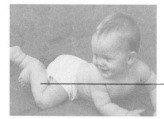

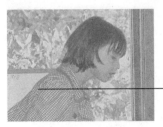

Part T W O

Normal Development

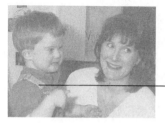

Part THREE

Pediatric Disorders

8 Cerebral Palsy, *113*
JOYCE A. WANDEL

9 Mental Retardation, *127*
DONNA NEWMAN

10 Psychosocial Disorders, *139*
SUSAN STOCKMASTER

11 Other Common Pediatric Disorders, *159*
GRETCHEN EVANS PARKER

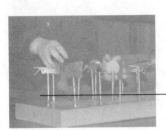

Part FOUR

Occupational Therapy Process

Pediatric SKILLS
for Occupational
Therapy Assistants

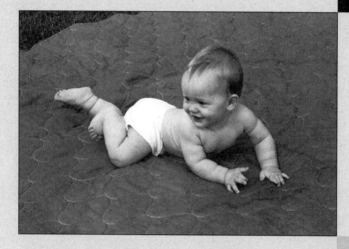

Overview

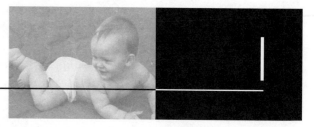

Scope of Practice

JEAN W. SOLOMON

PAULA MURRILL

CHAPTER *Objectives*

After studying this chapter, the reader will be able to accomplish the following:

- Recognize eight subject areas in which entry-level certified occupational therapy assistants should have general knowledge
- Define a practice model
- Describe the biomechanical, sensorimotor, and rehabilitative practice models
- Describe the four levels at which registered occupational therapists supervise certified occupational therapy assistants
- Define service competency and give examples of the way it may be obtained

| KEY TERMS | CHAPTER OUTLINE |

During the past 20 years, significant changes have occurred in the provision of pediatric occupational therapy services.[10] Numerous federal laws have been implemented that expand the services available to infants, children, and adolescents who have special needs or disabilities (see Chapters 4 and 16). Approximately 20% of all certified occupational therapy assistants (COTAs) work in a variety of pediatric settings. Occupational therapy (OT) practitioners also provide pediatric services in medical settings, such as outpatient clinics, and community settings, such as the home or a day-care center.[11] Because numerous practitioners work with infants, children, and adolescents, both entry-level registered occupational therapists (OTRs) and COTAs must have a solid foundation in pediatrics.

The American Occupational Therapy Association (AOTA) has identified several subject areas that should be included in any pediatric occupational therapy curriculum.[14] An entry-level OT practitioner should have knowledge in the following areas:

1. *Normal development:* Children with special needs or atypical development patterns should be recognized and treated (see Chapters 5, 6, and 7).
2. *Importance of families in the occupational therapy process:* Families are the most consistent participants on the pediatric team (see Chapter 2).
3. *Specific pediatric diagnoses:* Pediatric occupational therapy practitioners must determine which tools and methods are most appropriate for assessment and intervention (see Chapters 8 through 11).
4. *Occupational therapy practice models (or approaches):* Assessment and intervention information should be organized into a meaningful plan (see Chapters 12 through 15 and 17).
5. *Assessments appropriate for a specific child with a specific disability or diagnosis:* Practitioners must be able to accommodate numerous types of diagnoses (see Chapters 8 through 12).
6. *Age-appropriate activities:* Pediatric occupational therapy practitioners should be able to vary therapy activities to suit the age of the child (see Chapters 6, 7, and 13 through 17).
7. *Differences among systems in which occupational therapy services are provided:* Therapy should be tailored to specific settings. For example, a child who is receiving services in a public school system should have therapy goals and objectives that are educationally relevant, whereas a child who is receiving services as an inpatient in a hospital should have medically necessary goals (see Chapters 2 through 4).
8. *Assistive technology:* Pediatric occupational therapy practitioners should be able to work effectively with infants, children, and adolescents who have disabilities or special needs (see Chapter 16).

AOTA'S "UNIFORM TERMINOLOGY FOR OCCUPATIONAL THERAPY"

The third edition of **AOTA's "Uniform Terminology for Occupational Therapy"** was published in 1994. The purpose of this document is to give occupational therapy practitioners a common language. Three major categories comprise "Uniform Terminology for Occupational Therapy": (1) occupational performance areas, (2) components, and (3) contexts. Occupational performance areas include activities of daily living (ADLs), play and leisure activities, and work and productive activities (see Chapters 7, 13, and 14). Performance components include sensorimotor components, cognitive integration and cognitive components, and psychosocial skills and psychological components (see Chapters 6, 15, and 17). Performance contexts include temporal aspects and the environment (see Chapter 5).[7]

SELECTED OCCUPATIONAL THERAPY PRACTICE MODELS

A **practice model** is a frame of reference that is used to direct an occupational therapy process. It helps the occupational therapy practitioner identify problems and develop solutions.[8] Current practice models are based in the teachings of classical theorists such as Freud, Erikson, and Piaget and have evolved over time to incorporate concepts of human occupation, activity analysis, goal-directed activity, and environmental adaptation. Three such practice models are the biomechanical, sensorimotor, and rehabilitative practice models. Practice models are seldom used individually and are usually used in combination with other models. For example, a practitioner may use both sensorimotor and rehabilitative approaches while working with a child who has cerebral palsy (see Chapters 8, 13, and 15).

[handwritten: orthopedic problem, ① assess physical limitations, ② ↑ ROM, ③ prevent or reduce contract]

Biomechanical Approach

Sarah is a 14-month-old infant who suffered a left brachial plexus injury (that is, damage to the nerves that control arm movement) during birth. Sarah is seen by an OTR once every 2 weeks. Chris, a COTA, visits Sarah twice a week to work on the goals that have been established by the OTR in collaboration with Sarah's family. Sarah's long-term occupational therapy goals include (1) increasing the active range of motion (AROM) in her left arm, (2) increasing the functional strength in her left arm, and (3) increasing her ability to use her left arm during age-appropriate activities such as playing with a toy or self feeding. Sarah's treatment sessions with Chris usually last 30 minutes. A typical therapy session is shown in the following daily progress note, or SOAP note. (See Box 1-1 and Chapter 3 for additional information on SOAP notes.)

BOX 1-1

The SOAP Note Format of Documentation

S (SUBJECTIVE)
Information from client or family concerning feelings or beliefs

O (OBJECTIVE)
Therapist's observations or evaluations of client's performance

A (ASSESSMENT)
Summary of therapist's interpretation of client's progress and analysis of current treatment plan

P (PLAN)
Plan of action for continued treatment, including any modifications to current treatment plan

S

Sarah's mother said that Sarah enjoys the range of motion (ROM) exercises she does each day. She especially enjoys singing the "Row, row, row your boat" song, which Chris had suggested that she sing during the stretching exercises.

O

Sarah was seen for a 30-minute therapy session in her home. Sarah's mother and older brother were present for the entire session. Active and passive range of motion of Sarah's left arm were assessed. Activities included having Sarah bear weight on her extended (straightened) left arm while reaching for toys with her right arm. She then reached for toys with her left arm while bearing weight on her right arm. Sarah also played with a shape sorter, using her left arm to stabilize the toy and her right arm to place the shapes into the sorter.

A

Sarah actively participated in the activities throughout the session. Her ability to sustain weight on her left arm with minimal physical assistance has improved. She is now able to reach for toys above her head, which indicates improved left shoulder AROM.

P

Chris will continue seeing Sarah twice a week and work toward achieving the previously stated goals.

Chris is using the **biomechanical approach** to treat Sarah. The biomechanical approach is a practice model used with children who have orthopedic (that is, bone, joint, or muscle) problems such as hand injuries, or lower motor neuron disorders (disorders of nerve connections outside of central nervous system [CNS]), such as brachial plexus injuries. The goals of the biomechanical approach are to (1) assess physical limitations on the client's ROM, muscle strength, and endurance; (2) improve ROM, strength, and endurance; and (3) prevent or reduce contracture and deformities.[8] The biomechanical approach focuses on the specific physical limitations on occupational performance components that interfere with the client's ability to engage in the performance areas of ADLs, play and leisure activities, and work and productive activities.

[handwritten: Uses sensory input to change muscle tone + movement patterns in kids]

Sensorimotor Approach

Amy is a 4-year-old child who has been diagnosed with spastic right hemiplegia cerebral palsy. A brain lesion caused abnormal muscle tone on the right side of her body, which prevents her from properly using her right arm and leg. She is receiving outpatient occupational therapy services at the local hospital, and her mother usually brings her to the clinic. Amy recently had a phenol alcohol nerve block—an injection into the nerves that innervate the arm—to help reduce the increased flexor tone in her right arm. Because of the recent changes in Amy's right arm, Brenda, the OTR, is currently providing all of the direct occupational therapy services. Brenda's sessions with Amy typically last for 45 minutes. A typical therapy session is shown in the following daily SOAP note.

S

Amy's mother said that she has noticed Amy's arm is easier to wash since Amy received the nerve block. She has also noticed that Amy's right elbow is straighter.

O

Amy arrived this morning eager to work on the therapy ball. She performed activities on the therapy ball while lying on her stomach and bearing weight on her elbows, followed by bearing weight on her extended arms. Brenda performed tapping—using the fingertips to deliver successive, light blows to the muscle belly—over the triceps to facilitate full extension (straightening) of Amy's elbow. (The triceps muscle is primarily responsible for elbow extension.) Amy participated in bilateral hand activities, such as buttoning large buttons and creating pictures using finger paint. When necessary, the wrist extensor muscles were stroked to encourage maintenance of a functional wrist position (for example, wrist extension while grasping) during the bilateral tasks.

A

Amy's ability to use her right arm has improved, as shown by her ability to button five large buttons while her wrist is extended.

P

Brenda will continue to work with Amy on the previously stated goals.

Brenda is using a **sensorimotor approach** to treat Amy. This type of approach involves the use of sensory input to change muscle tone and movement patterns in infants, children, and adolescents who have CNS damage.[8] Several types of sensorimotor approaches are used by occupational therapy practitioners (see Chapter 15). Because the use of the sensorimotor approaches requires skill and experience, entry-level OTRs and COTAs should be closely supervised while using these types of approaches.

Rehabilitative Approach

Timmy is a 6-year-old child whose left arm is amputated below the elbow as the result of a car accident 2 years ago. Timmy goes to a Shriners hospital in another town for the fitting and training in the use of his prosthesis, or artificial limb. He has outgrown his old prosthesis and is meeting with Dan, a COTA, to work on using and caring for his new artificial arm and to learn activities that will improve his ability to use it functionally. A typical therapy session is shown in the following daily SOAP note.

S

Timmy said that his new arm feels good.

O

Timmy was seen in the occupational therapy department for prosthetic training and home and family instruction on its care. The department's Prosthetic Checklist was used during the session. Timmy's father was shown how to don and doff the stump sock and new artificial arm. Timmy practiced using his new arm during dressing and undressing activities. He also practiced using the artificial arm as a stabilizer during paper and pencil tasks.

A

The new artificial arm fits well. Timmy is able to engage in age-appropriate functional activities while using his prosthesis.

P

Timmy is being discharged from Shriners Hospital.

Dan is using the **rehabilitative approach** to treat Timmy. The rehabilitative approach is used after an injury or illness to return a person to the highest possible level of functional independence as well as teach any compensatory methods that may be needed to perform certain activities.[8] Because many children are born with disabilities, occupational therapy practitioners are in some cases required to teach new skills (habilitate) instead of teach previously known skills (rehabilitate). However, for cases in which a child acquires a disability after birth, a rehabilitative approach is appropriate. The methods used during rehabilitation and habilitation include the following:

1. Self-care evaluation and training
2. Acquisition and training in the use of assistive devices

3. Prosthetic use training
4. Wheelchair management training
5. Architectural and environmental adaptation training
6. Acquisition and training in the use of augmentative communication devices and assistive technology
7. Play assessment and intervention

An occupational therapy practitioner who is using a rehabilitative or habilitative approach focuses on skill acquisition in the occupational performance areas of ADLs, play and leisure skills, and work and productive activities.

THE OCCUPATIONAL THERAPY PROCESS

The occupational therapy practitioner uses the practice models to plan and implement occupational therapy services. The process begins when a referral for occupational therapy services is made by a physician, teacher, or other concerned professional. The OTR decides whether the referred client should be screened, which helps the OTR determine whether the client will benefit from occupational therapy services. If the screening shows that the client will benefit from occupational therapy services, then an evaluation is done. The OTR decides the areas to be evaluated and assigns portions of the evaluation to the COTA. The evaluation process helps the OTR identify the client's strengths and weaknesses. Long-term goals and short-term objectives are established based on the OTR's interpretation of the assessment. In collaboration with the COTA, the OTR develops an intervention plan based on the goals and objectives. The plan is implemented and modified based on the client's progress and periodic reassessments. The client is discharged when all of the goals and objectives are met or the OTR determines that services should be discontinued. (For a more detailed discussion of the occupational therapy process, see Chapters 12 and 13.)

OTR AND COTA ROLES

The OTR is responsible for all aspects of the occupational therapy process and supervises the COTA. The extent to which the COTA is supervised by the OTR depends on a variety of factors including the knowledge, skill, and experience of the COTA. Regardless, OTRs and COTAs are both considered occupational therapy practitioners, and therefore they share the responsibility for communicating with each other about their clients.[7]

QUALIFICATIONS, SUPERVISION, AND SERVICE COMPETENCY

Entry-level COTAs must meet basic qualifications to practice in the field of occupational therapy. As they gain experience by working with OTRs, require less supervision and gradually become more competent providing occupational therapy services.

Qualifications

Entry-level COTAs meet specific qualifications, which include having successfully completed course work in an AOTA-accredited school and having passed the certification examination administered by the National Board for Certification in Occupational Therapy (NBCOT). In addition, COTAs must meet specific requirements established by an occupational therapy regulatory board in their state and obtain a license if required by state law.

Supervision

Four levels of supervision have been delineated by AOTA: close, routine, general, and minimal. Close supervision is direct, daily contact between the COTA and OTR at the work site. Routine supervision is direct contact between the COTA and OTR at the work site at least every 2 weeks and interim contact through other means such as telephone conversations or e-mail messages. General supervision is a minimum of direct contact 1 day per month and interim supervision as needed. Minimum supervision is supervision on an "as needed" basis. It is important to note that individual state occupational therapy regulatory agencies may require stricter guidelines than those established by AOTA. Stricter state guidelines supersede the AOTA guidelines.[2,3,5,6]

The level of supervision COTAs require varies with their level of expertise. AOTA defines three levels of expertise: entry, intermediate, and advanced. COTAs' progress from one level to another is based on their acquisition of skills, knowledge, and proficiency, not on their years of experience. Entry-level COTAs are typically new graduates or entering into a new practice setting. Intermediate-level COTAs have acquired a higher level of skill through experience, continuing education, and involvement in professional activities. Advanced-level COTAs have specialized skills and may be recognized as experts in particular area of practice. Although the extent to which a particular COTA is supervised varies according to the individual, the level of supervision generally falls into one defined by AOTA based on the COTA's expertise. An entry-level COTA requires close supervision, an intermediate-level COTA requires routine or general supervision, and an advanced-level COTA requires minimum supervision (see Table 1-1).[9]

Service Competency

Levels of supervision are closely related to establishing service competency. AOTA's definition of service competency

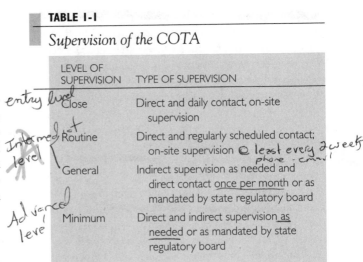

TABLE 1-1

Supervision of the COTA

LEVEL OF SUPERVISION	TYPE OF SUPERVISION
Close	Direct and daily contact, on-site supervision
Routine	Direct and regularly scheduled contact; on-site supervision
General	Indirect supervision as needed and direct contact once per month or as mandated by state regulatory board
Minimum	Direct and indirect supervision as needed or as mandated by state regulatory board

(Handwritten annotations: "entry level" by Close; "Intermediate 1st level" by Routine, "@ least every 2 weeks phone - email"; "Advanced level" by Minimum)

is ". . . the determination, made by various methods, that two people performing the same or equivalent procedures will obtain the same or equivalent results."[2,3,5,6] Service competency is a means of ensuring that two individual occupational therapy practitioners will have the same results when administering a specific assessment, observing a specific performance area or component, or providing treatment. Communication between COTAs and OTRs is an essential part of the entire occupational therapy process but is especially important when establishing service competency. OTRs must be sure that they and the COTAs are performing assessments and treatment procedures in the same way. Once an OTR has determined that a particular COTA has established service competency in a certain area, the COTA may be allowed to perform an assessment or treatment procedure (within the parameters of that particular area) without close OTR supervision. Ensuring service competency is an ongoing, mutual learning experience.

AOTA has specific guidelines for establishing service competency. For standardized assessments and treatment procedures that require no specific training to administer, the OTR and COTA both perform the procedure. If they obtain equivalent results, the COTA can be allowed to administer subsequent procedures independently. For assessments and treatment procedures requiring more subjective interpretations, direct observation and videotaping are valuable tools that can be used to establish service competency. These tools allow practitioners to observe a client performing a particular task and compare their individual interpretations of the performance. Likewise, an OTR can videotape a client, have a COTA watch the tape, and compare and contrast the observations that have been made. If the OTR and COTA consistently have similar interpretations, the COTA has established competency in observing and interpreting the particular area of performance.[2,3,5,6] Specific examples of establishing service competency follow.

Videotaping

Chris is the previously mentioned COTA who used the biomechanical approach to treat Sarah's brachial plexus injury. Before working with Sarah, Chris watched a videotape of his supervising OTR treating another child who had a brachial plexus injury. He discussed the tape with the OTR, which revealed that he understood the treatment procedures used. Sarah's next therapy session, which was led by Chris, was videotaped. The OTR watched the tape and observed that Chris carefully positioned the child and successfully carried out the treatment plan. The OTR determined that Chris had established the service competency needed to treat Sarah. The OTR and Chris agreed that as part of an ongoing learning process they would videotape one of Sarah's treatment sessions each month.

Cotreatment

Amy is the previously mentioned 4-year-old who was diagnosed with cerebral palsy and recently received a nerve block to decrease flexor tone in her right arm. Brenda, the OTR, has been treating her since the nerve block was performed. Recently Brenda asked Richard, a COTA, to assist her with treating Amy. Richard prepared for cotreatment by reading about nerve blocks and carefully observing Brenda and Amy's one-on-one treatment session. Richard asked pertinent questions and expressed a keen interest in working with Amy. After several successful cotreatment sessions in which Brenda and Chris obtained equivalent outcomes from the treatment procedures used, Brenda assigned Amy's case to Richard. Richard now only receives general supervision from Brenda because he demonstrated service competency while working with Amy.

Observation

Dan, a COTA, used the rehabilitative approach to treat Timmy, the six year old who sustained a below elbow amputation. Prior to becoming a COTA Dan volunteered regularly at the Shriners hospital. He observed many clients being fitted with prostheses. After graduation he was hired to work in the OT department at the hospital. As a COTA he worked closely with the OTR who developed treatment plans for clients with injuries similar to Timmy's. Dan also observed and assisted in administering the department's Prosthetic Checklist; a checklist designed to assess prosthetic care, application and use. Dan began working with Timmy when the child was fitted for his first prosthesis at the age of 3. The OTR observed Dan administer the Prosthetic Checklist and determined that her findings were equivalent to Dan's. When Timmy was fitted with a new prosthesis, the OTR was confident Dan could independently complete the checklist accurately. Dan had demonstrated service competency in administering the assessment.

SUMMARY

This chapter presented an overview of pediatric OT practice with particular focus on the COTA. Areas of proficiency for the entry-level COTA are followed by a discussion of the biomechanical, sensorimotor and rehabilitative practice models. The roles of the OTR and COTA are defined along with a discussion of the COTA's qualifications and levels of supervision. Service competency and means of establishing service competency are presented. Finally, specific examples illustrate how the practice models, levels of supervision, and service competency are used in the delivery of occupational therapy services.

References

1. American Occupational Therapy Association: *Revision of guidelines for pediatric curriculum content for occupational therapy*, Bethesda, Md, 1998, The Association.
2. American Occupational Therapy Association: Entry-level role delineation for registered occupational therapists (OTRs) and certified occupational therapy assistants (COTAs), *Am J Occup Ther* 44:1091, 1990.
3. American Occupational Therapy Association: Guide for supervision of occupational therapy personnel, *Am J Occup Ther* 48:1045, 1994.
4. American Occupational Therapy Association: *Guidelines for curriculum content in pediatrics*, Bethesda, Md, 1991, The Association.
5. American Occupational Therapy Association: Occupational therapy roles, *Am J Occup Ther* 47:1087, 1993.
6. American Occupational Therapy Association: Supervision guidelines for certified occupational therapy assistants, *Am J Occup Ther* 44:1089, 1990.
7. American Occupational Therapy Association: Uniform terminology for occupational therapy, *Am J Occup Ther* 48:1047, 1994.
8. Early MB: *Physical dysfunction skills for the occupational therapy assistant*, St Louis, 1998, Mosby.
9. Punwar AJ: *Occupational therapy: principles and practice*, ed 2, Baltimore, 1994, Williams & Wilkins.
10. Rainville EB, Cermack SA, Murray EA: Supervision and consultation for pediatric occupational therapists, *Am J Occup Ther* 50:725, 1996.
11. Steib PA: Top employment settings for COTAs, *OT Week* 10(17):18, 1996

Recommended Reading

Kramer P, Hinojosa J, editors: *Frames of reference for pediatric occupational therapy*, Baltimore, 1993, Williams & Wilkins.

Neistadt ME, Crepeau EB, editors: *Willard & Spackman's occupational therapy*, ed 9, New York, 1998, Lippincott.

REVIEW *Questions*

1. List and describe five content areas that a pediatric occupational therapy practitioner needs to have knowledge in while working with children and adolescents.
2. What is a practice model? Why are practice models useful to occupational therapy practitioners?
3. What are the primary concerns that occupational therapy practitioners have while using the biomechanical practice model?
4. What are the primary concerns that occupational therapy practitioners have while using the sensorimotor practice model?
5. What are the primary concerns that occupational therapy practitioners have while using a rehabilitative practice model?
6. What is service competency? How is it established?

SUGGESTED *Activities*

1. In small groups, list and discuss daily living and play activities that you think would be appropriate while working with Sarah, Amy, and Timmy. How do the chosen activities relate to the biomechanical, sensorimotor, and/or rehabilitative practice models?
2. Interview a COTA or OTR who works in pediatrics. The focus of the interview should be supervision and service competency. Questions might include:
   (a) Which courses in school have been most useful to you as a pediatric OT practitioner?
   (b) How many years of clinical experience do you have?
   (c) What is the level of supervision that you receive (COTA) or give (OTR)? What are the means by which this occurs?
   (d) How is service competency established between the OTR and the COTA in your workplace?

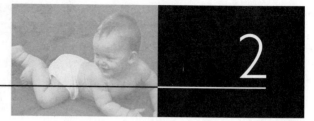

Family Systems

PAMELA J. WINTON

ROBERT E. WINTON

CHAPTER *Objectives*

After studying this chapter, the reader will be able to accomplish the following:

- Describe the reason it is important for an occupational therapy practitioner to have knowledge of and skills related to working with families
- Understand the way a therapy program for a child can have an impact on the family unit
- Describe key concepts from family systems and life cycle theories and the role of these concepts in intervention with children
- Recognize and appreciate that all families have unique ways of adapting and coping with life events, and effective therapy builds on these existing coping strategies
- Describe several communication strategies that an occupational therapy practitioner can use to promote family-professional partnerships

KEY TERMS	CHAPTER OUTLINE

Margarita Sanchez is a 3-year-old child who has been diagnosed with pervasive developmental delays and mild to moderate cerebral palsy. She lives in a small apartment with her paternal grandmother, great aunt, parents, and three siblings (who are 11 months, 5 years, and 6 years). When the occupational therapy (OT) practitioner, Heather McFall, arrives for a routine visit, she learns that Margarita's mother has not been working with Margarita on the toilet training program that was discussed during the last visit. Heather had recommended that they start the program because she thought it was important that Margarita be toilet trained in time to begin a public school prekindergarten program in the fall. After some discussion, it becomes apparent that in the winter, Mrs. Sanchez is unable to deal with the wet, soiled clothes that invariably accompany a toilet training program. After talking more, Heather and Mrs. Sanchez agree to wait until the weather gets warmer to begin toilet training. During their conversation, Heather also realizes that she needs to plan a time for the Sanchez family to visit the prekindergarten classroom and see what they think of the program. Although Heather is enthusiastic about the academic and social experience that Margarita would have in the classroom, Mrs. Sanchez seems hesitant and uncharacteristically quiet when they talk about the program. Heather has learned that Mrs. Sanchez becomes quiet when she has reservations about an idea.

As Heather leaves the apartment she thinks about her relationship with the family and how it has developed during the 2 years she has been working with Margarita. In the beginning of the relationship, Heather was often frustrated by Mrs. Sanchez's seeming disinterest in or ability to follow through with some of the home programming ideas that Heather introduced. Heather had fretted and fumed and tried to help Mrs. Sanchez see the importance of taking Margarita's needs seriously and devoting the necessary time to therapy.

Heather remembers a breakthrough in their relationship. She had arrived at the Sanchez apartment one hot day feeling faint. Mrs. Sanchez insisted that she stretch out on the family couch and brought her a cool drink made with herbs and lemon. During the 15 to 20 minutes Heather reclined on the couch, she saw the Sanchez family in a new light.

The Sanchez women were deftly preparing a special meal for a church dinner while simultaneously caring for the young children who were in the way in the crowded kitchen area. Although Heather did not understand Spanish, which Mrs. Sanchez always spoke with her mother, she noticed the obvious warmth, affection, and good humor in the interactions among the children and adults. Mrs. Sanchez had been pleased that the cold drink revived Heather's color and began to tell her about the church festival and the children's pageant that would be part of the festivities. As Heather lay there watching the scene, she realized why the adaptive high chair she had unsuccessfully tried to

incorporate into the therapy plan remained unused in a crowded corner. The children were running in and out of the kitchen, snacking on the fresh ingredients that were part of the dishes being prepared. These "snacks" were lunch. Heather saw that an adaptive high chair would simply be in the way in a crowded kitchen and definitely would not fit into their lunch routine. Margarita was in a child car seat on the counter where the food was being prepared. Mrs. Sanchez sang little songs and made visual and physical contact with Margarita while fixing the food. She also gave Margarita tastes of things as she cooked. As Heather watched the bits and pieces of chicken, rice, and mashed beans go into Margarita's mouth, she had worried about the possibility of Margarita choking, and Margarita's position in the car seat was not ideal. However, Heather realized that unless the adaptive high chair could be conveniently blended into the meal routine, it would never be used and might interfere with the way the family operated. She also realized that Margarita was getting a good variety of textures and nutrients in the food she was being given in the somewhat haphazard process that made up meal time in the Sanchez family.

On that significant day, Heather left the Sanchez apartment with a much better understanding of Margarita and her family. During the next home visit, Heather, Mrs. Sanchez, and Mrs. Sanchez's mother worked on positioning Margarita properly in the car seat during feedings in a way that would minimize the risk of choking.

THE IMPORTANCE OF FAMILIES

The story of Margarita and her family underscores the reason it is important for occupational therapy practitioners to understand family systems. Box 2-1 contains the key reasons using a family-centered approach is recommended in early intervention when working with young children who have disabilities.

Families have a *significant* environmental influence on a young child's life and development. As evident in the

---

BOX 2-1

Reasons Families are Important

- A family has a significant environmental influence on a young child's life and development.
- Interventions with children inevitably impact the family.
- Laws and current service delivery models promote a family-centered approach.
- Professional organizations, including AOTA, have identified areas of competency and created recommended guidelines for working with families.

previous story, the majority of Margarita's time is spent with her family. If her family members are not convinced of the benefits of therapy or are unable to find time to carry out the intervention plan, Margarita simply will not improve. As interventionists, occupational therapy practitioners enter children's lives for a fairly short time and then leave. Family members are the "constants" in most children's lives. When possible, collaboration and trust are key ingredients for intervention success with families. Supporting families in their parenting role is critical; they need confidence and competence to nurture and educate their children.

CLINICAL *Pearl*

Developing a trusting and collaborative relationship with families is one of the key ingredients for intervention success.

Interventions with children inevitably impact family life, therefore they are most effective when the family is included and invested in the development of the treatment plan. Margarita's story reveals the importance of thinking about the family as a whole while designing intervention plans. Margarita's therapist learned the importance of this concept when she struggled with getting the family to use the adaptive high chair. By observing the family meal time and considering their customs and routines, Heather was able to understand why the adaptive equipment that she thought would help Margarita was not being used. Heather's strategy of discussing meal time feeding and safety issues with Mrs. Sanchez and her mother and collaborating with them on developing a plan was an effective way to ensure that the plan fit into the family's daily routines and was a plan that the family would try to carry out.

The family-centered approach is also the focus of many current laws and health care delivery models. The passing of Public Law 99-457 in 1986 (IDEA, Part C) is considered revolutionary because of the law's emphasis on the central role a family plays in interventions with young children. This law and its subsequent interpretations have altered the way services for young children are planned and delivered. Some of the highlights of the early intervention component of the law include the following: (1) families are mandated coleaders on state-level advisory boards that make recommendations about the way service systems are designed; (2) family concerns, resources, and priorities guide the development of individual intervention plans; (3) families play an important role in children's assessments and evaluations; and (4) families have

BOX 2-2

AOTA *Guidelines for Curriculum Content in Pediatrics*

ACADEMIC AND LEVEL I FIELDWORK
Family Systems Theory
The way families operate as units, the impact of diverse cultures and child-rearing patterns on family life, and differences in child rearing

Family Life Cycle
Critical stages of family life and parenting

Family Ecology
The way family systems operate in society, including in immediate community, state, and federal systems

Effects of Disabilities on Families
The emotional and social impact of an infant's, a toddler's, a child's, or a youth's disability on the parents' and family's life

Effects of Family and Environment on Children with Disabilities
The impact of different family styles and environments on an infant, a toddler, a child, or a youth with disabilities

Role of Occupational Therapy
The occupational therapist's role in helping a family assess their concerns and priorities for intervention; the use of self-report instruments in occupational therapy

LEVEL II PEDIATRIC FIELDWORK (FOR ENTRY-LEVEL PRACTICE)
Rapport
The way to establish rapport with caregivers; the occupational therapist's role as a partner in treatment planning

Collaboration
Strategies for having collaborative consultations with infants, toddlers, children, or youths with disabilities and caregivers

Modified from American Occupational Therapy Association Commission on Education: *Guidelines for curriculum content in pediatrics,* Bethesda, Md, 1991, The Association.

certain rights to confidentiality, record keeping, notification, and other procedures related to the programs and agencies that serve their children. The law ushered in additional changes that ultimately benefit families, such as promoting interdisciplinary and interagency collaboration. It was clear that collaboration was needed among agencies and disciplines when numerous stories surfaced about families receiving conflicting advice and recommendations from various health care professionals about their children's disabilities.[6]

Professional organizations, including the American Occupational Therapy Association (AOTA), have identified particular areas of competency and recommended certain guidelines to emphasize the importance of practitioners having the skills and knowledge to work effectively with families.[1] The dramatic changes in the relationships between families and professionals catalyzed by Public Law 99-457 and the increased focus on the importance on families in all human service organizations have not developed overnight. The existing workforce has had to develop new collaboration and communication skills. University and community college training programs have had to retrain their faculties and upgrade their curricula to prepare students adequately for the newly defined pediatric roles (Box 2-2). Professional organizations have supported the changes by creating recommended practice guidelines and areas of competency.

CURRENT ISSUES AFFECTING OCCUPATIONAL THERAPY PRACTITIONERS AND FAMILIES
Changes in Policies and Service Delivery Models

As mentioned previously, policies and legislation passed during the last 10 years have affected service delivery models and recommended occupational therapy practices. The resulting changes have included emphasis on the following approaches to service delivery:

- Interdisciplinary and family-centered approaches are used when planning and implementing interventions.
- Children who have disabilities are included in regular education settings.
- Therapists act as consultants, providing pediatric treatment that is integrated into the children's regular routines instead of using "pull out therapy"* (Figure 2-1).

Expansion of Practitioners' Roles

Recent changes in service delivery and implementation have resulted in an expansion of the occupational ther-

---

*"Pull out therapy" is therapy that is not provided in the context of a child's daily routine.

apy practitioners' roles. Their duties now also include the following:

- Assessing family interests, priorities, and concerns
- Observing and gathering information about the daily routines of the child and family and in the classrooms
- Gathering and sharing information with families about development and intervention strategies
- Implementing therapy in collaboration with parents, caregivers, and general educators

Demographic Changes in the U.S. Population

In addition to changes in laws, policies, and recommended practices, the demographic makeup of the children being served has also changed. It is estimated that by the year 2080, the majority of Americans will be persons of color.[4] In contrast, although the U.S. population is becoming more diverse, members of professional organizations such as AOTA and the American Speech and Hearing Association (ASHA) are predominately Caucasian.[1,3]

Implications for Practice

The myriad changes taking place in the occupational therapy environment affect service delivery and implementation in numerous ways, including the following:

- Occupational therapy practitioners are more likely than ever to be working with children and families whose cultural background and home language is different than their own. They may need to use translators or interpreters. They must develop the ability to appreciate and respect cultural differences, which may mean developing an awareness of their own cultural identity, inherent biases and values, and knowledge of other cultures.
- Young children who have disabilities are more likely than ever before to be in regular early childhood and educational programs. Occupational therapy practitioners must be able to embed therapy into the daily routines of the home, child care setting, and regular education setting and must develop expertise in consulting with day-care providers, families, and other specialists.
- Occupational therapy practitioners need the knowledge and skill to work as members of interdisciplinary teams, which requires interpersonal, communication, and collaboration skills.
- Occupational therapy practitioners must obtain information on a wide range of community-based programs and services, both specialized and generic,

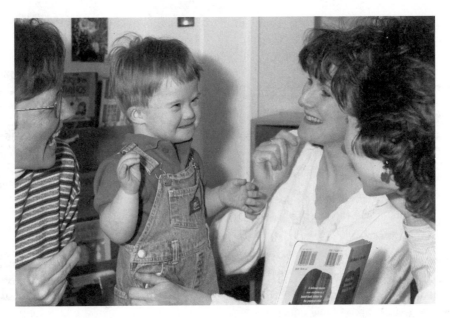

FIGURE 2-1 Therapist working with mother, child, and early childhood teacher at a day-care center. This is an example of interdisciplinary collaboration and embedding therapy into the daily routine. (Courtesy Don Trull.)

to meet the individualized needs of the various families and children with whom they work.

FAMILY SYSTEMS THEORY

Description

Family systems theory is a core framework for guiding interactions with families. It is a group of ideas that describe the many ways that individuals in families are connected across time and space,* and its implications about the families with whom practitioners work are far reaching. Developing and increasing an understanding of the family as a system significantly affects the way practitioners working with families perceive their roles, determine which potential outcomes are positive, and perceive family changes. The core concepts of the family systems theory are provided in Box 2-3.

Implications for Practice

A major goal in working with families is establishing a trusting relationship. One of the first steps in establishing trust is to identify what the family hopes to accomplish. Families sometimes simply have a basic desire to help their children grow and develop. Regardless of whether a fam-

ily's goals are vague, it is important to the determine the way they perceive their situation and priorities.

> **CLINICAL** *Pearl*
>
> The first step in a successful intervention is identifying what the family hopes to accomplish.

> **CLINICAL** *Pearl*
>
> Intervention efforts should begin with a clarification of the way a family perceives their situation and defines their priorities, regardless of how unfocused their goals may seem.

The second step in building a trusting relationship is developing strategies for accomplishing the family's goals. The strategies should be developed in collaboration with the family to ensure adherence to the family's beliefs, daily living patterns, and **rules.** In the story about Margarita, Heather began the intervention process by working with the mother, which was the appropriate way to begin establishing a trusting relationship. However, she may have inadvertently violated the **boundary** and **hierarchy** of the parental **subsystem** when *she* determined the

---

*The definition of *family* in this chapter is inclusive: ". . . two or more people who regard themselves as a family and who perform some of the functions that families typically perform. These people may or may not be related by blood or marriage and may or may not usually live together."[7]

BOX 2-3

Family Systems Theory Concepts

RULES AND HIERARCHIES

Like all systems, family systems are organized by "rules," which define order and hierarchy, or who has power and authority. The rules may be ones that are spoken and well known by the family, but they may also be unspoken and, in some cases, known only subconsciously. An example of a *spoken* rule is something like, "No one eats until after the blessing." Examples of unspoken rules include no one kids around or laughs when Dad is home, Mom must speak to all visitors first, and the children may not reveal any particular information to visitors unless Mom has given permission with a nonverbal cue.

SUBSYSTEMS

Families are made up of subunits that have distinct functions and relationships. Individual family members can belong to multiple subsystems; for example, a mother is part of a spousal subsystem and a parental subsystem.

BOUNDARIES

The unique behaviors, emotions, and topics of discussion—which are all governed by rules—associated with a family system define the family's external boundary. Similar unique rules define the internal boundaries of the family's subsystems; for example, parents who do not discuss parenting disagreements in front of the children have established a parent-child internal boundary. Boundaries can be rigid, allowing little involvement from outsiders. An example of a family with rigid external boundaries would be one in which the father does not allow anyone outside of the family to see him lose his temper or cry, and no one outside the family knows that the mother is a heavy drinker. Boundaries can also be permeable, allowing frequent involvement from outsiders. An example of a family with permeable boundaries would be one in which the parents seek the advice and counsel of a very close family friend for parenting issues. Boundaries can also be clear (for example, parents saying, "We do not have time for Susie's occupational therapy appointment right now.") or diffuse (for example, Susie not being present for her appointments and vague excuses being made by the parents).

timeline for Margarita's toilet training and *she* determined that a high chair should be used during meals. Instead, Heather could have simply presented these options to Mrs. Sanchez and left the decision to her, thereby leaving the parental subsystem hierarchy unruffled. The father, grandmother, and aunt might also have been significant members of the parental subsystem. Because Heather had failed to include them in the planning process, she may have created additional resistance to change. Fortunately, Heather's fainting spell reestablished the hierarchy, and Mrs. Sanchez was able to reassume her role as she "mothered" Heather. Heather was unintentionally forced out of her professional role, which had actually only been used to provide a useless high chair and frustration. Heather's illness temporarily made her a "help seeker" and allowed Mrs. Sanchez to be a "help giver." This changed her relationship with the Sanchez family and simultaneously gave her an opportunity to see them functioning in their daily routine, which led to an appreciation of their strengths.

Margarita's story shows a serendipitous reestablishment of hierarchy. It also shows a common professional occurrence, which is the professional role clashing with existing family hierarchies and violating family boundaries. This can significantly limit the chances of success. The paradox is that families desire professional expertise and assistance. It is hard to resist the temptation to take

a directive role and tell a family exactly what to do. A family may accept guidance with every intention of following through; however, the likelihood of a family following a plan is slim unless the plan is carefully constructed to fit within existing family routines, beliefs, and daily living patterns. The best way to tailor a plan to a specific family is to develop a relationship with them, observe, and listen. If a practitioner is able to develop a trusting relationship with a family, then the family is more likely to take advantage of the practitioner's expertise. Ironically, practitioners who give up some of their professional power are often able to make the most of their professional skills and expertise.

CLINICAL *Pearl*

The likelihood that families will follow through with intervention plans depends on the extent to which the plans are constructed to fit within families' existing routines, beliefs, and patterns of family life.

Occupational therapy practitioners should also be aware that developing a trusting relationship with families takes time. It takes longer to establish trust with families who have rigid external boundaries than with families who have more permeable boundaries. Differences in backgrounds and heritages also influence how quickly and easily relationships are formed.

FAMILY LIFE CYCLE

Description

Another concept covered in AOTA's guidelines is the family **life cycle.** Like individuals, families go through normal or typical developmental phases. No consensus exists on the number of phases that should be considered, which is not surprising considering that family development is a flowing process and not a discontinuous series of steps. Critical stages of the family life cycle are those involving life transitions: birth, marriage, leaving home, and death.

Perhaps one of the most important points about the phases of the life cycle is the fact that moving from one phase to another causes stress and requires the family to adapt. Life cycle changes bring about changes in needs, interests, roles, and responsibilities for each family member. For instance, becoming a parent entails learning a whole new set of skills and alters the relationship between the parents and among the parents and their extended family and friends. Families often need extra support from friends, neighbors, or extended family members during life cycle transitions.

Children who have disabilities often have special needs and undergo numerous stressful life cycle events. These events may include being unexpectedly hospitalized for a lengthy period, undergoing unusual and sometimes painful treatments, and becoming involved in special education and early intervention programs. These events often involve new relationships with numerous different professionals. Forming new relationships, especially when individual choice is not involved (which is what happens when a practitioner is assigned a case), can be stressful. In Margarita's story, the arrival of an occupational therapy practitioner into the Sanchez household created a certain degree stress until the family began to trust her. She then became an honorary supportive family member, which helped balance out the stress.

Watching a child miss the typical milestones that usually take place in a child's life can create stress for a family. For instance, the realization that a child has not started walking or talking by the appropriate age can be very stressful for a family. In Margarita's case, the fact that Margarita's younger 11-month-old sister began to walk while the 3-year-old Margarita had not caused her family some anguish.

Because certain events, such as frequent hospitalizations and participating in occupational therapy intervention or not reaching important milestones, are not nor-

mative **life cycle events** (that is, not usual or expected transition events), families have fewer people with whom to share their experiences. For instance, parents of adolescents often find it helpful to share "war stories" with other families about adolescent transition events, such as teaching an adolescent to drive. The majority of parents of adolescents can relate to the challenges and triumphs associated with this event. Research has shown that sharing experiences and getting support from family, friends, and neighbors is an effective strategy for dealing with stress.[6] However, few parents can relate to **nonnormative life cycle events,** such as the experience of raising a child who will never be able to walk.

Implications for Practice

The life events that have been described are somewhat arbitrary, obviously overlap, and are grossly inadequate representations of the wide range of family experiences that exist. Cultural factors can also affect how these events and life stages are perceived and experienced. For instance, is it acceptable for an adult child to be living with parents? For many Caucasian families, this situation would be considered a failure, whereas for many Latino families, this situation is the norm. It is the tendency of practitioners to attach meaning to the phases of the family life cycle, and the meanings are usually rooted in our own background, beliefs, and experiences. This tendency can potentially put practitioners at odds with certain families. An example of this is shown in the previously mentioned case of Margarita. Heather wanted Margarita to attend the prekindergarten program connected with the public schools because she thought it would enhance Margarita's social and cognitive development. However, the Sanchezes consider it unusual for children to attend any school at such a young age. Their 6-year-old son attends a neighborhood parochial school that has several bilingual nuns on the staff; the Sanchezes know and trust the school. Enrolling Margarita in a public school, especially an unfamiliar one, before the age of 6 is not a priority for the family.

Being sensitive to family transition events (normative and nonnormative) and providing extra support at these times (if desired by the family) is also important. Events such as the death of a parent, launching of an older child, or job transition can all take time and attention away from intervention efforts. Consider the big picture when working with a family.

During nonnormative transition events, families sometimes find it extremely helpful to be connected with other families of children who have disabilities. They can share information, similar experiences, and methods of coping. "Parent-to-parent programs" exist in many communities, and research has demonstrated their helpfulness.[7]

FAMILY ADAPTATION
Description

In what ways do families adapt to unexpected events, such as the birth of a child who has developmental delays? Crises, which are brought on by overwhelming stress, are not *always* negative. Families are living systems that evolve in response to internal events (for example, illness, death, birth, emancipation) and external events (for example, loss of job, a move to another city, occupational therapy practitioner involvement). Like all living things, families are generally adaptive by nature. Although serious crises can precipitate alcoholism, separation or divorce, or family violence, in some cases they can enable rapid positive changes, such as recommitment to a marriage or resolution of a long-standing conflict. For many years, research on families of children with disabilities was focused on family dysfunction, stress, and pathology. However, in recent years, research revealed what some families had been saying for years: despite the stress caused by their child's disability, dealing with the disability strengthened the family or changed it in some positive way.[8]

Families react and adapt to crises in individualized and unique ways. Family **adaptation** is affected by the interaction of family **resources** (for example, time, money, friends) and family perceptions (the way events are defined).

Social support plays an extremely important role in family and individual well-being. For families of children with disabilities, the informal support of family, friends, and neighbors appears to be more important than the formal support received from professionals and institutions. Of course, an important factor is the way families define their resources. In the previously mentioned Sanchez family, the extended family is a source of positive support for Margarita's parents, whereas in other families, having a mother-in-law and aunt living in the home could be a source of additional stress.

In addition, the way families define and understand a particular event, such as the birth of a child with a disability, is an important component of family adaptation. Specific **perceptual coping strategies** are listed in Box 2-4.

At times, therapists get impatient with families who seem to be ignoring or minimizing problems. Although being judgmental in these situations is tempting, these families are using their own coping strategies. Families adapt as a whole, and this adaptive capacity should be supported. Occupational therapy practitioners should not assess a given situation and assign direct responsibility to any specific factor. For example, a practitioner cannot accurately assume that George, a 6-year-old who cannot tie his shoes, would be able to if he had only started occupational therapy work at age 3. Too many other variables are relevant. For example, family financial demands, time constraints, and emotional strain may have been significant when George was 3. Beginning occupational ther-

---

BOX 2-4

Perceptual Coping Strategies

PASSIVE APPRAISAL
Ignoring a problem and hoping it will go away

REFRAMING
Redefining a situation in ways that make it more manageable

DOWNWARD COMPARISON
Identifying a situation that is worse than your own

USE OF SPIRITUAL BELIEFS
Using philosophical or spiritual beliefs to make sense of and find meaning in a situation

---

apy at that age could have forced George's father, who had overcome drinking and spousal abuse problems, to regress. In turn, this could have caused George to regress and lose his toileting skills. No individual, not even an occupational therapy practitioner, can conceive of all potential positive outcomes and all the ways to achieve these outcomes. Families and occupational therapy practitioners have attitudes and biases about causes of problems and possibilities of overcoming them. Regardless, the adaptive potential of a family as a whole is unlimited, and remembering this can help families and occupational therapy practitioners achieve the best possible outcomes.

Implications for Practice

When meeting a family for the first time, it is important to be curious and interested in the unique ways that the family has been adapting to their child's disability—the ingenious ways that they cope in their daily lives. In the previously mentioned story about Margarita Sanchez, this inadvertently happened when Heather became ill and had to watch the family carry out their daily routine.

CLINICAL *Pearl*

When meeting a family for the first time, it is important to express curiosity and interest in the unique ways that they are adapting to their child's disability without judging and evaluating.

It is also important to utilize and support existing resources in families' lives. Occupational therapy practitioners sometimes get so excited about specialized support services that they forget about generic support services, such as churches, neighborhood playgrounds, and community recreation centers, that are closer to home. If occupational therapy practitioners are not careful, their clients may suddenly realize that they have lost touch with neighbors and friends because of the time spent taking their children to specialized programs far from home. They could end up as part of a specialized world inhabited mainly by professionals.

Families must carry out daily tasks to perform the basic family functions.* Family routines must be considered when home therapy programs are developed, otherwise time-consuming programs maybe prescribed that simply cannot be done within the parameters of the daily household routines and time schedule.

ESSENTIAL SKILLS FOR SUCCESSFUL INTERVENTION WITH FAMILIES

For occupational therapy practitioners, having good communication skills is equally as important as having the proper knowledge to treat a client. Some essential communication skills include the following:

- *Solution-focused curiosity and interest:* People generally have an extremely positive response to practitioners who are nonjudgmentally interested in them and their situations. The focus should be on strengths, achievements, and desires rather than on the traditional problems and deficits. This "solution focus" allows the practitioner to support the adaptive potential of the family and accept its current state. Using the previous story about the Sanchez family as an example, Heather could have asked Mrs. Sanchez, "What have you found works best for feeding Margarita?" rather than "What problems do you encounter when feeding Margarita?"
- *Contract development:* A family who has requested or been referred for occupational therapy services has some goal, even if only a vague goal, that they hope the services will help accomplish. The practitioner may have a very different idea of what the goal should be. Collaborating with the family to clarify and develop a common set of goals, or verbal **contract,** helps practitioners efficiently and effectively develop the treatment plan. For example, after introducing herself, Heather could have asked Mrs. Sanchez about Margarita and what she hoped to accomplish by

getting involved with the early intervention program. Asking, "What are Margarita's biggest problems?" or stating, "I think we should work on toileting so that Margarita is ready for kindergarten" could slow the development of a relationship between Heather and the Sanchez family. Carefully eliciting and acknowledging the family's wishes would create a solid basis for working with them. Heather could say something like, "So, you aren't sure about what you want to accomplish, but no matter what we do, Mrs. Sanchez, you want Margarita to feel like she is a part of the whole family." If Mrs. Sanchez nodded and smiled, Heather would know that she had identified the primary goal to be reached (or contract to be followed) with the Sanchez family.

CLINICAL *Pearl*

When talking with families, ask "how" questions rather than "why" questions. Ask them to describe rather than explain situations. Instead of trying to establish some sort of linear cause and effect relationship between different factors, try simply to understand the relationships among events, people, and situations.

- *Acknowledgment:* "Solution-focused curiosity and interest" and "contract development" are skills that are grounded in the central communication tool known as **acknowledgment,** a tool that practitioners can use to assure their clients that what they are saying is being heard and understood. Occupational therapy practitioners can acknowledge the clients with whom they are speaking by providing appropriate feedback. Feedback can be verbal repetition or confirmation of the clients' statements (for example, "So you have lived here for 5 years" or "I see"), nonverbal body movements (for example, nodding the head, sitting forward with an interested expression), or paraverbal cues (for example, "uh-huh" or "mm-hmm").
- *Time management:* An occupational therapist's arrival and departure are the most important moments of contact with a family. At both times the practitioner should be solution focused or future oriented. When arriving at the home, the practitioner is attempting to establish or reestablish a positive rapport with the family. After discussing any relevant events that have taken place since the previous visit, the practitioner creates or restates an agreed-on contract to guide activities during the current visit. When departing from the home, the practitioner and family identify events that will or may take place before the next visit, as well as

---

*Family functions include activities related to education, recreation, daily care, affection, economics, and self-identity.[7]

discuss a potential contract for the next visit. It can be difficult and frustrating for a practitioner to leave after a visit in which little progress has been made. In such a case, it is often helpful to leave the family with some "homework" relating to their goal—to look for and note circumstances that relate to their defined goal—so that the practitioner can use the information as a stepping stone in the next session. For example, imagine that a family wants their daughter to be able to zip a zipper, but the goal seems unreachable and little progress is being made. Their occupational therapy practitioner could ask them to pay attention to the circumstances under which their daughter attempts to touch or play with the zipper. The visit can then end on a more positive note, with the family having a smaller goal on which to focus.

SUMMARY

Family systems theory provides a useful framework for thinking about families and the ways in which they operate. The challenges and triumphs of parenting a child who has disabilities are similar to other challenges and triumphs that all families face, regardless of whether they have children with disabilities. An important factor in whether families can successfully adapt to these challenges is the strength and support of their relationships with other key individuals. An occupational therapy practitioner is one of these key players—a person who has the opportunity to make a difference in the life of a family through a sensitive, individualized intervention approach.

References

1. American Occupational Therapy Association: *AOTA 1995-96 member update*, Bethesda, Md, 1996, The Association.
2. American Occupational Therapy Association Commission of Education: *Guidelines for curriculum content in pediatrics*, Bethesda, Md, 1991, The Association.
3. American Speech-Language-Hearing Association: *We can do better: recruiting, retaining, and graduating African-American students*, 1995, The Association.
4. Bacharach S: *Education reform: making sense of it all*, New York, 1990, Medina.
5. Dunst C, Trivette C, Deal A: *Enabling and empowering families: principles and guidelines for practice*, Cambridge, Mass, 1988, Brookline Books.
6. Simons R: *After the tears: parents talk about raising a child with a disability*, San Diego, 1987, Harcourt Brace.
7. Singer G et al: A multi-site evaluation of Parent-to-Parent programs, *J Early Intervention*, 1998.
8. Turnbull AP, Turnbull HR: *Families, professionals, and exceptionality: a special partnership*, ed 3, Englewood Cliffs, NJ, 1997, Prentice Hall.

Recommended Reading

McWilliam PJ, Winton PJ, Crais ER: *Practical strategies for family-centered intervention*, San Diego, 1996, Singular Press.
McWilliam PJ, Bailey DB: *Working with children and families: case studies in early intervention*, Baltimore, 1993, Paul Brookes.
Turnbull AP, Turnbull HR: *Families, professionals and exceptionality: a special partnership*, ed 3, Englewood Cliffs, NJ, 1997, Prentice Hall.

REVIEW *Questions*

1. What are three current societal trends that impact the work of the occupational therapy practitioner? Describe the impact of these trends on occupational therapy pediatric practice.
2. Describe three key concepts related to family systems theory and the implications of these concepts for occupational therapy practitioners.
3. Explain the reason nonnormative transition events may be more stressful than normative events.
4. Using the information provided on family systems and family adaptation, explain the reason it is important to individualize therapy programs for children and families.
5. What are four communication strategies that could be used during the initial home visit with a family?

SUGGESTED *Activities*

1. Spend some time with a child with disabilities in the child's natural environment (e.g., home, neighborhood). Observe the various activities taking place. Keep a list of the ways different therapy activities could be embedded in these routines. Imagine the way therapy concepts could be introduced to the parents and then implemented. Write these ideas down.
2. Talk with families of children with disabilities and with occupational therapy practitioners. Ask each group to describe characteristics of an occupational therapy practitioner that they think are important. Take notes and summarize their comments. Compare the comments of the two groups. Create a personal list of the skills and competencies of an effective occupational therapy practitioner.

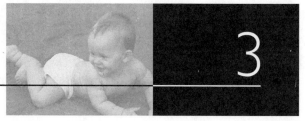

Medical System

DAWN B. OAKLEY

KATHLEEN LOGAN-BAUER

CHAPTER *Objectives*

After studying this chapter, the reader will be able to accomplish the following:

- Identify and discuss the key components (that is, settings and key members) of a pediatric medical system
- Differentiate among pediatric acute, subacute, long-term care and home care medical settings
- List five commonly assessed areas of function in a pediatric, medical-based occupational therapy evaluation
- Differentiate among the multidisciplinary, transdisciplinary, and interdisciplinary styles of collaboration
- Discuss the role of treatment and documentation in a pediatric medical system
- Discuss medical reimbursement issues and payment options for pediatric medical services
- Identify three important challenges faced by a medical-based pediatric practice

KEY TERMS	CHAPTER OUTLINE

MEDICAL CARE SETTINGS

A medical system includes many team members, including children, families, specialists, generalists, nurses, physicians, physical therapists, recreational therapists, speech and language pathologists, and occupational therapists. A *pediatric medical care system* is a group of individuals (professional, paraprofessional, and nonprofessional) who form a complex and unified whole dedicated to caring for children who are ill (Box 3-1). To a beginning allied health care professional, this environment may seem overwhelming at first.

Comprehensive pediatric medical care includes a continuum of various settings. Pediatric medical care is provided in one of five settings: a neonatal intensive care unit (NICU), a step-down nursery or pediatric intensive care unit (PICU), a subacute setting, the home, or a residential, or long-term care, facility.

BOX 3-1

Key Pediatric Medical Terms

CARDIOLOGIST
A physician specializing in the treatment of heart disease.

CIVILIAN HEALTH AND MEDICAL PROGRAM OF THE UNIFORMED SERVICES (CHAMPUS)
CHAMPUS provides supplemental benefits to those in the uniform services direct medical care system. The program pays for medical care given by civilian providers to eligible persons, who include retired members of the United States uniformed services and their dependents, dependents of deceased members of the military, and dependents of members of the North Atlantic Treaty Organization (NATO) when the NATO member is stationed in or passing through the United States on official business. The CHAMPUS program is spelled out in 32 CFR, section 199. The program is administered by the Department of Defense.

CIVILIAN HEALTH AND MEDICAL PROGRAM OF THE VETERANS ADMINISTRATION (CHAMPVA)
The federal program administered by the Defense Department of Veterans Administration that provides care for the dependents of totally disabled veterans. Care is given by civilian providers.

DEVELOPMENTAL PEDIATRICIAN
A pediatrician with specialized training in the developmental milestones of typical childhood development

GENETICIST
A person who specializes in genetics

HMO/PPO
Health maintenance organization, preferred provided organization

MEDICAID
The federal program that provides health care to indigent and medically indigent persons (i.e., those who cannot afford to pay their medical bills and qualify for Medicaid for medically related services). Although partially federally funded, the Medicaid program is administered by the states, in contrast to Medicare, which is funded and administered at the federal level by the Health Care Financing Administration (HCFA). The Medicaid program was established in 1965 by an amendment to the Social Security Act under a provision entitled *Title XIX—Medical Assistance*.

NEONATALOGIST
A pediatrician with 3 years of advanced education who specializes in the treatment of neonates and premature infants

NEUROLOGIST
A physician who specializes in nervous system diseases

OPHTHALMOLOGIST
A physician who specializes in the treatment of eye disorders

Modified from Slee V, Slee D: *Slee's health care terms,* ed 3, St Paul, 1996, Tringa Press; Thomas CL, editor: *Taber's cyclopedic medical dictionary,* ed 18, Philadelphia, 1997, FA Davis.
Continued

BOX 3-1

Key Pediatric Medical Terms—cont'd

ORTHOPEDIST

A specialist in orthopedics

PEDIATRICIAN

A physician who specializes in the diagnosis and treatment of illnesses and dysfunctions of children

PEDIATRIC NURSE PRACTITIONER

A registered nurse who provides primary health care to children (e.g., Jane Grey, R.N., P.N.P). Special preparation is required.

PHYSIATRIST

A physician who specializes in physical medicine

PHYSICAL THERAPY ASSISTANT

A technical health care worker trained to carry out physical therapy procedures under the supervision of a physical therapist

PULMONOLOGIST

A physician who is trained and certified to treat pulmonary diseases

RADIOLOGIST

A physician who uses x-rays or other sources of radiation for diagnosis and treatment

REGISTERED PHYSICAL THERAPIST

A health care worker who has successfully completed an accredited physical therapy education program and passed a licensing examination. A registered physical therapist is legally responsible for evaluating, planning, conducting, and supervising a physical therapy program using rehabilitative and therapeutic exercise techniques and physical modalities.

SPEECH AND LANGUAGE PATHOLOGIST

An individual who is educated and trained to plan, direct, and conduct programs to improve the communication skills of children and adults with language and speech impairments caused by physiological factors, articulation problems, or dialect. A speech and language pathologist can evaluate programs and may perform research related to speech and language problems.

Modified from Slee V, Slee D: *Slee's health care terms*, ed 3, St Paul, 1996, Tringa Press; Thomas CL, editor: *Taber's cyclopedic medical dictionary*, ed 18, Philadelphia, 1997, FA Davis.

Neonatal Intensive Care Unit

The NICU is needed for infants who have complicated births. The goal of the NICU team is to address the **acute,** or extremely severe, symptoms or conditions of an infant to so that the infant can become physiologically stable (i.e., maintain a stable body temperature, heart rate, and respiratory rate).

The medical status of NICU clients is closely monitored by the medical team. A neonatologist serves as the leader of the NICU team (Figure 3-1). In addition to conducting a neonatal assessment, the neonatologist consults the other medical team professionals about the specific needs of the infant. The following conditions may indicate that an infant should be admitted to the NICU: cyanosis— an infant who turns blue because of insufficient oxygen; bradycardia—a heart rate of less than 100 beats per minute (bpm); low birth weight (LBW)—a weight of less than 2500 g; very low birth weight (VLBW)—a weight of less

than 1500 g; or extremely low birth weight (ELBW)— a weight of less than 750 g. When presented with an infant who has one or more of these conditions, additional medical team members should take part in consultations and provide additional examinations. Pulmonologists (lung specialists), cardiologists (heart specialists), gastroenterologists (digestive specialists), and respiratory therapists are examples of the additional medical team members who may be needed to address the needs of infants in the NICU.

Pediatric Intensive Care Unit

After an infant meets certain physiological requirements, the infant is moved out of the NICU. If the medical team determines that the infant still requires some form of hospital-based medical care, the infant can be transferred to a step-down nursery or pediatric intensive care unit (PICU) (Figure 3-2). In addition to continuing to address

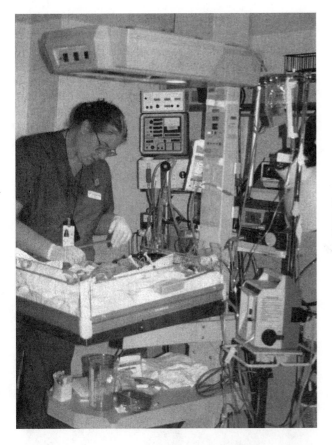

FIGURE 3-1 The NICU can be an overwhelming environment. (From Parham LD, Fazio LS: *Play in occupational therapy for children,* St Louis, 1997, Mosby.)

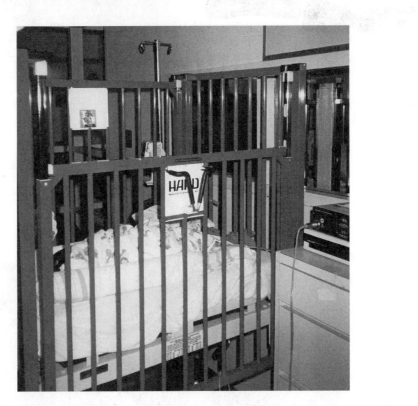

FIGURE 3-2 Infants are transferred to a step-down nursery or PICU when they have the ability to maintain satisfactory physiological functioning. (Courtesy Dawn B. Oakley and Kathleen Logan-Bauer, Bayside, New York.)

the acute symptoms infant, the goals of the PICU team are to attempt to wean the infant from external sources of medical support, and when applicable, provide sensorimotor stimulation. As the infant is moved from one unit to another, certain additional team members may be required, whereas the services of certain other members may no longer be needed. For example, in the PICU, the infant's medical team leader is no longer a neonatologist, it is a pediatrician.

Subacute Setting

After being released from a step-down nursery or PICU, an infant may be able to go home, but may be required to move to a **subacute** (Figure 3-3) setting. The medical needs of a given infant, as well as the desires of the infant's primary caregivers, have an impact on this decision. The goals of the subacute team are to provide appropriate medical treatment while continuing to wean the infant off medical supports and to continue carrying out developmentally based therapeutic interventions.

Home

As an infant's status improves, discharge plans are formulated. The issue of where the infant goes after being discharged is discussed with the infant's primary caregivers. Going home is the ultimate goal of infants in acute, step-down nursery, and subacute settings. Once at home, the goals are to facilitate caregiver and infant bonding and promote the continued acquisition of developmentally appropriate skills.

The medical needs of infants who have been discharged and gone home are handled on an outpatient basis. They receive medical care through scheduled clinic

and outpatient hospital-based visits (Figure 3-4). The infant's nursing, therapy, and equipment needs are coordinated by a community **home care** agency. Home care agencies are to monitor their client's medical needs and provide and coordinate home-based therapeutic services. The age of the client determines where services are pro-

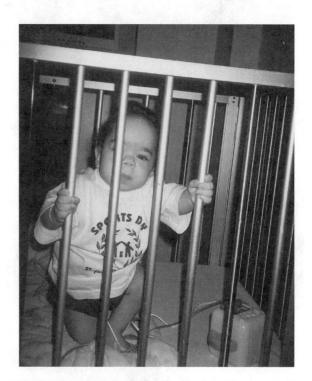

FIGURE 3-3   As infants become medically stable, they are discharged and transferred to a subacute or home care setting. A commercially available device is often all that is necessary to monitor the infants when they are alone. (Courtesy Dawn B. Oakley and Kathleen Logan-Bauer, Bayside, New York.)

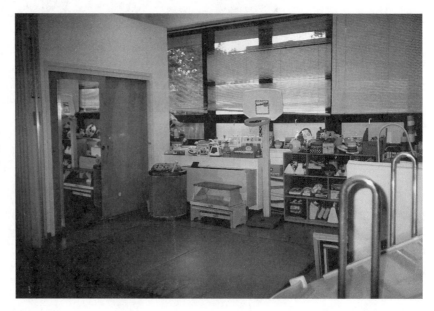

FIGURE 3-4   Occupational therapy outpatient hospital-based clinic. (Courtesy Dawn B. Oakley and Kathleen Logan-Bauer, Bayside, New York.)

vided. Infants and young children usually receive home-based services. As children mature, any additional needed therapy services may be provided in an outpatient clinic or community-based school setting.

CLINICAL *Pearl*

Practitioners must respect families' values, beliefs, and customs while providing home-based occupational therapy services for children.

Long-Term Care Facility

During discharge planning, some primary caregivers decide that they are unable to handle their child's specific medical needs. In these cases, residential or **long-term care** facilities are options. The goals of the long-term care team are to provide appropriate medical care and carry out appropriate therapeutic interventions. An example of a therapeutic intervention is providing sensorimotor stimulation to prevent the development of contractures and prevent or minimize losses in range of motion.

MOVING THROUGH THE MEDICAL SYSTEM CONTINUUM

The extent to which a child is involved in the medical system continuum can change significantly as the child's circumstances change. For example, a child may be admitted to an acute care facility because of an acute illness. The child may be subsequently discharged and return home but then be admitted to a long-term care facility because of extenuating circumstances at home. This is just one example of the way a child's involvement in the pediatric medical care system can change. The following case study follows the progression of one child through the pediatric medical care settings.

CASE *Study*

Daniel was born after 33 weeks gestation by a cesarean section with vacuum extraction because of fetal distress. At birth, he was limp and cyanotic with a heart rate of less than 100 bpm. No respiratory effort was noted at birth. Daniel's birth weight was 2900 g. He required mechanical ventilation for the first 3 days of life. Daniel was weaned to nasal continuous positive airway pressure (CPAP) from days 3 to 18. He was reintubated on day 25 for gastrostomy tube placement.

Three days after his gastrostomy tube placement, Daniel was transferred to a step-down nursery. After the transfer, consultation requests were made to the staff geneticist, a physiatrist, and rehabilitation services.

After Daniel had spent 30 days in the step-down nursery, the medical team and his parents determined that he should be discharged and transferred to a subacute facility. The responsibility of Daniel's treatment was assumed by the subacute facility.

The medical team and Daniel's parents decided that he was ready to be discharged and return home after he spent 1 year as an inpatient at the subacute facility. Daniel's care was transferred from inpatient, medical-based care to outpatient, home-based medical care.

As noted in the case study, when a pregnant mother has an emergency delivery, some degree of pediatric medical care is often required to treat birth-related trauma. In addition, children may need pediatric medical care for accidental injuries, neurological and musculoskeletal traumas, and complications resulting from genetic defects.

ROLE OF OCCUPATIONAL THERAPY IN THE PEDIATRIC MEDICAL SYSTEM

CLINICAL *Pearl*

Childhood is filled with many typical developmental stages and events. The normal developmental progression can be negatively affected by atypical experiences and events, such as a prolonged hospitalization.

The prolonged hospitalization of an infant or child is not a normally occurring event. A hospitalization of more than a few days puts a typical child at risk for some degree of developmental delay. For example, to develop meaningful social and emotional bonds, infants and children need to be comforted and held by other human beings. Children and infants who are hospitalized typically are not held as often as those who are not in a hospital. These children and infants could have difficulty developing the social and emotional skills needed for successful interactions with members of their families and schools.

The perceived or actual presence of developmental deficits warrants the provision of occupational therapy and other rehabilitative services. Perceived deficits are deficits that may not yet be present but are known to be associated with a particular condition such as Down syndrome. Perceived deficits can also be temporary developmental delays resulting from atypical experiences and events. The fundamental principle of occupational therapy is to promote optimal performance in each of the developmental areas: gross motor, fine motor, cognitive, and activities of daily living (ADLs). Pediatric medical-based occupational therapy practitioners use play activities to facilitate the acquisition of age-appropriate developmental skills.

Role of the Occupational Therapy Practitioner

Medical-based occupational therapy practitioners are either registered occupational therapists (OTRs) or certified occupational therapy assistants (COTAs). OTRs are responsible for providing the overall framework for medical-based services. Collaboration between the two types of occupational therapy practitioners is essential and is facilitated by the COTA's knowledge of the OTR's responsibilities, which include conducting **screenings** and **evaluations,** formulating and carrying out daily treatment plans, and documentation. COTAs responsibilities include formulating and carrying out daily treatment plans and documentation. COTAs also assist with or conduct portions of the pediatric medical-based screening and contribute to the pediatric medical-based evaluation.

After receiving a referral from a physician, the medical-based pediatric screening and evaluation are usually completed by the OTR within 24 and 72 hours, respectively. The screening and evaluation are conducted using formal and informal measurement tools as well as clinical and parental observations. Throughout the assessment process, a medical-based practitioner should be aware that factors such as time, the severity of the illness, and the overall stress associated with being in a hospital environment may mask a child's true abilities in a given performance area.

The deficits that are identified during the screening and evaluation are addressed in a medical treatment plan. An OTR usually formulates the long-term goals and short-term objectives that guide the treatment plan. The medical treatment plan is developed by an OTR or OTR and COTA. The medical treatment plan is an outline of the activities and tasks that are used during treatment sessions.

The occupational therapy practitioner initiates occupational therapy treatment only when the medical stability of a child has been determined. The medical stability is used to determine the manner in which services are provided and how often they are provided. The goals in the treatment plan should be gradually integrated into the child's environment. Treatment strategies should increase, not decrease, the child's functional level.

Role of the COTA

As mentioned previously, medical-based pediatric occupational therapy services are provided to promote the optimal function of hospitalized children. COTAs are prepared to play a role in the provision of these services. The responsibilities of the COTA are dictated by the facility in which services are being provided. Typical responsibilities of a COTA include conducting an initial developmental screening, collaborating with another practitioner on an evaluation, planning treatment, updating goals, and collaborating with another practitioner on developing a discharge plan.

The following discussion of the role of the COTA in a pediatric medical care setting follows the course outlined in the previous case study. Daniel's medical care was initiated in the hospital and continued after he was discharged and sent home.

Neonatal Intensive Care Unit

NICU-based treatment is performed only by highly qualified allied health professionals. The therapists who work in the NICU are required to have advanced education and certification in NICU-based treatment. For example, therapists in the NICU must have a thorough knowledge of life signs, which are key indicators of the infant's status (for example, color, respiration rate, body temperature, extremity movement). Changes in these indicators are noted by the therapist through sight, hearing, and touch.[8] A role for the COTA in the provision of NICU services has not been identified.[1] If a practitioner would like to work with this special client population, the practitioner should obtain the necessary education and certification required to ensure that treatment is provided safely and appropriately.

Step-Down Nursery and Pediatric Intensive Care Unit

Providing treatment in a step-down nursery or PICU also requires related experience to ensure the provision of the most appropriate treatment. However, unlike in the NICU, COTAs with appropriate educational training may be able to receive on-the-job training, which qualifies them to assume a role in providing medical service in the step-down nursery and PICU.[1]

Additional education and on-the-job training are necessities for COTAs in the step-down nursery and PICU because the infants and children admitted to these units may still have significant medical problems. A COTA working in one or both of these settings usually participates in the screening, evaluation, and treatment of the clients. COTAs should be aware that the initiation of a screening or treatment may distress a step-down nursery or PICU client. During the initiation of any screening or treatment procedures, COTAs should be sensitive to indications of distress and prepared to respond appropriately.

During the initial screening and assessment, the COTA is introduced, or oriented, to the client's case. Each client is evaluated to establish a functional physiological baseline (for example, respiratory rate, heart rate, oxygen saturation level). Clients must constantly be evaluated during daily treatment sessions to ensure they remain within the physiological range that was established according to their baseline functioning level.

Subacute, Long-Term Care, and Home Care Settings

COTAs must be trained in medical-based pediatric therapy to provide services in the subacute, long-term care, and home care settings. The difference between working in one of these settings and a step-down nursery or PICU is that an experienced COTA practitioner may not be required to work under the direct supervision of an OTR in these types of settings. The clients in these settings are typically more medically stable than those in the NICU, step-down nursery, or PICU. However, COTAs working in these settings should be familiar with the signs of physiological distress and prepared to respond properly.

TEAM COLLABORATION

Team collaboration is important in any medical setting, but it plays a particularly essential and integral part of medical and therapeutic intervention in a pediatric medical setting. Before initiation of a therapeutic intervention, practitioners should consult with the doctors and nurses assigned to the client's care. Practitioners should frequently obtain updates on the status of their clients. Areas of particular importance include medications, physiological stability, nutritional status, and sleep patterns. Practitioners can obtain information from the medical team from written reports and during rounds and team meetings.

Consultations among medical team members facilitate team collaboration. Team members may use one of four types of collaborative styles: **multidisciplinary, interdisciplinary, transdisciplinary,** or "individual versus group" sessions[9] (Table 3-1).

TABLE 3-1

Methods of Team Collaboration

APPROACH	DESCRIPTION
Multidisciplinary	The multidisciplinary approach evolved from a medical model in which multiple professionals evaluated the child and made recommendations.[10] Professionals who use this type of approach may be directly or indirectly involved with the child and family but do not necessarily consult or interact with each other. Assessment, goal setting, and direct intervention may be carried out by each professional with minimal integration across disciplines.[3]
Interdisciplinary	The interdisciplinary approach to treatment is cooperative and interactive. A team comprising professionals from several disciplines (who are often at the same location) have frequent, direct involvement with the child and collaborate with each other on the child's program. Although evaluations are performed independently by discipline, program planning is carried out by group consensus, and goals are set collaboratively with professionals and parents. This approach allows the child and family to receive coordinated services and benefit from the expertise of professionals from several disciplines.[5]
Transdisciplinary	Although the transdisciplinary approach involves collaboration among various disciplines, one team member is usually designated to intervene directly, and the other team members act as consultants. This approach was developed on the basis that families benefit more from having their intervention program provided by one primary professional rather than multiple professionals. All team members contribute to assessment and program planning, and then the designated person implements the plan while consulting with other members of the team. Therefore the transdisciplinary model enables health care professionals to perform tasks that are normally outside the scope of practice of their discipline. Implementation of this model requires professionals to be comfortable with role release, or relinquishing some or all of their professional duties to another professional. During this process, team members must share information and exchange responsibilities.[7]
"Individual Versus Group" Sessions	The "individual versus group" sessions approach is used to encourage frequent team member collaboration. It allows for informal and impromptu communication between two or three team members. During the team collaborations, information is exchanged about the child's status. Specific information is shared so that members can compare notes, which in turn serves to improve the treatment approaches of the members of the individual disciplines.[9]

Modified from Case-Smith J, Allen AS, Pratt PN: Arenas of occupational therapy services. In Case-Smith J, Allen AS, Pratt PN, editors: *Occupational therapy for children*, ed 3, St Louis, 1996, Mosby.

BOX 3-2

Medical-Based Occupational Therapy Evaluation

ST. MARY'S HOSPITAL FOR CHILDREN INITIAL OCCUPATIONAL THERAPY EVALUATION

Name: Kevin   Unit: CUW
DOB: 7/13/80   Sex: Male
Medical Record #: 12345
Diagnosis: Duchenne's muscular dystrophy
2/28/98: Doctor's orders received. Full evaluation with recommendations to follow.

MEDICAL HISTORY

Kevin is a 17-year- 8-month-old male with Duchenne's muscular dystrophy. On 3/21/96, he underwent a spinal fusion and multiple tendon releases. He was subsequently placed in two long-leg casts with bars. Kevin was born at 36 weeks gestation and weighed 5 lb, 5 oz. Kevin was a healthy child until he was diagnosed with Duchenne's muscular dystrophy at age 5.

GENERAL OBSERVATIONS

Kevin is a thin, frail male who has an overall decreased affect. He has a scar from spinal surgery that extends from approximately T1/T2 to his coccyx. He is able to verbalize his needs by speaking in a soft, high-pitched voice. Kevin is able to visually track objects in all planes. He is seated in a reclined wheelchair with his lower extremities elevated and in a spica cast.

GROSS MOTOR FUNCTION

Kevin has hypotonicity throughout his trunk and upper extremities. He is unable to transition from a prone to a supine position or a supine to a prone position. Kevin requires significant assistance to maintain a sitting posture. He exhibits pectus excavation, bilateral scapular winging, a kyphotic posture, and bilateral rib flaring.

UPPER EXTREMITY FUNCTION

Passive range of motion (PROM) is WNL. Goniometric active range of motion (AROM) measurements are as follows (*WNL*, within normal limits):

	R	L
Shoulder flexion	No ROM at either shoulder; uses compensatory techniques (e.g., climbs arms on chest)	
Elbow flexion	Flexes both elbows in a gravity-eliminated plane	
Wrist extension	0-30 degrees	0-25 degrees
Wrist flexion	0-60 degrees	0-55 degrees
Ulnar deviation	0-30 degrees	WNL
Radial deviation	0-20 degrees	WNL
Supination	WNL	WNL
Pronation	WNL	WNL

(Courtesy Kathleen Logan-Bauer, Bayside, NY.)

CLINICAL *Pearl*

For a transdisciplinary team to be effective, the team members must trust and respect each other so that they are comfortable with role release (that is, relinquishing certain professional duties to other team members).

DOCUMENTATION

The ability to clearly document the events that occur in a pediatric medical setting is crucially important. Documentation is used for many purposes including updating others on clients' status, justifying the necessity of services, and explaining requests for supplies and reimbursements.

A practitioner who works in a pediatric medical care system should know the types of documentation that ex-

BOX 3-2

Medical-Based Occupational Therapy Evaluation—cont'd

A functional muscle test was performed with Kevin positioned in a semireclined wheelchair at approximately 60 degrees (*DIP*, distal interphalangeal; *PIP*, proximal interphalangeal):

Elbow flexion	P+	P
Elbow extension	P+	P+
Pronation	F+	P/P+
Wrist extension	F+/G−	F−
Wrist flexion	F+/G−	P+
DIP flexion	G	P+
PIP flexion	G	P+

Gross grasp and pinch strengths follow:

	R	MEAN	L	MEAN
Gross grasp	5.1 lb	108 lb	2.2 lb	93 lb
3-jaw-chuck	0 lb	23.8 lb	0 lb	23.4 lb
Lateral pinch	0 lb	23.5 lb	0 lb	22.9 lb
Pincer grasp	0 lb	17 lb	0 lb	16.1 lb

Stereognosis, temperature, pain and proprioceptive/kinesthetic awareness are intact.

COGNITIVE/PERCEPTUAL FUNCTION

Kevin is able to state his address, telephone number, and birthday. With constant verbal prompts, he is able to independently assemble a 25-piece puzzle. Kevin has a low attention span and poor overall endurance.

Formal cognitive and perceptual testing place Kevin in the ninth percentile rank of his peers. He has notable deficits in the areas of: visual memory, visual-spatial relationships, and visual figure-ground relationships.

ADL

Kevin depends on staff for all of his self-care activities. He attempts to help dress himself when prompted. He demonstrates the ability to independently button three small buttons. However, he complains of finger pain when asked to unbutton the small buttons. Kevin is able to hold and eat a sandwich that is placed into his hand. He places his hand on his upper chest and bends his neck to eat the sandwich. Kevin requires elbow support to bring a spoon to his mouth. He requires a flexible straw to drink.

EQUIPMENT

Kevin is currently positioned in a reclining wheelchair with elevated leg rests. A power wheelchair has been ordered by his school therapist. He wears a body jacket when he sits at an angle of more than 45 degrees. A bilateral forearm orthosis was suggested for Kevin to allow him to eat more independently, but he was resistant to the idea.

SUMMARY/RECOMMENDATIONS

Kevin is a 17-year- 18-month-old male who has Duchenne's muscular dystrophy. He has decreased muscle tone and strength, which interferes with his ability to function independently. This therapist recommends that Kevin receive occupational therapy services.

ist and reasons these documents are necessary. A medical-based screening or assessment is usually the first type of document a practitioner is required to complete. An initial screening may be used to determine whether a thorough evaluation is needed. In some medical care settings, a more detailed assessment is the second step in the documentation process. In other medical care settings the assessment is the first document completed by a practi-

tioner. Screenings and evaluations usually comprise some if not all of the following sections: medical history, general observations, gross motor function, fine motor function, visual and perceptual function, cognitive function, sensory function (when applicable), ADL function, summary and recommendations, frequency, long-term goals, and short-term goals. Box 3-2 contains an example of a medical assessment that outlines a client's strengths and weaknesses. The information is used to establish baseline functioning, thereby delineating the parameters for improvement.

A specific example of a standardized pediatric assessment is the WeeFIM (UB Foundation Activities, Inc, Queens, NY.)[13] The WeeFIM is a functional assessment that is used to describe a child's performance during essential activities; it is used to measure which activities children can actually carry out, not what they may be capable of doing. The assessment can be used to clarify a child's functional status, provide information for team conferences, facilitate goal planning, and provide information on burden of care issues, which are issues relating to person who is meeting the child's basic needs, (that is, eating, bathing, dressing, grooming, transferring, moving, and toileting).[12,13] The WeeFIM also provides a common, uniform language for practitioners to use when measuring and documenting the severity of disabilities and outcomes of pediatric rehabilitation and habilitation. It allows practitioners to measure disability types as well as determine the amount of help a certain child needs to perform basic skills. The assessment is conducted using direct observations or interviews of the caregiver and can be used for pediatric inpatients and outpatients (Box 3-3) (although it is not meant to be used as the only diagnostic tool).

CLINICAL *Pearl*

The WeeFIM is a tool that can be used for efficient assessments and documentation of progress.

After the initial screening or assessment has been completed, the practitioner notes the child's progress and changes in the status over time. The progress is recorded in the form of a daily note, weekly progress note, or monthly progress note in a narrative or **SOAP note** format (see Chapter 1). The acronym "SOAP" stands for subjective information, objective (what is done), assessment (effect of treatment), and plan (what will be done). (See *Physical Dysfunction: Practice Skills for the Occupational Therapy Assistant* [which is listed in the references] for a clear, concise description of common medical documentation.[6])

Progress notes are important for justifying service implementation and continuation of services and for discharge planning. A practitioner should record the therapeutic interventions and the child's responses to them clearly and concisely (see Chapter 12).

When a child's therapy program includes a piece of specialized medical equipment, the practitioner must doc-

---

BOX 3-3

WeeFIM Instrument Rating Guidelines

INPATIENT
Within 72 Hours of Admission
WeeFIM admission assessment must be completed.

Within 72 Hours of Discharge
WeeFIM discharge assessment must be completed.

Within 80 to 180 Days of Discharge
WeeFIM follow-up assessment must be completed. Interim WeeFIM assessments (between admission and discharge) may be performed at facility's discretion.

OUTPATIENT
During Initial Contact
WeeFIM admission assessment must be completed. Additional WeeFIM assessments may be performed at facility's discretion.

At Time of Discharge
WeeFIM discharge assessment must be completed.

Modified from Uniform Data Systems for Medical Rehabilitation: *WeeFIM system workshop,* Queens, NY, 1988, UB Foundation Activities.

---

ument the reason. Insurance sources may be reluctant to provide equipment for children in inpatient medical care settings. A child's insurance source may approve or deny a request based on a practitioner's ability to justify the necessity of the requested item. The necessity of a certain piece of equipment can be justified by identifying the ways in which it will benefit the child's level of functioning. Some examples of functions that should be discussed are respiratory, cardiac, musculoskeletal, esophageal, and gastrointestinal functions; benefits related to the child's safety should be discussed as well. An example of a letter of justification is shown in Box 3-4. The letter includes information on the way the requested equipment will improve the child's ability to function in the areas of respiration, trunk control (musculoskeletal function), endurance (cardiac and respiratory function), and swallowing and digestion (physiological function).

REIMBURSEMENT

Medical-based treatment is reimbursed by a variety of sources including private insurance companies, Medicaid, the Civilian Health and Medical Program of the Uniformed Services (CHAMPUS), the Civilian Health and Medical Program of the Veterans Administration (CHAMPVA), health maintenance organizations (HMOs), and preferred

Letter of Equipment Justification

RE: FRANKIE
DIAGNOSIS: SEVERE TRACHEOMALACIA, GASTROESOPHAGEAL REFLUX, AND SUPRAVENTRICULAR TACHYCARDIA
MEDICAID #: FG12345U
DOB: 7/12/96

To whom it may concern:

Frankie is a 10-month-old male who had severe tracheomalacia, gastroesophageal reflux, and supraventricular tachycardia at birth. He has decreased head and postural control as well as a tracheotomy.

Current equipment: Currently Frankie does not have any equipment.
Equipment ordered: One Panda stroller with swivel-front wheels, a combined sun/rain hood, and foot straps.
Justification: Frankie is an active, alert, and oriented 10-month-old male with decreased head and trunk control, affecting his ability to assume and maintain independent upright postural sets. Frankie's inability to maintain an upright and erect posture places him at risk for occluding his tracheotomy and limits his ability to achieve his full respiratory capacity. These limitations affect his endurance and gas exchange.

A Panda stroller will assist Frankie with maintaining a neutral posture, which will facilitate his mechanical efficiency and therefore improve his endurance for maintaining an upright position. Improving his endurance will increase his upper extremity usage, which will foster the acquisition of age-appropriate fine motor skills. The stroller will help prevent bony deformities and joint contractures, thereby preventing the need for future surgeries. Frankie's ability to swallow and digest will also be improved if he can maintain a neutral position. A neutral position allows Frankie to use gravity to help him carry out the previously stated functions.

Thank you in advance for your assistance with this matter.

_____ Therapist's Signature

_____ Therapist's Signature

_____ Physiatrist's Signature

(Courtesy Nechama Karman, Dawn B. Oakley, Queens, NY, 1996.)

provider organizations (PPOs) (see Box 3-1). Many of these sources require specific documentation to justify the services rendered. An occupational therapy practitioner should be aware of the general billing requirements and documentation for each source. For example, private insurance companies, HMOs, and PPOs require frequent documentation to justify the initiation and continuation of services. In certain instances, specific clinics and vendors must be used. A hospital social worker or case manager is the best source of information regarding insurance requirements and coverage.

Another reimbursement source is charitable organizations. Many charitable organizations do not give money to a particular child. They are usually not-for-profit companies or organizations that raise funds to be given to other not-for-profit organizations. A charitable organization makes a donation to a pediatric institution or agency who then deposits the donation into an appropriate general fund. The agency then determines the way to distribute these funds to pay for specific expenses of individual children.

CHALLENGES FOR OCCUPATIONAL THERAPY PRACTITIONERS WORKING IN THE MEDICAL SYSTEM

Three major areas present unique challenges for occupational therapy practitioners in medical care system settings. The first is the number specialties that are included in the pediatric medical care system. In addition to rehabilitative services (e.g., occupational therapy, physical therapy, speech therapy), a variety of specialized services comprise the system, including radiology technicians, medical laboratory technicians, audiologists, pharmacists, dietitians, orthotists, and recreational therapists. A medical-based occupational therapy practitioner has to become familiar with the specific pediatric disciplines and their roles in the medical institution. This knowledge will further facilitate the team collaboration process that was discussed previously.

The second challenging area is medical terminology. A medical-based occupational therapy practitioner has to be familiar with the extensive medical terminology typically used in pediatric medical settings. The terminology can initially seem overwhelming. However, study of the basic word roots and common diagnoses used in pediatric medical practice can help practitioners develop of this much needed knowledge base. A good reference source for medical terminology is *Mosby's Medical, Nursing, and Allied Health Dictionary.*[2]

The third challenging area, which is related to the challenge of learning medical terminology, is continuing education. A medical-based practitioner should obtain additional education and become certified in advanced pediatric practice skills such as sensory integration or neurodevelopmental treatment. The medical field is a dynamic system, and practitioners who would like to maintain a role within this system must keep up with developments in current assessment techniques, treatments, and medical equipment.

SUMMARY

The pediatric medical care system is composed of individuals dedicated to caring for ill children. The five major settings in the pediatric medical care system are the NICU, step-down nurseries or the PICU, subacute settings, residential or long-term care settings, and home-based care settings. Specific goals are addressed in each of these settings. Depending on their needs, infants or children are transferred from one setting to another for treatment.

Because a long-term hospitalization is not a typical event in an infant's or a child's life, it can hinder their development. As early as 1947, this fact prompted members of the medical community to identify a role for hospital-based occupational therapy services. Although practice in certain settings requires an advanced level of skill, medical-based occupational therapy services can generally be carried out by competent OTRs or COTAs.

Medical-based occupational therapy services should be provided in a way that promotes team collaboration, whether be it institution specific or facility specific. The four most common team collaboration approaches are multidisciplinary, transdisciplinary, interdisciplinary, and "individual versus group" sessions.

Appropriate documentation facilitates the collaboration process. Although documentation requirements vary based on the regulations of each institution, commonly required forms of documentation include screenings, evaluations, treatment plans, progress notes, letters of justification, and discharge summaries. An occupational therapy practitioner may be required to complete one or more of these documents. A practitioner's ability to clearly document medical-based objectives and progress has a direct

impact on an institution's reimbursement rate and clients' ability to receive requested services and equipment.

The complex nature of the pediatric medical system poses a unique challenge for medical-based occupational therapy practitioner in that they must possess more than the basic occupational therapy skills. In addition, practitioners need to have a working knowledge of the pediatric medical specialties, be able to use and interpret pediatric medical terminology, and stay informed about the frequent changes in the pediatric health care environment.

References

1. American Occupational Therapy Association: COTA *information packet (a guide for supervision)*, Bethesda, 1995, The Association.
2. Anderson KN, Anderson LE, Glanze WD: *Mosby's medical nursing, and allied health dictionary*, ed 9, St Louis, 1998, Mosby.
3. Bruder M, Bologna T: Collaboration and service coordination for effective early intervention. In Brown W, Thurman SK, Pearls LK, editors: *Family-centered early intervention with infants and toddlers: innovative cross-disciplinary approaches*, Baltimore, 1993, Brookes.
4. Case-Smith J, Allen AS, Pratt PN: Arenas of occupational therapy services. In Case-Smith J, Allen AS, Pratt PN, editors: *Occupational therapy for children*, ed 3, St Louis, 1996, Mosby.
5. Case-Smith J, Wavrek B: Models of service delivery and team interaction. In Case-Smith J, editor: *Pediatric occupational therapy and early intervention*, Boston, 1993, Andover Medical.
6. Jabri J, Dreher JM: Documentation of occupational therapy services. In Early MB, editor: *Physical dysfunction: practice skills for the occupational therapy assistant*, Baltimore, 1998, Mosby.
7. Lyon S, Lyon G: Team functioning and staff development: a role release approach to providing integrated educational services for severely handicapped students, *J Assoc Severely Handicapped* 5(3):250, 1980.
8. Oakley D, Bauer-Logan K: *Early intervention symposium*, St. Mary's Hospital for Children, Queens, NY, 1996.
9. Oakley D, Bauer-Logan K: *Traumatic brain lecture series*, St. Mary's Hospital for Children, Queens, NY, 1995.
10. Peterson NL: *Early intervention for handicapped and at-risk children*, Denver, 1987, Love.
11. Slee V, Slee D: *Slee's health care terms*, ed 3, St Paul, 1996, Tringa Press.
12. Thomas CL, editor: *Taber's cyclopedic medical dictionary*, ed 18, Philadelphia, 1997, FA Davis.
13. Uniform Data System for Medical Rehabilitation: *WeeFIM system workshop*, Queens, NY, 1988, UB Foundation Activities.

REVIEW *Questions*

1. When might a child be transferred from one medical setting to another medical setting?
2. Which functional areas are assessed in a pediatric, medical-based occupational therapy evaluation?
3. In what ways do the multidisciplinary, transdisciplinary, and interdisciplinary models of collaboration differ?
4. In what ways could a medical practitioner's documentation impact the treatment and equipment needs of a child?
5. Why is continuing education an important aspect of medical-based practice?

SUGGESTED *Activities*

1. Create three examples of narrative and SOAP notes based on three observations of children in a natural setting (e.g., school yard, playground).
2. Purchase and review flash cards of common medical terminology roots.

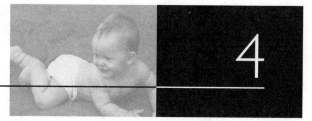

Educational System

SHARON KALSCHEUER SUCHOMEL

CHAPTER *Objectives*

After studying this chapter, the reader will be able to accomplish the following:

- Identify the federal laws that govern provision of education services to children with disabilities
- Explain the procedure to develop an individual family's service plan
- Explain the formation and function of an individual education program team
- Compare and contrast the roles of the occupational therapist and occupational therapy assistant in the school setting
- Discriminate between clinical and educational occupational therapy services using federal and professional practice guidelines

KEY TERMS

Due process

Related services

Individuals with Disabilities Education Act

Individual educational programs

Referral network

Early intervention team

Individual educational program team

Exceptional educational need

Individual family's service plan

Role delineation

CHAPTER OUTLINE

PRACTICE SETTINGS

FEDERAL LAWS

Education of Handicapped Act (Public Law 94-142)

Rehabilitation Act and the Americans with Disabilities Act

Public Law 99-457

Individuals with Disabilities Education Act

IDENTIFICATION AND REFERRAL

EVALUATION

ELIGIBILITY

INDIVIDUAL FAMILY'S SERVICE PLAN AND INDIVIDUAL EDUCATIONAL PROGRAM

TRANSITIONS

RIGHTS OF PARENTS AND CHILDREN

OTR AND COTA ROLES

CLINICAL MODELS VERSUS EDUCATIONAL MODELS

SUMMARY

It is estimated that one third to one half of practicing occupational therapists work with children, and public school systems are the second largest employers of occupational therapists.[3] Despite these statistics, occupational therapy practitioners often find that they work alone, without other practitioners, and with a limited support network. This is especially true in rural areas where one practitioner may provide therapy services to several small school districts or a cooperative educational service area. When occupational therapy services are provided in an educational setting, therapists, educators, and families must radically shift their usual ways of thinking.[7] Being a member of an educational team requires practitioners to broaden their focus to the ways children function in their families, communities, and schools. This mode of thinking contrasts significantly with the traditional medical model of "evaluate and treat," which focuses on children and their disabilities or limitations.[6] To be an effective member of the educational or family service plan team, the practitioner must possess the specialized technical skills of an occupational therapy practitioner as well as have knowledge of the educational system and current special education laws and regulations.[3,7] Practitioners must be able to apply their occupational therapy knowledge and intervention skills to a school setting while communicating effectively with parents* and educators.

PRACTICE SETTINGS

As noted previously, the majority of pediatric occupational therapy practitioners work in public school settings. Some practitioners work in community programs serving infants and children from birth to 3 years, or the "birth to three" population (see Chapter 3). Birth to Three programs can be home based or facility based, with the agencies who are responsible for the program varying from state to state. In some states the Department of Health and Social Services is the responsible agency, whereas in other states the public school system assumes responsibility for providing early intervention services.[13]

FEDERAL LAWS

Pediatrics is the only area of practice in which occupational therapy services are mandated by law.[3] Box 4-1 summarizes the laws that have an impact on occupational therapy services in public school systems.

---

*In this chapter the term *parent* is used generally and refers to the legal guardian who is the child's primary caregiver and is responsible for the child's well being. For example, the parent may be a grandparent, aunt or uncle, or even a friend of the family.

BOX 4-1

Summary of Federal Laws Impactin[g] Occupational Therapy in Education

1973
Public Law 93-112, Section 504 of the Rehabilitation Act
- Discrimination against people with disabilities when offering services is prohibited.

1975
Public Law 94-142: Education for All Handicapped Children Act (Renamed Education of the Handicapped Act [EHA])
- All children have the right to a free and an appropriate public education.

1986
Public Law 99-457, Part H (Added to EHA)
- Birth to Three services should be equal in all states and counties.

1990
Americans with Disabilities Education Act
- In areas of public services, discriminatory practices against individuals with disabilities by employers is prohibited.
- EHA is renamed the Individuals with Disabilities Education Act (IDEA)

1997
- IDEA is revised (IDEA-R).
- Part H of IDEA-R is renamed Part C.

Education of Handicapped Act (Public Law 94-142)

The Education of Handicapped Act (EHA) (Public Law 94-142) requires schools to provide free appropriate public education (FAPE) to all children from birth to 21 years.[4,7,8] Children with disabilities have the right to have their educational programs geared toward their unique needs, regardless of the nature, extent, or severity of their disabilities. Provisions under this law guarantee children the right to be educated in the least restrictive environment (LRE) and to receive other services that may be required for them to benefit from their education program. The law also outlines parents' and children's rights and explains their legal course of action (that is, their right to **due process**) when the right to a free, appropriate public education is hindered.

TABLE 4-1

Comparison of IDEA and IDEA-R

FORMER IDEA	IDEA-R
TEAM NAMES	
M-team (multidisciplinary team)	IEP team
REGULAR EDUCATION TEACHERS	
Other than students with learning disabilities, not involved with special education students	Participation on IEP teams
MEETINGS	
Number of Meetings	
Two meetings: (1) an M-team meeting to determine eligibility and (2) a separate IEP and placement meeting to determine services and program	One meeting
Placement Meeting	
Possible parental involvement	Required parental involvement
REPORTS	
M-team summary with minority report (If a member of the team disagrees with the eligibility findings, the member can submit a dissenting report.)	Single report of IEP team's determination of eligibility; no minority report
CONSENT	
Not required for reevaluation	Parental consent for reevaluations
MEDIATION	
Not available	Mediation (A voluntary process in which an impartial person helps schools and families reach agreements on issues relating to the identification evaluation, educational placement of the child, and provision of a free appropriate public education without going through a due process hearing.)
SPECIAL NEEDS TERMINOLOGY	
Handicapping condition, or handicap	Disability
PARENTS' RIGHTS	
Sent 6 times	Sent 3 times

Least restrictive environment

The right to be educated in the LRE means that a child with a disability should be educated in a regular classroom whenever possible.[4,8] The child is also entitled to have the opportunity to interact with peers who do not have disabilities. Previously, students with disabilities were placed in special schools with other students who had disabilities, or they were placed in self-contained classrooms without an opportunity to interact with other peers.

The LRE guidelines have provided the impetus for the development of the mainstreaming and inclusion models (that is, models in which children with disabilities are able to spend some time in regular classrooms). School personnel determine whether a child with disabilities can receive an appropriate education in a regular classroom with the aid of support services and necessary modifications. If the decision is made to remove the child from the general education program, the team must consider whether the child has spent as much time as possible in regular classrooms. The spirit of the EHA is to require schools to provide an entire continuum of services to students with special needs.[1,5,8] For some children, this may be placement in a regular classroom that has been modified to meet their needs (for example, one that has been equipped with positioning devices). For other children, this may be placement in a regular classroom that allows them to go to a resource room for assistance from a special education or resource teacher. Some children need specialized instruction from a special education teacher and spend the majority of the day in the self-contained classroom but go to a regular classroom for certain classes or activities.

Related services

According to the EHA, schools are required to provide special services, or **related services,** to a child if those services are necessary for the child to benefit from the special education program. Related services include transportation, physical therapy, occupational therapy, speech therapy, assistive technology services, psychological services, school health services, social work services, and parent counseling and training.[4,8]

Rehabilitation Act and Americans with Disabilities Act

The educational rights of children with disabilities are protected by two additional federal laws: Section 504 of the Rehabilitation Act (which was passed in 1973) and the Americans with Disabilities Act (ADA)(which was passed in 1990).[1,8,9,10] Section 504 of the Rehabilitation Act stipulates that any recipient of federal aid (including a school) cannot discriminate when offering services to people with disabilities. The ADA made the law more specific by prohibiting discriminatory practices in areas relating to employment, transportation, accessibility, and telecommunications. A student with a disability who is not eligible for special education services but has difficulty participating in and benefiting from a regular educational program may be eligible for receiving related services. To be eligible the student must have a condition that ". . . substantially limits one or more major life activities," with learning being a major life activity.[1]

Public Law 99-457

Public Law 99-457 was passed in 1986. This added Part H (which is now known as Part C) to the EHA. Part C outlines a national program to assist each state in establishing a system of services for children with developmental delays from birth to three years and their families.[13] Before the passage of Public Law 99-457, services available

to this population were not consistent among counties and states.

Individuals with Disabilities Education Act

In 1990, EHA was renamed the Individuals with Disabilities Education Act (IDEA). It was subsequently revised in 1997 and is now known as the IDEA-R. The revisions include sweeping changes in the identification, evaluation, and implementation of **individual educational programs** (IEPs).[16] Table 4-1 contains a comparison of the IDEA and the IDEA-R.

Although specific policies, procedures, and timelines for Birth to Three programs vary from those of the public school setting, both systems follow a similar framework that includes the following steps: identification and referral, evaluation, determination of eligibility, and development of the IEP or individual family's service plan (IFSP), and transitions.

IDENTIFICATION AND REFERRAL

The parents are often the first individuals to become concerned about their child's development or school performance. Clinics, Birth to Three programs, and school districts may conduct public screenings to identify children who may be eligible for early intervention or school special education services. In addition, a **referral network,** which includes parents, doctors, nurses, health professionals, schools, day-care centers, clinics, and any other organization that comes into contact with children is used to identify eligible children.[13] If any member of the network has a concern regarding a child's development, a referral is made to the appropriate agency (for example, a Birth to Three program, public school system). Once a referral is made, the responsible agency determines whether a screening or evaluation is needed.

EVALUATION

After a referral is received and parental consent to evaluate is obtained, an evaluation team is formed. In the Birth to Three program, it is called an **early intervention team,** or EI team.[13] In the public school setting, the evaluation team was previously called a "multidisciplinary team," or "M-team." According to the IDEA-R, it is now called an **individual educational program team,** or IEP team.[4,8] In Birth to Three programs and the school system, the evaluation team comprises parents, agency coordinators, and at least two professionals who are skilled in assessing and creating programs for children with special needs (one of whom must be knowledgeable in the child's suspected area of need).[16] In other words, if it is suspected that a child may need fine motor skills assistance, an occupational therapist would be on the team. If the child may need cognitive skills assistance, an early childhood or special educator would be on the team. If there are concerns about the child's speech and language development, a speech therapist would be on the team. The team members are responsible for evaluating a child's development in their area of expertise and determining whether that child is eligible to receive special services. Evaluators should remember that the evaluation only measures the child's abilities at that particular time. It is therefore critical to consider the viewpoint of the parents—the individuals who have a broad sense of the child's abilities in different settings and are able to further identify the child's strengths and needs. Reevaluations are conducted if conditions warrant reevaluation or the child's parents or teachers request a reevaluation. The school district is also required to consider reevaluating these children at least every 3 years.

ELIGIBILITY

After the child's evaluation, the EI or IEP team determines the child's eligibility. To be eligible for services from a Birth to Three program, a child must have a diagnosed condition that is likely to result in developmental delays or must have an already established 25% delay in a particular area. Examples of diagnosed conditions include Down syndrome, autism, cerebral palsy, vision and hearing impairments, birth defects, and chronic or progressive conditions. Children are also eligible if the team determines they have a 25% developmental delay in one or more of the following areas: cognitive, physical or motor, communication, social or emotional, and adaptive behavior or self-help.[1,13]

In the public school system, eligibility for services is based on **exceptional educational need** (EEN). The IEP team must consider all of the information obtained through evaluation to determine whether the child has a disability or condition that handicaps the child.[4,8] The team must also determine whether presence of that condition interferes with the child's ability to participate in an educational program and whether related services are required for that child to benefit from an educational program. The presence of a disability does not necessarily mean that a child cannot participate in the educational program nor does it mean that the child has an EEN. For example, consider Mary, an 8-year-old girl with a diagnosis of cerebral palsy-left hemiplegia. She is currently in the second grade. Her parents requested an evaluation through the school district, so the school district conducted an IEP team evaluation and meeting to determine whether she was eligible for occupational therapy services. The results of the evaluation revealed that Mary has age-

appropriate learning and thinking skills (cognition), has age-appropriate communication skills, can independently walk and move around the building, and can independently perform classroom tasks (for example, printing, managing materials). Mary interacts well with her teacher and classmates and is an active participant in the classroom. The occupational therapy practitioner reports that Mary has mild spasticity in her left upper extremity, decreased control (isolation and precision) of her left upper extremity, and difficulty with bilateral tasks, but she successfully compensates for these factors and can participate in all classroom activities. The IEP team determines that Mary has a disability (because she has been diagnosed with cerebral palsy), but it does not interfere with her ability to receive an appropriate education. Therefore an EEN does not exist, and occupational therapy services are not required for Mary to participate in and benefit from her educational program. If Mary's family thinks she would benefit from occupational therapy services to address issues related to her muscle tone, range of motion (ROM), fine motor skills, and bilateral coordination skills, they can seek occupational therapy services in a clinic on an outpatient basis. This may require a physician's orders, and they should investigate whether occupational therapy services are covered under their health plan. In addition, for a child to be eligible to receive occupational therapy services in the public school setting, the services and goals must be educationally relevant.

INDIVIDUAL FAMILY'S SERVICE PLAN AND INDIVIDUAL EDUCATIONAL PROGRAM

The **individual family's service plan** (IFSP) is a plan and a process. The plan is a written description and reflection of the process. The IFSP is the result of a collaboration between the parents and the Birth to Three program professionals. It includes the family's goals for the child and the way the agency is going to provide the needed services (Box 4-2).[13] Families must sign the IFSP before services can be provided. The family can agree to accept all or only a portion of the recommended services. The child and family only receive the services that they want. IFSP reviews are conducted at least every 6 months.

For school-age children (that is, 3 years to 21 years), the process just described is referred to as *developing the IEP*. An IEP is a plan (a written document) as well as a process. The IEP team consists of the child's parent or parents, at least one regular education teacher, at least one special education teacher or special education provider, a representative of the school district who is knowledgeable about the general curriculum, an individual who can interpret instructional implications of evaluation results (that is, the way certain factors may affect the child's ability to learn), and related services personnel. The child may be present when appropriate, and the family may invite anyone they wish to have present. When developing the IEP, the IEP team considers the extent of the child's educational needs.[4,16] The IEP is reviewed at least annually but may be reviewed more frequently if requested or deemed necessary. The format of the IEP may vary. Box 4-3 contains information that must be included in an IEP. (See the Chapter 4 Appendix for a sample IEP form.)

BOX 4-2

Components of an IFSP

The format of the written plan may differ from program to program, but an IFSP must contain the following information:
- Child's current level of development
- Summaries of evaluation reports
- Family's concerns
- Desired outcomes (goals)
- Early intervention services and supports necessary to achieve outcomes
- Frequency of, method for providing, and location of services
- Payment arrangements (if any)
- Transition plan

TRANSITIONS

Children undergo a variety of transitions as they grow and develop from infancy to 21 years of age. Their services and programs change as they enter and leave Birth to Three programs and the public school systems. A transition plan includes the steps that should be taken to support children and their families as they go through these changes, making the transitions smooth and successful. As children enter and exit various programs, transition planning is used to link them up with different agencies, helping clarify the agencies' roles and the services they will provide during and after the children's transitions.[13]

RIGHTS OF PARENTS AND CHILDREN

The IDEA-R includes outlines of several procedural safeguards for children with disabilities and their parents. These procedures are detailed in the United States Code of Federal Regulations, Title 34, Subtitle B, Chapter III, Part 300. In brief the safeguards include notifying parents of all proposed actions, obtaining a consent to evaluate, allowing parents to attend IEP team meetings, and pro-

---

BOX 4-3

Components of an IEP

- Statement of child's present levels of educational performance, including the way the child's disability affects the child's involvement in the general curriculum or age-appropriate activities
- Statement of measurable, annual goals, including short-term objectives related to increased involvement and progress in the general curriculum and other educational needs such as social and extracurricular needs
- Description of special education and related services and supplementary aids and services
- Description of program modifications or supports to be used by school personnel to enable the child to attain goals; be involved and progress in general curriculum, extracurricular, and nonacademic activities; and be educated and participate in activities with other children, both with and without disabilities
- Explanation of the extent to which the child will not participate in the regular classroom and in IEP activities with children who do not have disabilities
- Statement of any individual modifications needed for the child to participate in formal assessments of student achievement (for example, statewide or districtwide tests)
- Projected date for beginning services and educational modifications; anticipated frequency, location, and duration of services
- Transition services, including linkages with other agencies
- Statement of the way progress toward annual goals is measured
- Descriptions of methods to regularly inform parents of child's progress (at least as often as parents of children without disabilities are informed)

viding the right to an independent evaluation and the right to appeal school decisions in front of an impartial hearing officer.[8,11,12] The IDEA requires school districts to inform parents of their rights in a written format.

OTR AND COTA ROLES

OTRs and COTAs have related but distinct roles in the educational setting. A successful partnership between the two ensures effective and efficient use of training and potential, encourages creativity, and promotes professional growth and respect.[2] All occupational therapy services provided in the educational setting must comply with federal and state regulations. Additionally, professional standards of practice help OTRs and COTAs with **role delineation** in the educational setting. The occupational therapy practitioners must work together to provide the best possible service to the child.

Occupational therapy staff members are either employed directly by the local educational agency (school district), or services are contracted through a local hospital, health agency, or private practice therapist. Occupational therapy practitioners employed by the local educational agency must comply with the supervision and employment practices of the school district's administration structure. If the occupational therapy services are contracted through a hospital or health agency, the occupational therapy practitioners are considered employees of the particular institution or agency and can therefore be supervised by another therapist employed by that organization. Supervision guidelines and expectations should be closely coordinated between the employing institution and the local educational agency. In either situation, all licensing or state regulations regarding caseload and supervision standards must be followed.[2,4]

The OTR is legally responsible for all aspects of the occupational therapy process. COTAs are responsible for providing services within their established level of competence. Professional supervision is a partnership that requires communication and mutual responsibility to clarify competencies and responsibilities. The practice standards established by the AOTA delineate levels of supervision. The required level of supervision depends on many factors, such as the COTA's level of experience and service competency, the complexity of the evaluation and therapy methods used, and the current practice guidelines and regulations of the state or local educational agency. OTRs must always remember that they are ultimately responsible for service performance.[2] If an OTR is not comfortable with a COTA's performance of a particular task, the task should not be delegated to the COTA. Likewise, a COTA who is not comfortable performing a certain task is responsible for communicating this concern to the supervising OTR.

Each of the practitioners has a role in screening and evaluation, IEP formation, treatment planning, and intervention. During the evaluation, OTRs determine which data are collected and the tools and methods to be used. COTAs can observe and assist with data collection by making clinical observations and administering and scoring tests within their service competency level. OTRs are responsible for analyzing, interpreting, and reporting information verbally and in writing. During the IEP formation, OTRs contribute to the IEP process and are part of the IEP team. COTAs assist with developing goals and may attend the IEP meeting (under the direction of an OTR) to report findings and recommendations. COTAs do not interpret findings or negotiate changes in levels of service or goals. COTAs are responsible for communicating their observations, ideas, and suggestions for interpretation or changes to OTRs. The role of COTAs in the intervention phase is to demonstrate service competency performance skills to the OTR and engage students in activities related to the intervention goals (following initial direction from an OTR). COTAs work with students on activities such as printing, cutting with scissors, using a keyboard, lunch room skill activities, and managing clothing for toileting or recess. COTAs also work with teachers and other school personnel on appropriate positioning of the student and determining which materials or methods can be used in the classroom to increase the student's ability to participate successfully. COTAs are responsible for informing OTRs of changes in the student's environment and providing current data regarding the student's performance.[2]

CLINICAL MODELS VERSUS EDUCATIONAL MODELS

As stated previously, providing occupational therapy services in an educational setting requires a shift in thinking and a change in philosophy. This process can be difficult for therapists and complicate communication with educators and families. Occupational therapists are traditionally trained under a medical model and therefore think of services for children in a framework based on dysfunction and its underlying components. According to the medical model, environmental factors that can support or hinder a child's performance are not a primary concern. The focus of a medical model is remediation of underlying components of dysfunction and removal of pathological processes so that development can continue.[6,7] In other words, the problem is identified through an evaluation and is then treated. Practicing occupational therapy according to an educational model requires therapists to have a broader view of children and their performance. A child's abilities are described in terms of functional ability (rather than disability) in the educational environment and the ability to meet classroom demands. The focus of treatment in an educational model is on developing the skills necessary to function within a particular environment.[4,7]

Consider the previous example of Mary, the 8-year-old girl with left-sided hemiplegia. Using a medical model, an occupational therapist might address muscle tone, ROM, strength, and isolated muscle control for fine motor skills. If Mary were being assessed using an educational model, her abilities would be assessed in terms of the demands of the classroom and her ability to function within the classroom. Occupational therapy services may be recommended if Mary's printing skills are not commensurate with her grade level expectations; she has behavioral or social issues; or she has difficulty handling materials, cutting with scissors, or performing other activities that are expected of a typical second grade student. The occupational therapy practitioner may treat Mary directly and address performance components such as tone, ROM, and bilateral hand skills with the intent of improving the functional skill of cutting with scissors. The occupational therapy practitioner may also suggest adaptations to the environment and alter the methods or materials that the teacher is using in the classroom.

Although a medical model can be used in a school setting, the desire to mainstream children with disabilities into regular classrooms, the requirement to provide services in a natural LRE, and the fact that occupational therapy services must be educationally relevant have caused occupational therapy practitioners to rethink their philosophy about the most appropriate frame of reference in an educational setting.[7] In recent years, educational agencies and third-party payers have increased their requests for occupational therapists to use outcome-based assessments and practices in pediatric therapy. Therapists are being asked to not only identify and treat problem areas but also to qualify functional performance and consider factors other than neuromuscular and psychosocial processes, such as the child's potential for improvement, social skills, environmental demands, and family priorities.[6,7]

CLINICAL *Pearl*

Occupational therapy services should be provided in the classroom whenever possible. An informal exchange of ideas and effective intervention strategies naturally evolve among team members when the occupational therapy practitioner works with children in their classrooms.

Federal, state, and local educational agency regulations can help establish guidelines for the provision of occupational therapy services in the school system.[4,14,15] Box 4-4 contains questions that can assist therapists with determining whether a child needs occupational therapy services in the school setting and what level of service is recommended. Answering these questions helps practitioners clarify their recommendations and the role of occupational therapy in the educational setting. The fourth and fifth questions are probably the most important for distinguishing between clinical and educational services and determining the appropriate level of service that is to be provided. Having an EEN designation and significantly delayed skills does not necessarily mean that a child should receive occupational therapy services in school, a fact that is especially true for older students with severe cognitive deficits. Their needs (for example, working on functional skills such as self-care) can and should be ad-

---

BOX 4-4

Determining the Need for Occupational Therapy in the School

1. *Does the child have an EEN?* Because occupational therapy is a related service, the child must have an EEN or qualify under Section 504 of the Rehabilitation Act to be eligible to receive services provided by the school system.
2. *Does the evaluation indicate the need for occupational therapy services?* The evaluation can consist of standardized tests, portfolio reviews, classroom and school environment observations, and consultations with parents and teachers.
3. *Does the child demonstrate a significant delay in motor, sensory or perceptual, psychosocial, or self-help skills in comparison with established norms of other children of the same age?* A significant delay is one that is greater than one standard deviation below the norm and affects school performance.
4. *Is occupational therapy a related service that may be required for the child to benefit from and participate in an educational program?* Factors that affect the answer to this question include the child's program, other related services received, demands of the classroom, child's level of function, and potential for improvement or skill development.
5. *Does the child require the specialized skills of an occupational therapy practitioner, or can tasks and interventions be carried out by other personnel?* For example, a teacher may be able to help a child learn eating skills by using adaptive equipment provided by an occupational therapy practitioner.

dressed in their educational program. Rather than working with one particular student, the occupational therapy practitioner can serve as a consultant to the teacher and classroom staff by helping them resolve particular situations or making recommendations regarding methods and materials. The occupational therapy practitioner may become more directly involved if a student's skills deteriorate or the practitioner thinks that a short period of direct service will help the student become more independent. Although the IEP team is responsible for determining the need for and level of services, the COTA assists the OTR by providing current data and observations.

CLINICAL *Pearl*

Remember that the teacher is the manager of the classroom. The occupational therapy practitioner's presence should not disrupt the classroom routine.

SUMMARY

Practicing occupational therapy in an educational system, whether it is a school system or a Birth to Three program, is a unique challenge for occupational therapy practitioners. They must possess the technical knowledge and skills of their discipline as well as be knowledgeable about development, family systems, learning theory, community resources, and current federal and state regulations. Although federal regulations exist that dictate broad policies, occupational therapy practitioners must keep abreast of the state department of regulations and local education agency procedures where they practice to ensure compliance in all areas.

Other challenges include communicating and working as a team. The occupational therapy practitioner must be able to translate occupational therapy knowledge into the lay language of educators and families. In Birth to Three programs, therapists must be able to successfully function as part of a team that values parent involvement and family-centered services. This may mean family needs take precedence over therapy or that therapy must be incorporated into a family's daily routines. In the public school system, it may involve adapting interventions so that they can be provided in a busy, crowded classroom. It may also involve teaching skills to other professionals and paraprofessionals so that they can provide the services.

Providing occupational therapy services in an educational system requires occupational therapy practitioners to be flexible and holistic. They must analyze children in terms of their ability to fill normal and valued roles in the school, family, community, and society rather than in terms of their deficits in performance components and performance areas. Only then can occupational therapy practitioners provide the best services for children.

References

1. American Occupational Therapy Association: *Occupational therapy services for children and youth under IDEA*, Rockville, Md, 1997, The Association.
2. American Occupational Therapy Association: Roles of occupational therapists and occupational therapy assistants in schools, *AJOT* 41:798, 1987.
3. American Occupational Therapy Association Pediatric Curriculum Committee: *Guidelines for curriculum content in pediatrics*, Rockville, Md, 1991, The Association.
4. Bober P, Corbett S: *Occupational therapy and physical therapy. A resource and planning guide*, Madison, Wis, 1996, Wisconsin Department of Public Instruction.
5. *Daniel RR v State Board of Education*, 874 F 2d 1036, 1989.
6. Haley S, Coster W: *Pediatric evaluation of disability inventory*, Boston, 1992, New England Medical Center Hospitals.
7. Hinojosa J, Kramer P: *Frames of reference for pediatric occupational therapy*,1993, Williams & Wilkins.
8. Martin E, Martin R, Terman D: The legislative and litigation history of special education, *Future Child* 6:25, 1996.
9. Public Law 101-336, Americans with Disabilities Act, 1990.
10. Public Law 101-476, Individuals with Disabilities Education Act, 1990.
11. *United States Code of Federal Regulations*, title 34, subtitle B, chapter III, part 290.
12. *United States Code of Federal Regulations*, title 34, subtitle B, chapter III, part 300.
13. Wisconsin Birth to Three Program: *Families are the foundation of Wisconsin's birth to three program*, Madison, Wis, 1993, Department of Health and Social Services.
14. Wisconsin Department of Public Instruction PI 11.24.
15. Wisconsin Department of Public Instruction Rules [s.115.83(1)(a)].
16. Wisconsin Department of Public Instruction website: *www.dpi.state.wi.us*.

Recommended Reading

Hanft B, Place P: *The consulting therapist: a guide for OTs and PTs in schools*, Tucson, 1996, Therapy Skill Builders.

REVIEW *Questions*

1. What are some of the federal laws that impact the provision of occupational therapy services in the public school system?
2. Which factors determine whether a child is eligible to receive occupational therapy services in a school setting?
3. In what ways do therapy services provided according to an educational model differ from therapy services provided according to a medical model?
4. In what ways do the roles of an occupational therapist and an occupational therapy assistant differ in a school setting?

SUGGESTED *Activities*

1. Visit a public school and observe the various programs and environments that have been developed for students with special needs, such as a learning disabilities resource room and self-contained classroom.
2. Be politically aware and active. Keep abreast of local, state, and federal law changes. Participate in public hearings and contact legislators when laws affecting the provision of therapy services are being debated.

CHAPTER 4 APPENDIX

INDIVIDUALIZED EDUCATION PROGRAM   Page ____ of ____

Name of Student		Date of Birth	Gender	Grade	Ethnicity (if parents choose to identify)	
Parent or legal guardian		Address		City	Zip Code	Telephone

District of residence	District of placement	For students transferring between public agencies within the state: Date IEP adopted _____ Name & title of district representative _____

A statement for each of the following, with amount, frequency, location and duration (if different from IEP ending date below):

- Special education

- Supplemental aids & services   ☐ Yes   ☐ No   (If yes, describe (a) the aids, services and other supports that are provided to or on behalf of the child in regular education classes or other educational related settings and (b) program modifications or supports for school personnel that will be provided.)

- Related services   ☐ Yes   ☐ No   (If yes, specify)

  ☐ Audiology   ☐ Psychological services
  ☐ Counseling   ☐ Recreation
  ☐ Educational interpreting   ☐ Rehabilitation counseling services
  ☐ Medical services for diagnosis & evaluation   ☐ School health services
  ☐ Occupational therapy   ☐ Transportation
  ☐ Orientation and mobility   ☐ Other (specify): _____
  ☐ Physical therapy   ☐ Other (specify): _____

Projected beginning and ending date(s) of IEP services and modifications _____ to _____
                                                                           month / day / year   month / day / year

Physical education   ☐ Regular   ☐ Specially designed
Vocational education   ☐ Regular   ☐ Specially designed

An explanation of the extent, if any, to which the child will not participate with children in the regular class and in extracurricular and other nonacademic activities:

Name of Student	Page ____ of ____

Are transition services required? ☐ Yes ☐ No

If yes and student is age 14, a statement of instruction (e.g., courses) and educational experiences necessary to prepare the student for postschool outcomes:

If yes and student is age 16 (or younger if appropriate), include required transition activities within the goals and objectives/benchmarks, related services, and agency responsibilities, and complete the Summary of Transition Services.

Consideration of special factors:

A. Does the child's behavior impede his/her learning or that of others? ☐ Yes ☐ No

If yes, list positive behavioral interventions, strategies, and supports to address that behavior:

B. Does the child have limited English proficiency? ☐ Yes ☐ No

If yes, describe the language needs that relate to this IEP:

C. If visually handicapped, does the child need Braille instruction? ☐ Yes ☐ No ☐ Not applicable

If no, justify:

D. Does the child have communication needs? ☐ Yes ☐ No

If yes, describe:

Is the child deaf or hard of hearing? ☐ Yes ☐ No

If yes, did you consider the following?

- The child's language and communication needs ☐ Yes ☐ No

- Opportunities for direct communication with peers and professional personnel in the child's language and communication mode ☐ Yes ☐ No

- Necessary opportunities for direct instruction in the child's language and communication mode ☐ Yes ☐ No

E. Does the student need assistive technology services or devices? ☐ Yes ☐ No

If yes, specify particular devices or services including frequency, location, and duration details:

CHAPTER 4 APPENDIX—cont'd

Name of Student	Page ____ of ____

Will the student reach the age of majority within 1 year, or has the student already reached the age of majority? ☐ Yes ☐ No

If yes, documentation that student has been informed of his/her rights which will transfer at age of majority:

Does the child require extended school year (ESY) services to receive a free and appropriate public education (FAPE)? ☐ Yes ☐ No

Will the student participate in statewide assessments? ☐ Yes ☐ No

☐ With modifications/accommodations (describe):

If no, state why the assessment is not appropriate for the student and what, if any, alternate assessments will be used:

Will the student participate in districtwide assessments? ☐ Yes ☐ No   If yes, list_____

☐ With modifications/accommodations (describe):

If no, state the reason the assessment is not appropriate for the student and what, if any, alternate assessments will be used:

Date of IEP meeting:	Date of IEP review:	Documentation of efforts to involve the parents in the IEP meeting:
IEP meeting participants	**IEP meeting participants**	
LEA representative/title	LEA representative/title	1. _____
Regular education teacher/title	Regular education teacher/title	_____
Special education teacher/title	Special education teacher/title	_____
Parent/guardian	Parent/guardian	2. _____
Child (if appropriate)	Child (if appropriate)	_____
Related services provider/title	Related services provider/title	_____
Interpreter	Interpreter	3. _____
Private school representative	Private school representative	_____
Community agency representative	Community agency representative	_____
Other/title	Other/title	
Other/title	Other/title	
Other/title	Other/title	

Name of Student	Page ____ of ____

Present level of educational performance, including how the child's disability affects the child's involvement and progress in the general curriculum (for preschool children, how the disability affects participation in appropriate activities). Consider the strengths of the child, the concerns of the parents for enhancing the education of the child, and the results of the initial or most recent evaluation of the child.

Measurable annual goal

Procedures for measuring progress toward the annual goal

Procedures for notifying parents of the child's progress toward the annual goal at least as often as parents are informed of the progress of children without disabilities.

Benchmarks or short-term objectives necessary to monitor the progress in general curriculum and disability-related educational needs throughout the school year.

Short-Term Objectives	Objective criteria (quantitative measure)	Evidence of accomplishment (how measured)	Evaluation schedule	Objectives Met	Not met

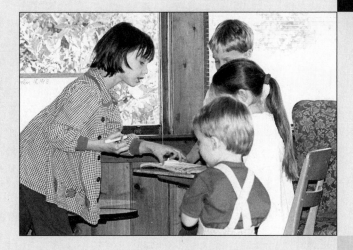

Part TWO

Normal Development

Principles of Normal Development

JEAN W. SOLOMON

CHAPTER *Objectives*

After studying this chapter, the reader will be able to accomplish the following:

- Explain the importance of knowing and understanding characteristics of typical development while working in the pediatric occupational therapy arena
- Discuss the relationship between typical development and the performance contexts
- Define and briefly describe the periods of development
- Describe the general principles of development
- Apply the general principles of development and justify a developmental sequence of skill acquisition in the occupational performance components or areas

KEY TERMS   CHAPTER OUTLINE

Sally is a certified occupational therapy assistant (COTA) who is employed by the local public school system. She has been assigned a new client, a 3-year-old girl named Amy. The supervising OTR has begun the occupational therapy evaluation and has requested that Sally schedule a visit to assess the child's self-care and play skills to determine whether the child is functioning at the appropriate age level in these areas. Sally realizes that to accurately assess Amy's skills relative to her chronological age, she needs to review normal development definitions and principles.

The occupational therapy practitioner must understand the process of typical development. The sequence of skill acquisition in relation to occupational performance components and areas is the foundation for occupational therapy assessment of and intervention with children who have special needs. The sequence of skill acquisition is predictable in the normally developing child.[1] The occupational therapy practitioner's knowledge of normal development guides the order of expectations and choice of activities for children who are not developing typically. In atypical development, delays in performance component skills may make it difficult or impossible for a child to perform activities of daily living (ADLs), engage successfully in play activities, or acquire functional work and productive skills. The occupational therapy practitioner identifies deficits in the occupational performance components (for example, sensorimotor and neuromusculoskeletal domains) that interfere with a child's functional independence. The practitioner relies on knowledge of typical development to assist the child with developing useful, functional skills.

GENERAL CONSIDERATIONS

An occupational therapy practitioner who is attempting to grasp the basis of normal development must consider general pediatric terms, the predictable sequence of skill acquisition in normal development, the principles of development, and the relationship between development and performance contexts. An understanding of the general terms used by pediatric therapists is necessary for effective communication. The pediatric therapist also needs to know the predictable sequence of skill acquisition in a typically developing child. The occupational therapy practitioner must understand the relationship between typical development and the occupational performance contexts as delineated in the American Occupational Therapy Association's (AOTA's) "Uniform Terminology for Occupational Therapy."[3]

Definition of Terms

A basic understanding of the generic terms used by pediatric practitioners who work in pediatrics helps practitioners and other individuals working in the area of pediatrics to communicate effectively. **Normal** is defined as that which occurs habitually or naturally.[2] In this chapter normal is used interchangeably with **typical** in the discussions of development. **Development** is the act or process of maturing or acquiring skills ranging from simple to more complex.[2] **Growth** is maturation of a person.[2] Because development and growth are so closely defined, these terms are used interchangeably in this chapter (Box 5-1).

Predictable Sequence of Skill Acquisition

Normal development of skills in the occupational performance components and areas occurs in a predictable sequence.[1,4,5,7] The occupational therapy practitioner uses knowledge of typical development while working with children who have special needs to identify the areas in which there are deficits and develop a plan to improve their ADL, play, and work skills. Although developmental checklists and other tools may help a practitioner identify the presence and absence of certain skills, understanding the process of how and why children are able to develop these skills is more useful in the clinical setting. For example, an occupational therapy practitioner could use an observational checklist to determine whether a child can independently finger feed. A practitioner who has knowledge of normal development and its predictable sequence of events would know that children usually learn to eat with their fingers before learning to eat with a spoon. Therefore if a child is not yet finger feeding, the practitioner would not introduce spoon feeding (depending on the circumstances). Knowledge and understanding of normal development guides the occupational therapy practitioner in the treatment planning process.

Relationship Between Typical Development and Performance Contexts

Occupational therapy practitioners need to understand the relationship between typical development and AOTA's **performance contexts.** Because normal development events are sequential and predictable,[1,4,5,7] the chronologi-

---

BOX 5-1

Definition of Normal Development

Normal development is defined as the natural process of acquiring skills ranging from simple to complex.

cal age of the child (that is, how old the child is) impacts the child's skill development level in the occupational performance components and areas. Although practitioners obviously cannot change the age of a child, they can offer age-appropriate activities during intervention sessions. Being familiar with age-appropriate activities helps occupational therapy practitioners choose tasks for therapy sessions with children. For example, a practitioner may use colored blocks while performing fine motor and sorting activities with a 3-year-old child, but blocks are not suitable for use in a session with a 14-year-old adolescent. It would be more appropriate to have the adolescent use objects like coins for fine motor and sorting activities.

Although normal development is predictable and sequential, the rate of skill acquisition varies among children. This variability greatly depends on the environmental contexts delineated in AOTA's "Uniform Terminology for Occupational Therapy" (Box 5-2). The environmental aspects include physical, social, and cultural factors.[3]

The physical, or nonhuman, aspects of the environment[3] impact the rate of skill acquisition in both performance components and areas. For example, if a child lives in a climate that requires warm clothing, the child will learn to don and doff a sweater or a coat more quickly than a child who lives in a temperate climate. A child who lives in a two story house will more likely learn to ascend and descend stairs before a child who lives in a single story house.

The social environment, or the availability and anticipation of behaviors by significant others,[3] influences the rate of skill acquisition in the performance components and areas. An infant who is breastfed will not acquire the ability to drink from a bottle or cup as quickly as an infant who is bottle fed. An infant who is carried frequently may not develop gross motor and mobility skills as quickly as an infant who is allowed to move around on the floor or in a playpen.

The cultural environment, which comprises customs, beliefs, activity patterns, and behavior standards,[3] also in-

fluences the rate of skill development in the performance components and areas. Anticipation of behaviors refers to an individual's expectation of repetition of a daily schedule (for example, waking up, eating, bathing, dressing—in that order) or consistency of cause and effect behaviors (for example, washing the dishes and cleaning the room causing the mother to be pleased with the child). An adolescent who has parents that believe only adults should be employed may develop work skills later in life than an adolescent whose parents believe that summer and after-school jobs are appropriate and should be encouraged. In certain cultures, using eating utensils is not the adult norm. Children in this type of cultural environment may never learn to use a fork or spoon.

Studying the process of normal development allows practitioners to learn about its predictable sequences and contextual variability. Although this knowledge is important, having the skills to solve problems related to the developmental process is more useful than memorizing the sequences of skill acquisition within the performance components and areas. Carefully studying this chapter and participating in the suggested activities gives practitioners an excellent basis for using the problem-solving approach with the developmental process. One framework to use when studying development is one based on the generally accepted periods of development. Another framework involves the general principles used by therapists while working in pediatrics.

PERIODS OF DEVELOPMENT

Periods of development are intervals of time during which a child increases in size and acquires specific skills in the performance components and areas.[2] Pediatric occupational therapy practitioners work with children of varying chronological ages. The following normal developmental periods are used as the basis for comparison in subsequent chapters dealing with normal development (Box 5-3).

Gestation and Birth

Gestation refers to the developmental period of the fetus or unborn child in the mother's uterus. The gestational period begins with conception and ends with birth.[2] The gestational period is also referred to as the *prenatal* or *before birth period*.[2] Gestation typically lasts 40 weeks.[2] The birthing process is also known as the *perinatal* (around birth) *period*. The perinatal period varies greatly in duration for a variety of reasons (which are beyond the scope of this book). The perinatal period ends when the infant is able to independently sustain life without placental nutrients from the mother. The postnatal, or after birth, period is the immediate interval of time following birth. During the postnatal period, the infant is known as a *neonate* or *new baby birth*.[2]

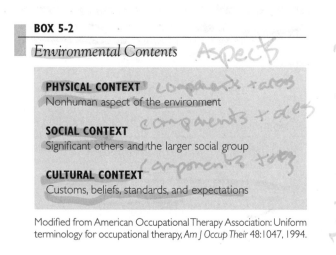

BOX 5-2

Environmental Contents

PHYSICAL CONTEXT
Nonhuman aspect of the environment

SOCIAL CONTEXT
Significant others and the larger social group

CULTURAL CONTEXT
Customs, beliefs, standards, and expectations

Modified from American Occupational Therapy Association: Uniform terminology for occupational therapy, *Am J Occup Ther* 48:1047, 1994.

Infancy

Infancy is the period from birth through approximately 18 months of age.[8] Infancy is characterized by significant physical and emotional growth.[8] Normal infants grow considerably in height and weight during the first 18 months of life.[8] They develop sensory and motor skills, and by 18 months of age, they are walking, talking, and performing simple self-care tasks such as eating with a spoon, drinking from a cup, and undressing.

Early Childhood

Toddlers and preschool children are in the period of early childhood, which begins at 18 months of age and lasts through 5 years of age.[2,8] During the early childhood period, children become increasingly independent and establish more of a sense of individuality.

Middle Childhood

Middle childhood begins at 6 years of age and lasts until puberty, which begins at approximately 12 years of age in females and 14 years of age in males.[8] Children in this developmental period spend the majority of their time in educational settings.

Adolescence

Adolescence is the period of physical and psychological development that accompanies the onset of puberty. Puberty is a stage of maturation in which a person becomes physiologically capable of reproduction. Adolescence is marked by hormonal changes and their resulting challenges.[2] Adolescence ends with the onset of adulthood (usually 21 years of age) when individuals begin to function independently of their parents.[2]

Occupational therapy practitioners use the periods of development as reference points while working with children with special needs. Knowledge of sequences of development within each period is used as a guide for the occupational therapy process. (See Chapters 6 and 7 for a detailed discussion of specific skills gained in the performance components and areas during each period of development.) Practitioners need to know the general principles of development to understand the reasons children gain skills predictably and sequentially.

PRINCIPLES OF NORMAL DEVELOPMENT

The general **principles of development** are widely accepted in the various pediatric disciplines (Box 5-4). The following principles are tools used by occupational therapy practitioners to solve problems during the pediatric occupational therapy process.

- **Normal development is sequential and predictable.** The rate (speed) and direction (vertical or horizontal) of development vary among children, but the sequence remains the same.[1,4,5,7] For example, normally developing infants acquire head control before trunk control (an example of vertical development). Head and trunk control are necessary for infants to sit independently. Infants learn to roll, then sit, then creep, and finally walk. The sequence is the same for all children. However, each child acquires these skills at a unique rate of speed.

- **Maturation and experience affect a child's development.**[4,5,6,] Maturation and experience influence the rate and direction of normal development. Maturation is the innate, or natural, process of growth and development,[2] and experience is a result of interac-

---

BOX 5-3

Periods of Development

GESTATION AND BIRTH
From conception to the moment at which neonate can survive on its own without placental nutrients

INFANCY
From birth through 18 months of age

EARLY CHILDHOOD
From 18 months of through 5 years of age

MIDDLE CHILDHOOD
From 6 years of age until the onset of puberty (12 years of age for females and 14 years of age for males)

ADOLESCENCE
From puberty until the onset of adulthood (usually 21 years of age)

BOX 5-4

General Principles of Development

1. Development is sequential and predictable.
2. Maturation and experience affect development.
3. Development involves changes in the biological, psychological, and social systems.
4. Development occurs in two directions: horizontal and vertical.
5. Development progress in order in three basic sequences:
   - Cephalad to caudad
   - Proximal to distal
   - Gross to fine

tions with the environment. Although most developmental theorists agree that maturation and experience impact a child's development, their opinions about which one is the more significant vary.

- **Throughout the course of normal development, changes occur in the biological, psychological, and social systems.**[5] Therefore development is a dynamic and continuously changing process. Changes in the biological system include changes to the function and processes of internal structures.[8] Psychological system changes affect the emotional and behavioral characteristics of the individual.[8] Changes in the social system include factors that affect individuals in their immediate environment and society as a whole.[8] Changes occur in all three systems throughout the course of typical development. A change in one of the systems impacts the other two systems.

- **Development progresses in two directions: vertical and horizontal.**[5] As children progress through the various developmental levels related to the specific performance components or areas, they are progressing vertically. For example, in the performance area of ADLs, children learn to eat with their fingers before they learn to eat with a spoon. This is an example of a vertical progression. As children learn to roll, then crawl, then creep, and then walk, they are progressing vertically in the gross motor skills performance component. In both of the examples, development is occurring in a vertical direction within a specific performance component or area. Development that involves different performance components and areas is horizontal progression. A child who is simultaneously learning to finger feed, use a pincer grasp, and creep is progressing horizontally because several different performance components and areas (that is, ADLs, fine motor skills, and gross motor skills) are involved.

- **Motor development follows three basic rules.**
  1. *Development progresses cephalad to caudad, or head to tail.*[5] For example, head control develops before trunk control.
  2. *Development progresses in a proximal to distal direction, which means that children develop control of structures close to their body before they develop control of structures farther away from their body.*[4] For example, children develop shoulder control before hand control. The shoulder is closer (or more proximal) to the body than the hand (which is farther away, or more distal).
  3. *Development progresses from gross control to fine control, which means that children gain control of large body movements before they gain control of more refined movements.*[4] For example, children are able to catch a large ball using both arms and their body before they learn to catch a tennis ball with

one hand. They use the large arm muscles to catch a large, 8-inch ball and the small wrist and hand muscles to catch a tennis ball.

These general principles of development provide a framework for occupational therapy practitioners to use while solving developmental problems. The principles can be used to guide the treatment planning processes while working with children who have special needs.

SUMMARY

Normal development is sequential and predictable. Occupational practitioners rely on their knowledge and understanding of typical development while working with children who have special needs. Occupational therapy practitioners must also consider the relationship between normal development and AOTA's performance contexts.

The periods and general principles of development help to provide a framework for organizing and understanding information related to typical development. The periods include gestation and birth, infancy, early childhood, middle childhood, and adolescence. The general principles of development, which are widely used in the various pediatric disciplines, help occupational therapy practitioners plan evaluations and interventions while working with children who have special needs.

References

1. Alexander R, Boehme R, Cupps B: *Normal development of functional motor skills,* Tucson, 1993, Therapy Skills Builders.
2. *American heritage dictionary of the English language,* ed 3, New York, 1996, Houghton Mifflin.
3. American Occupational Therapy Association: Uniform terminology for occupational therapy, ed 3, *Am J Occup Ther* 48:1047, 1994.
4. Boehme R: *Improving upper body control: an approach to assessment and treatment of tonal dysfunction,* Tucson, 1988, Therapy Skill Builders.
5. Case-Smith J, Allen AS, Pratt PN: *Occupational therapy for children,* ed 3, St Louis, 1996, Mosby.
6. Kielhofner G: *Conceptual foundations of occupational therapy,* Philadelphia, 1997, FA Davis.
7. Kramer P, Hinojosa J: *Frames of reference for pediatric occupational therapy,* Baltimore, 1993, Williams & Wilkins.
8. Meyer WJ: Infancy, *Microsoft Encarta 98 encyclopedia,* Redmond, Wash, 1997, Microsoft.

Recommended Reading

Gilfoyle ZM, Grady AP, Moore, JC: *Children adapt,* ed 2, Thorofare, NJ, 1990, Slack.
Knoblock H, Pasamanick D, editors: *Gesell and Amatruda's developmental diagnosis,* ed 3, New York, 1975, Harper & Row.

REVIEW *Questions*

1. Explain the following terms: normal, typical, development, growth.

2. List and describe the periods of development.
3. List and describe the general principles of development.

SUGGESTED *Activities*

1. Visit a day-care center or playground to observe children playing. Notice the variety of approaches that are used by different children to accomplish the same task.

2. In small study groups discuss the general principles of development and then describe these principles in your own words. Give examples of these principles in relation to your own development.

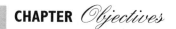

Development of Occupational Performance Components

DIANNE KOONTZ LOWMAN

CHAPTER *Objectives*

After studying this chapter, the reader will be able to accomplish the following:

- Describe significant physiological changes that occur at each stage of development
- Identify the sequences of gross motor and fine motor skill development
- Outline the stages of cognitive development defined by Piaget's theory
- Describe the issues in each phase of psychosocial development using the theories of Erikson and Greenspan

KEY TERMS

Performance components

Sensorimotor components

Cognitive integration and cognitive components

Psychosocial and psychological components

Primitive reflexes

Gross motor skills

Righting reactions

Equilibrium reactions

Fine motor skills

CHAPTER OUTLINE

INFANCY
Physiological
Sensorimotor
Cognitive and Language
Psychosocial

EARLY CHILDHOOD
Physiological
Sensorimotor
Cognitive and Language
Psychosocial

MIDDLE CHILDHOOD
Physiological
Sensorimotor
Cognitive and Language
Psychosocial

ADOLESCENCE
Physiological
Sensorimotor
Cognitive and Language
Psychosocial

SUMMARY

T
hree generations of family members have gathered for a family reunion. While looking at the grandmother's photograph album, conversation centers around how much the 2-year-old grandson looks like his father and grandfather did at the same age. The family is amazed to see how their bodies, sizes, proportions, and postures look similar, even though their clothing and environments are significantly different!

From birth through adolescence the child progresses through the periods of development (see Chapter 5). Development that occurs within each period is described in terms of physiological, sensorimotor, cognitive, and psychosocial domains. The occupational **performance components** comprise the **sensorimotor components, cognitive integration and cognitive components,** and **psychosocial skills and psychological components** (Box 6-1). Deficits in any of these components may interfere with the child's performance in the areas of self-care, play, and education. The normal developmental sequences are presented in this chapter to assist practitioners with identifying potential deficits or delays. Practitioners should note that sequences may vary, and physical, social, and cultural aspects of the environment may affect developmental progression.

As children follow a developmental sequence within an individual performance component, they are also developing in other performance components. For example, an 18-month-old toddler travels and explores indepen-

Acknowledgment: This chapter's author would like to thank the occupational therapy students in Virginia Commonwealth University's Department of Occupational Therapy for researching the material in this chapter and field testing the review questions and suggested activities.

dently, has a precise grasp, is beginning to use tools to solve problems, and demonstrates an understanding of the function of objects in play.

INFANCY

Phillip is an active and happy 1 year old. It is his first birthday party, and he is busy experimenting with his new toys. As family and friends watch, he attempts to sit on his push toy and make it move across the kitchen floor. When his older siblings offer help, he pushes them away because he wants to play alone.

Physiological

At birth the average weight of the newborn is 7 lb 2 oz, and the average length is between 19 and 22 inches. The appearance of the newborn may be characterized by covering comprising a layer of fluid called the *vernix caseosa;* a large, bumpy head; a flat, "board" nose; reddish skin; puffy eyes; external breasts; and fine hair called *lanugo* covering the body.[12] At 1 minute after birth, the newborn's physiological status is tested using the APGAR scoring system, which rates each of the following five areas on a scale of 0 to 2: color, heart rate, reflex irritability, muscle tone, and respiratory effort. Scores are computed 1 minute and 5 minutes after birth. The closer the score to 10, the better the condition of the newborn; scores of 6 or less indicate the need for intervention.[35]

The infant's first 3 months of life are characterized by constant physiological adaptations. Structural changes in the newborn's circulatory system include the expansion of the lungs and increased efficiency of blood flow to the heart. The developing central nervous system par-

BOX 6-1

Occupational Performance Components

SENSORIMOTOR COMPONENTS

Sensorimotor components involve the ability to receive input, process information, and produce output. The components are sensory, neuromusculoskeletal, and motor.

COGNITIVE INTEGRATION AND COGNITIVE COMPONENTS

Cognitive integration and cognitive components involve the ability to use higher brain functions. The components are level of arousal, orientation, recognition, attention span, initiation of activity, termination of activity, memory, sequencing, categorization, concept formation, spatial operations, problem solving, learning, and generalization.

PSYCHOSOCIAL SKILLS AND PSYCHOLOGICAL COMPONENTS

Psychosocial skills and psychological components involve the ability to interact in society and process emotions. The components are psychological, social, and self-management.

From American Occupational Therapy Association: Uniform terminology for occupational therapy, *Am J Occup Ther* 48:1047, 1994.

ticipates in the body's regulation of sleep, digestion, and temperature.[10]

Physical growth is dramatic—from birth until 6 months, infants experience a more rapid rate of growth than during any other time except gestation.[20] During the first year, infants triple their body weight and add 10 to 12 inches of height. Their body shape changes, and by 4 months the size of their heads and bodies are more proportionate. By 12 months, average infants weigh 21 to 22 lb and is 29 to 30 inches tall. During the second year of life, physical growth slows. By 24 months, average toddlers weigh about 27 lb and is 34 inches tall. The posture of toddlers is characterized by *lordosis* (forward curvature of the spine) and a protruding abdomen, a posture that toddlers retains well into the third year.[34]

At 4 months, sleep patterns begin to regulate, and some infants may sleep through the night. By 8 months the average infant sleeps 12 to 13 hours per day, but the range can vary from 9 to 18 hours per day. By 6 to 7 months the average infant acquires the first tooth, a lower incisor. As a result, saliva production increases, which leads to drooling. At approximately 8 months the upper central incisor teeth begin to surface, at 9 months the upper lateral incisors appear, and at 12 months the first lower molars surface.[29]

Sensorimotor

Brazelton[9] identified six behavioral states observed in the newborn: (1) deep sleep, (2) light sleep, (3) drowsy or semidozing, (4) alert, active awake, (5) fussy, and (6) crying. The infant's state should be noted when observing the way the infant responds to stimulation.[12]

Sensory skills

Newborns have vision at birth and can best see objects about 8 inches away, which is the typical distance between the caregiver's face and the infant.[30] By the first month of life an infant shows a preference for patterns and can distinguish between colors. By 3 months the infant's visual acuity develops enough to allow distinction between a picture of a face and a real face.[10] By 12 months the infant's visual acuity is about 20/100 to 20/50.[25]

Hearing is well developed in newborns and continues to improve as they grow. Newborns tend to respond strongly to their mother's voice.[26] During the first 2 months, infants respond to sound with random body movements. At 3 months, infants move their eyes in the direction of sound.[10] At 6 months, infants localize sounds to the left and right.[5] At birth, newborns are able to taste sweet, sour, and bitter substances. Between birth and 3 months, infants are able to differentiate between pleasant and noxious odors. Infants are very sensitive to touch, cold and heat, pain, and pressure; one of the most important stimuli for infants from birth to 3 months is skin contact and warmth.[28] Holding and swaddling the infant provide skin contact and maintain temperature.[12]

Gross motor skills

The newborn's body is characterized by physiological flexion, a position of extremity and trunk flexion.[8] This flexion tends to keep the infant in a compact position and provides a base of stability for random movements to occur. Movements of the newborn are characterized by a motion called *random burst* in which everything moves as a unit.[1] The newborn has numerous **primitive reflexes** that are genetically transmitted survival mechanisms. These automatic responses to stimuli help the newborn adapt to the environment. Primitive reflexes are controlled by lower levels of the central nervous system. As higher levels of the central nervous system mature, the higher systems inhibit the expression of the primitive reflexes. As infants learn about the environment, primitive reflexes are integrated into their overall postural mechanism with the more mature righting and equilibrium responses that dominate their movement.[36] Under stress, these reflexes may be partially present, but they are never obligatory in normal development. Some primitive reflexes are present at birth, whereas others emerge later in the infant's development (Table 6-1).

As shown in Table 6-2, infants' **gross motor skills** become gradually more complex as they develop.[1,8,12] Developing infants begin to combine basic reflexive movements with higher cognitive and physiological functioning to control their movements in the environment (Box 6-2). Between birth and 2 months, infants can turn their heads from side to side while in both the prone and supine positions. As physiological flexion diminishes, infants appear more hypotonic (have less muscle and postural tone), and the movements of each side of their body appear asymmetrical. The asymmetrical tonic neck reflex (ATNR) holds infants' heads to one side. By 4 months, infants can raise and rotate their heads to look at their surroundings. In the supine position (on the back), 4-month-old infants begin to bring their hands to their knees and can deliberately roll from the supine position to the side. The increased head and trunk control observed at this age is a result of emerging **righting reactions** and better postural control (see Box 6-2). At 5 months, infants can bring their heads forward without lagging when pulled to a sitting position. By 6 months, they can shift their weight to free extremities to reach for objects while in the prone position (on the stomach). In the supine position, 6-month-old infants can bring their feet to their mouths and are able to sit by themselves for short periods. At 7 to 8 months age, infants are able to push themselves from a prone position into a sitting position, roll over at will, and crawl on their stomachs. Be-

Text continued on p. 74

TABLE 6-1

Reflexes and Reactions

NAME OF REFLEX OR REACTION	POSITION (P) STIMULUS (S)	POSITIVE RESPONSE	AGE SPAN: AGE OF ONSET OR INTEGRATION	LACK OF INTEGRATION OR ONSET
ROOTING	P: Supine S: Light touch on side of face near mouth	Open mouth, turn head in direction of touch.	Birth to 3 mo	Interferes with exploration of objects and head control
SUCK/SWALLOW	P: Supine S: Light touch on oral cavity	Close mouth, suck, and swallow.	Birth to 2-5 mo	Interferes with development of coordination of sucking, swallowing, and breathing
MORO'S	P: Supine, head at midline S: Drooping head, more than 30 degrees extended	Arms extend and hands open, then arms flex and hands close; infant usually cries.	Birth to 4-6 mo	Interferes with head control, sitting equilibrium, and protective reactions
PALMAR GRASP	P: Supine S: Pressure on ulnar surface of palm	Fingers flex.	Birth to 4-6 mo	Interferes with releasing objects
PLANTAR GRASP	P: Supine S: Firm pressure on ball of foot	Toes grasp (flexion).	Birth to 4-9 mo	Interferes with putting on shoes because of toe clawing and gait and standing and walking, problems (for example, walking on toes)
NEONATAL POSITIVE SUPPORT Primary standing	P: Upright S: Being bounced several times on soles of feet (proprioceptive stimulus)	LE extensor tone increases and plantar flexion is present. Some hip and knee flexion or genu recurvatum (hyperextension of the knee) may occur.	Birth to 1-2 mo	Interferes with walking patterns and leads to walking on toes
ATNR	P: Supine, arms and legs extended, head in midposition S: Head turned to one side	Arm and leg on face side extension. Arm and leg on skull side flex (or experience increased flexor tone).	Birth to 4-6 mo	Interferes with reaching and grasping, bilateral hand use, and rolling

Modified from Alexander R, Boehme R, Cupps B: *Normal development of functional motor skills,* Tucson, 1993, Therapy Skill Builders; Bly L: *Motor skills acquisition in the first year: an illustrated guide to normal development,* Tucson, 1994, Therapy Skill Builders; Fiorentino MR: *Reflex testing methods for evaluating CNS development,* ed 2, Springfield, 1981, Charles C Thomas; Simon CJ, Daub MM: Human development across the life span. In Hopkins JL, Smith HD, editors: *Willard and Spackman's occupational therapy,* ed 8, Philadelphia, 1993, Lippincott.
LE, Lower extremity; *UE,* upper extremity; *ATNR,* asymmetrical tonic neck reflex; *STNR,* symmetrical tonic neck reflex; *TLR,* tonic labyrinthine reflex.

Continued

TABLE 6-I

Reflexes and Reactions—cont'd

NAME OF REFLEX OR REACTION	POSITION (P) STIMULUS (S)	POSITIVE RESPONSE	AGE SPAN: AGE OF ONSET OR INTEGRATION	LACK OF INTEGRATION OR ONSET
STNR	P: Quadruped position or over tester's knees S: 1. Flexed head 2. Extended head	1. Arms flex and legs extend (tone increases). 2. Arms extend and legs flex (tone increases).	Birth to 4-6 mo	Interferes with reciprocal creeping (children "bunny hop," or move arms and then legs in quadruped position) and walking
TLR	P: 1. Supine, head in mid-position, arms and legs extended 2. Prone S: Position (laying on floor); being moved into flexion or extension	1. Extensor tone of neck UE, and LE increase (when moved into flexion). 2. Flexor tone of neck, UE, and LE increases (when moved into extension).	Birth to 4-6 mo	Interferes with turning on side, rolling over, going from laying to sitting - position, and creeping In older children, interferes with ability to "hold in supine flexion" or assume a pivot prone position
LANDAU	P: Prone, held in space (suspension) supporting thorax S: Suspension (usually), also active or passive dorsiflexion of head	Hips and legs extend; UE extends and abducts. Elbows can flex. (Typically used to determine overall development.)	3-4 mo to 12-24 mo	Slows development of prone extension, sitting, and standing Early onset (1 mo): may indicate excessive tone or spasticity
PROTECTIVE EXTENSION UE Parachute, downward	P: Prone, head in mid-position, arms extended above S: Suspension by ankles and pelvis and sudden movement of head suddenly toward floor	Shoulders flex and of elbow and wrist extend (arms extend forward) to protect head.	6-9 mo, continues throughout life	Interferes with head protection
Forward, sideways, backward	P: Seated S: Child pushed: 1. Forward 2. Left, right 3. Backwards	Infant catches self in directions pushed: 1. Shoulder flexes and abducts; elbow and wrist extend (arms extend forward). 2. Shoulder abducts, elbow and wrist extend (arms extend to side). 3. Shoulders, elbows, and wrists extend (arms extend backward) to protect head.	6-9 mo, continues throughout life	Interferes with head protection when center of gravity displaced

Modified from Alexander R, Boehme R, Cupps B: *Normal development of functional motor skills*, Tucson, 1993, Therapy Skill Builders; Bly L: *Motor skills acquisition in the first year: an illustrated guide to normal development*, Tucson, 1994, Therapy Skill Builders; Fiorentino MR: *Reflex testing methods for evaluating CNS development*, ed 2, Springfield, 1981, Charles C Thomas; Simon CJ, Daub MM: Human development across the life span. In Hopkins JL Smith, HD, editors: *Willard and Spackman's occupational therapy*, ed 8, Philadelphia, 1993, Lippincott.
LE, Lower extremity; *UE,* upper extremity; *ATNR,* asymmetrical tonic neck reflex; *STNR,* symmetrical tonic neck reflex; *TLR,* tonic labyrinthine reflex.

TABLE 6-1

Reflexes and Reactions—cont'd

NAME OF REFLEX OR REACTION	POSITION (P) STIMULUS (S)	POSITIVE RESPONSE	AGE SPAN: AGE OF ONSET OR INTEGRATION	LACK OF INTEGRATION OR ONSET
STAGGERING LE Forward, backward, sideways	P: Standing upright S: Displacement of body by pushing on shoulders and upper trunk: 1. Forward 2. Backward 3. Sideways	Infant takes one or more steps in direction of displacements. UEs often also have a protective reaction, with elbow, wrist, and finger extending: 1. Shoulder flexes. 2. Shoulder abducts and extends. 3. Shoulder abducts.	15-18 mo, continues throughout life	Interferes with ability to catch self when center of gravity displaced; causes trips and falls
EQUILIBRIUM Sitting	P: Seated, extremities relaxed S: Hand pulled to one side or shoulder pushed	*Head righting: nonweight-bearing side*—trunk flexes; UE and LE abduct and internally rotate; and elbow, wrist, and fingers extend. *Head righting: weight-bearing side*—trunk elongates; UE and LE externally rotate; and elbow, wrist, and fingers extend and abduct.	7-8 mo, continues throughout life	Interferes with ability to sit or maintain balance when reaching for objects or displacing center of gravity
Standing	P: Standing upright, extremities relaxed S: Body displaced by holding UE and pulling to side	*Head righting: nonweight-bearing side*—trunk flexes; UE and LE abduct and internally rotate; and elbow, wrist, and fingers extend. *Head righting: weight-bearing side*—Trunk elongates; UE and LE externally rotate; and elbow, wrist, and fingers abduct and extend.	12-21 mo, continues throughout life	Interferes with ability to stand and walk and make transitional movements
EQUILIBRIUM OR TILTING Prone, supine	P: Prone or supine on a tilt board, extremities extended S: Board tilted to left or right	*Head righting: nonweight-bearing side*—Trunk flexes; UE and LE abduct; and elbow, wrist, hip, and knee externally rotate and extend. *Head righting: weightbearing side*—UE and LE internally rotate and adduct, and elbow, wrist, fingers, knees, and hips extend.	5-6 mo, continues throughout life	Interferes with ability to make transitional movements, sit, and creep

TABLE 6-2

Normal Development of Sensorimotor Skills

AGE	GROSS MOTOR COORDINATION	FINE MOTOR COORDINATION
BIRTH OR 37-40 WK GESTATION	Is dominated by physiological flexion Moves entire body into extension or flexion Turns head side to side (protective response) while in prone position Keeps head mostly to side while in supine position	Visually regards objects and people Tends to fist and flex hands across chest during feeding Displays strong grasp reflex but has no voluntary grasping abilities Has no voluntary release abilities
1-2 MO	Appears hypotonic as physiological flexion diminishes Practices extension and flexion Continues to gain control of head Moves elbows forward toward shoulders while in prone position Has ATNR with head to side while in supine position When held in standing position, bears some weight on legs	Displays diminishing grasp reflex Involuntarily releases after holding them briefly; has no voluntary release abilities
3-5 MO	Experiences fading of ATNR and grasp reflex Has more balance between extension and flexion positions Has good head control (centered and upright) Supports self on extended arms while in prone position; props self on forearms Brings hand to feet and feet to mouth while in supine position Props on arms with little support while seated Rolls from supine to prone position Bears some weight on legs when held proximally	Constantly brings hands to mouth Develops tactile awareness in hands Reaches more accurately, usually with both hands Palmar grasp Begins transferring objects from hand to hand Does not have control of releasing objects; may use mouth to assist
6 MO	Has complete head control Possesses equilibrium reactions Begins assuming quadruped position Rolls from prone to supine position Bounces while standing	Transfers objects from hand to hand while in supine position Shifts weight and reaches with one hand while in prone position Reaches with one hand and supports self with other while seated

Modified from Alexander R, Boehme R, Cupps B: *Normal development of functional motor skills,* Tucson, 1993, Therapy Skill Builders; Case-Smith J, Shortridge SD: The developmental process: prenatal to adolescence. In Case-Smith J, Allen J, Pratt PN, editors, *Occupational therapy for children,* ed 3, St Louis, 1996, Mosby; Clark GF: Oral-motor and feeding issues. In Royeen CB, editor: *AOTA self study series: classroom applications for school-based practice,* Rockville, 1993, American Occupational Therapy Association; Erhardt RP: *Developmental hand dysfunction: theory, assessment, and treatment,* ed 2, Tucson, 1994, Therapy Skill Builders.

TABLE 6-2

Normal Development of Sensorimotor Skills—cont'd

AGE	GROSS MOTOR COORDINATION	FINE MOTOR COORDINATION
6 MO—cont'd		Reaches to be picked up Uses radial palmar grasp; begins to use thumb while grasping Shows visual interest in small objects; rakes small objects Begins to hold objects in one hand
7-9 MO	Shifts weight and reaches while in quadruped position Creeps Develops extension, flexion, and rotation movements, which increase number of activities that can be accomplished while seated May pull to standing position while holding on to support	Reaches with supination Uses index finger to poke objects Uses inferior scissors grasp to pick up small objects Uses radial-digital grasp to pick up cube Displays voluntary release abilities
10-12 MO	Displays good coordination while creeping Pulls to standing position using legs only Cruises holding on to support with one hand Stands independently Begins to walk independently Displays equilibrium reactions while standing	Uses superior pincer grasp with finger tip and thumb Uses 3-jaw chuck grasp Displays controlled release into large containers
13-18 MO	Walks alone Seldom falls Begins to go up and down stairs	Displays more precise grasping abilities Precisely releases objects into small containers
19-24 MO	Displays equilibrium reactions while walking Runs using a more narrow base of support	Uses finger to palm translation of small object
24-36 MO	Jumps in place* Pedals tricycle*	Uses palm-to-finger and finger-to-palm translation of small object Displays complex rotation of small objects Shifts small objects using palmar stabilization Scribbles Snips with scissors

*From this point on, skills learned during the first 24 months are further refined.

Development of Coordinated Movement in Infancy

EXTENSION → FLEXION → LATERAL FLEXION → ROTATION

PRIMITIVE REFLEXES

Primitive reflexes are automatic movements that are usually stimulated by sensory factors and performed without conscious volition. Primitive reflexes cause the first involuntary movements to occur and allow for extension movements to emerge. Primitive reflexes are controlled at the lower levels of the central nervous system. As the higher levels (cerebral hemispheres) mature, the expression of the primitive reflexes is inhibited by these higher levels (that is, they seem to disappear).

RIGHTING REACTIONS

Righting reactions are postural reactions in response to changes of head and body position. Righting reactions bring the head and trunk back into an upright position. These reactions involve movements called *extension, flexion, abduction, adduction,* and *lateral flexion.*

EQUILIBRIUM REACTIONS

Equilibrium reactions are automatic, compensatory movements of the body parts that are used to maintain the center of gravity over the base of support when either the center of gravity or the supporting surface is displaced. These complex postural responses combine righting reactions with movements known as *rotation and diagonal patterns.* Essential for volitional movement and mobility, the use of righting reactions begins at 6 months and continues throughout life.

PROTECTIVE EXTENSION RESPONSES

Protective extension responses are postural reactions that are used to stop a fall or to prevent injury when equilibrium reactions fail to do so. These responses involve *straightening of the arms or legs* toward a supporting surface. Essential for mobility, use of protective extension reactions begins between 6 and 9 months and continues throughout life.

Modified from Alexander R, Boehme R, Cupps B: *Normal development of functional motor skills,* Tucson, 1993, Therapy Skill Builders; Bly L: *Motor skills acquisition in the first year: an illustrated guide to normal development,* Tucson, 1994, Therapy Skill Builders; Fiorentino MR: *Reflex testing methods for evaluating CNS development,* ed 2, Springfield, Ill, 1981, Charles C Thomas; Simon CJ, Daub MM: Human development across the life span. In Hopkins, JL, Smith, HD, editors: *Willard and Spackman's occupational therapy,* ed 8, Philadelphia, 1993, Lippincott.

tween 6 and 9 months, infants develops upper extremity protective extension reactions, which allow them to catch themselves when pushed off balance (Figure 6-1). From 7 to 21 months, infants develop **equilibrium reactions** that allow them to maintain their center of gravity over their base of support, reactions that are critical for transitional movements patterns (that is, movements from one position to another) and ambulation (see Box 6-2 and Figure 6-2). At 10 to 11 months, infants are practicing and enjoying creeping. By 12 months, they are learning to shift their weight and step to one side by cruising around furniture. At 13 or 14 months, most infants take their first steps, and between 12 and 18 months, they spend much of their time practicing motor skills by walking, jumping, running, and kicking. Mobility changes infants' perspectives on their environments. A chair is a one-dimensional object in the eyes of a 6 month old; it is only when the infant can finally climb over, under, and around the chair that the infant discovers what a chair really is.[19]

Fine motor skills

Between birth and 3 months, most interactions with the environment are through visual inspection. The grasp reflex allows the infant to have contact with objects placed in the hand. At 4 months the infant demonstrates visually directed reaching skills. At 5 months the infant can use a palmar grasp and an ulnar palmar grasp. The child's fingers on are placed on the top surface of an object. The fingers then press the object into the center of the palm toward the little finger (Figure 6-3, A). At 5 to 6 months, transferring objects from one hand to another is a two-step process (with the taking hand grabbing the objects deposited by the releasing hand before the releasing hand lets go). By 6 months the infant is coordinated enough to reach for an object while in a sitting or prone position. A 6-month-old infant uses a radial palmar grasp (in which the object is held between thumb and radial side of palm) (Figure 6-3, B) to transfer objects from hand to hand in a one-stage process (with the taking hand and releasing hand executing the transfer simultaneously). Grasp skills change significantly between 7 and 12 months. At 7 months the infant uses a radial digital grasp (holds objects between the thumb and fingertips), and the ability to voluntarily release an object begins to emerge. At about 9 months the infant learns to use an inferior pincer grasp (press the pad of the thumb to the pad of the

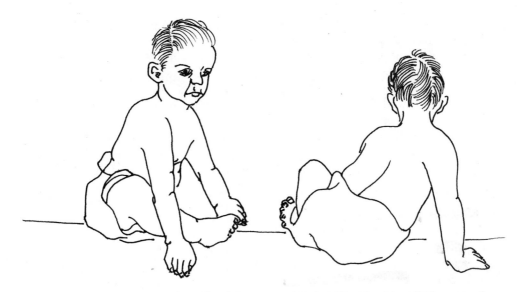

FIGURE 6-1 Equilibrium reactions allow infants to protect themselves by automatically moving forward and sideways after losing balance in a sitting position or from one position to a different position.

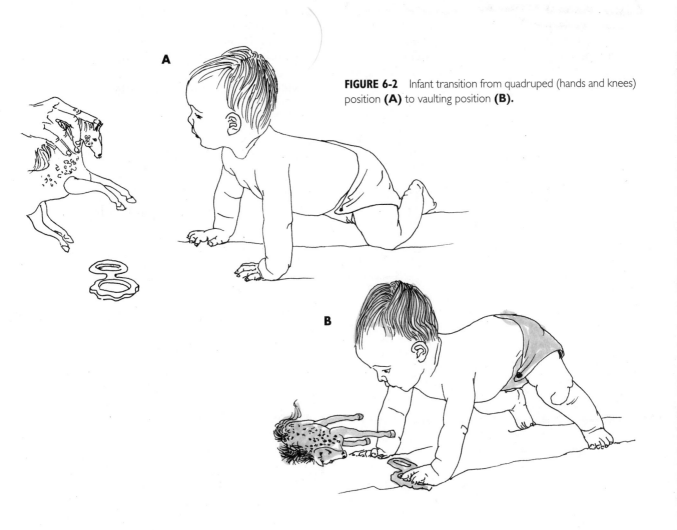

FIGURE 6-2 Infant transition from quadruped (hands and knees) position **(A)** to vaulting position **(B)**.

index finger) to pick up a small object. By 10 months the infant can release an object into a container. By 12 months the infant uses a superior pincer grasp (places the tip of the thumb to the tip of the index finger) (Figure 6-4) and consistently puts objects into containers. By 12 months the fine motor skills are developed enough to allow the infant to combine objects and explore their functional use. These skills facilitate the development of functional and symbolic play skills.[6,12,16]

Cognitive and Language

Piaget's stages of cognitive development

The infant's cognitive development can be described using Piaget's theory. Piaget stated that individuals pass through a series of stages of thought as they progress from infancy to adolescence. These stages are a result of biological pressures to adapt to the changing environment and organize structures of thinking. According to Piaget, cognitive development is divided into 4 stages: sensorimotor, preoperational, concrete operational, and formal operational. During the sensorimotor stage the infant develops the ability to organize and coordinate sensations with physical movements and actions. As shown in Table 6-3, the sensorimotor period has six substages.[20,28,31]

During the first stage, known as the *reflexive stage*, behavior is dominated by reflexes such as sucking and the palmar grasp. A rattle placed in an infant's hand is retained by the grasp reflex. Random motor movement causes the infant to accidentally shake the rattle. In the second stage, referred to as *primary circular reactions*, the infant repeats the reflexive movements and patterns simply for pleasure. During this stage an infant may accidentally get the fingers to the mouth and begin to suck on them. The infant then searches for the fingers again but has trouble getting them to the mouth because the coordination to do so has not been mastered. The infant repeats this action until the fingers get to the mouth. In the third stage, called *secondary circular reactions,* the infant begins to use voluntary movements to repeat actions that accidentally produced a desirable result. At this age an infant who accidentally hits a rattle with a foot while kicking would repeat the same kicking movement to reproduce the sound, thus creating a learned *scheme*, or mental plan, that can be used to reproduce the sound again. During the fourth stage, referred to as *coordination of secondary schemata,* several significant changes take place. The infant readily combines previously learned schemes and generalizes them for use in new situations. For example, the infant may visually inspect and touch a toy simultaneously. The

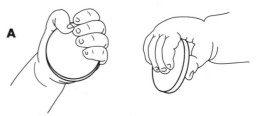

FIGURE 6-3 A, When using an ulnar palmar grasp, infant's fingers are on top surface of object, pressing it into center palm toward little finger. **B,** When using a radial palmar grasp, infant holds object between thumb and radial side of palm.

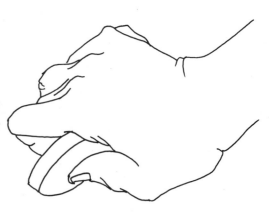

FIGURE 6-4 When using a superior pincer grasp, infant holds small object between tips of index finger and thumb. Wrist is slightly extended with ring and little finger curled into palm.

TABLE 6-3

Normal Development of Cognitive Skills

AGE	PIAGET'S SENSORIMOTOR PERIOD (BIRTH-2 YR)	COGNITIVE MILESTONES
BIRTH (37-40 WK GESTATION)	**REFLEXIVE STAGE**	Uses entire body during vocalizations Primarily uses abdomen to breathe Quiets in response to a voice Slowly follows moving objects visually (tracks)
1-2 MO	**REFLEXIVE STAGE (1 MO)** Begins displaying primitive reflexes Does not differentiate between self and objects or between sensation and action	Still closely associates all sounds with movement Still primarily uses abdomen to breathe; displays rhythmical breathing patterns while at rest Begins to explore environment by mouthing objects Stops all activity and experiences a change in breathing patterns while focusing on an object or person Has smoother visual tracking skills
3-5 MO	**PRIMARY CIRCULAR REACTIONS (2-4 MO)** Repeats reflexive sensory motor patterns for pleasure	Begins to put hand on bottle and find mouth Transitions from watching own hands to mouthing own hands Increases variety of sounds; has a less nasal cry Understands concept of object permanence: transitions from searching for only dropped objects to searching for partially hidden objects Pats bottle during feeding
6 MO	**SECONDARY CIRCULAR REACTIONS (5-8 MO)** Begins to show true voluntary movement patterns Repeats actions that create pleasurable sensations Has a primitive awareness of cause and effect	Calls out to get attention Repeats own sounds Uses increasingly varied sounds Increasingly disassociates sounds from movement Understands concept of cause and effect: repeats certain patterns of actions involving objects or people to achieve a particular result
7-9 MO		Puts objects in containers Copies movements such as banging objects together Begins to search for objects in containers Responds to word *no* Explores spatial concepts such as in/out and off/on by experimenting with different movements while playing

Modified from Case-Smith J, Shortridge SD: The developmental process: Prenatal to adolescence. In Case-Smith J, Allen J, Pratt PN, editors, *Occupational therapy for children,* ed 3, St Louis, 1996, Mosby; Maier HW: *Three theories of child development,* revised ed, New York, 1965, Harper & Row.

Continued

TABLE 6-3

Normal Development of Cognitive Skills—cont'd

AGE	PIAGET'S SENSORIMOTOR PERIOD (BIRTH-2 YR)	COGNITIVE MILESTONES
10-12 MO	**COORDINATION OF SECONDARY SCHEMATA (9-12 MO)** Begins to participate in object permanence problem-solving activities Begins to be capable of decentered thought (that is, realization that objects exist apart from self, in different contexts, and when out of sight)	Shows a desire for independence in motor development and skills Follows simple directions Uses objects to reach goal in independent problem-solving activities
13-18 MO	**TERTIARY CIRCULAR REACTIONS (12-18 MO)** Begins to use tools Searches for new schemes	Solves problems by trial and error Uses objects conventionally and begins to group Uses speech to name, refuse, call, greet, protest, and express feelings
19-24 MO	**INVENTIONS OF NEW MEANS THROUGH MENTAL COMBINATIONS (18-24 MO)** Begins to show insight Begins to purposefully use tools Mental representation is the hallmark of this stage Develops ability to use mental representation (that is, label and symbolically use mental schemes to present concepts)	Follows two-step directions Understands object permanence and engages in systematic searching Uses speech as a significant means of communication

Modified from Case-Smith J, Shortridge SD: The developmental process: Prenatal to adolescence. In Case-Smith J, Allen J, Pratt PN, editors, *Occupational therapy for children*, ed 3, St Louis, 1996, Mosby; Maier HW: *Three theories of child development*, revised ed, New York, 1965, Harper & Row.

major advancement during this period is the emergence of object permanence. The infant searches for an object that has disappeared. In addition the infant uses existing schemes to obtain a desired object. For example, the infant may pull a string to get an attached toy or object. During the stage called *tertiary circular reactions* the infant attempts a task repeatedly and modifies the behavior to achieve the desired consequences. The repetition helps the infant understand the concept of cause-and-effect relationships. Another important hallmark of this stage is the use of tools, such as using a cup to drink. During the last stage of the sensorimotor period, known as *inventions of new means through mental combinations*, the toddler begins using trial and error to solve problems. For example, the toddler learns that pulling on a tablecloth will bring down a plate of cookies to the floor. During the last stage the child also uses pretend play to create new roles for various objects. For example, stuffed animals that were previously used for teething or banging other objects are considered playmates (see Table 6-3).[20,28,31]

Language

Although Piaget's theory is defined in terms of sensorimotor learning, the development of language is closely related to cognitive development.[12] Undifferentiated crying characterizes the newborns' "language." By 3 months, their vocalizations are called *cooing* and are usually composed of pleasant vowel sounds. Around 4 months, infants begin to *babble*, or repeat a string of vowel and consonant sounds. From birth to 4 months age, infants are "universal linguists"—they are capable of distinguishing among each of the 150 sounds that comprise all human speech. By 6 months, infants recognize only the speech sounds of their native language.[24] By the age of 8 months, infants develop a sense of the existence of others, recognizing and imitating the actions of caregivers. They repeat sounds, which is know as *lallation* when the repetition is accidental and *echolalia* when the repetition is conscious. By 12 months, infants know between two and eight words and babble short sentences. Their vocabulary increases significantly during the second year. By 24 months, toddlers may have 50 to 200 words in their spoken vocabulary.[12]

TABLE 6-4

Psychosocial and Emotional Development

PERIOD	AGE (YEARS)	ERIKSON	GREENSPAN	TYPICAL BEHAVIORS
INFANCY	0-1	**TRUST VERSUS MISTRUST** Has needs gratified Gives to others in return Develops drive and hope	**SELF-REGULATION (0-3 MO)** Calms self Regulates sleep Notices sights and sounds Enjoys touch and movement	Has fussy periods to relieve stress Smiles Imitates gestures Uses special smiles for different people and events May experience joy and anger
			FALLING IN LOVE (2-7 MO) Is "wooed" by significant others Responds to facial expressions and vocalizations Attachment	Fears strangers (8 mo) Gives affection Learns about cause and effect Understands concept of object permanency
			PURPOSEFUL COMMUNICATION (3-10 MO) Displays reciprocal interactions when initiated by adult Initiates interactions	

Courtesy Jayne Shepherd. Modified from Erikson EH: *Childhood and society*, ed 2, New York, 1963, WW Norton; Greenspan, SI: *Playground politics: understanding the emotional life of your school-aged child*, Reading, Mass, 1993, Addison-Wesley; Greenspan S, Greenspan N: *First feelings: milestones in the emotional development of your baby and child*, New York, 1985, Viking Penguin.

Psychosocial

The **psychosocial** development of newborns begins with the earliest emotional connections and interactions with their caregivers. The development of this emotional connection, or feeling of love, between newborns and their caregivers was first examined in the context of attachment, or the development of affectionate ties on the part of the infant to the mother. Ainsworth[3] outlined four stages in the development of infants attachment to their caregivers:

1. *Initial attachment:* At 2 to 3 months, infants exhibit undiscriminating social responses.
2. *Attachment-in-the-making:* By 4 to 6 months, infants begin to discriminate among familiar and unfamiliar persons.
3. *Clear-cut, or active, attachment:* By 6 to 7 months, infants attach more to one primary caregiver, seeking proximity to and contact with that caregiver.
4. *Multiple attachments:* After 12 months, infants attach to persons other than their primary caregivers.

Another facet of the infant and caregiver relationship is called *bonding*. Bonding is characterized by behaviors such as stroking, kissing, cuddling, and prolonged gazing. These behaviors serve two functions: expressing affection and sustaining an interaction between caregivers and infants. By the time infants are 1 month, most parents are attuned to them and are able to interpret their cries and comfort them; in other words a *goodness of fit*, or match between infants' temperaments and their environments, exists between infants' needs and their caregivers' reactions. Caregivers also begin to recognize the early indicators of changes in their infants' temperaments and know ways to calm them or prevent overstimulation.[3,9,28]

Two theories of psychosocial and emotional development in infancy are highlighted in Table 6-4. According to Greenspan,[23] the first stage is called *self-regulation and interest in the world*. During the first few months after birth the infant is focused on organizing the internal and external worlds, and the primary caregivers' job is to help the infant regulate these influences. Around the second or third month the infant moves into the *falling in love* stage, the stage in which the infant forms strong attachments to the primary caregivers. The infant responds to the facial expressions and vocalizations of the caregivers with smiles and coos.

TABLE 6-4

Psychosocial and Emotional Development—cont'd

PERIOD	AGE (YEARS)	ERIKSON	GREENSPAN	TYPICAL BEHAVIORS
EARLY CHILDHOOD	1-3	**AUTONOMY VERSUS SHAME AND DOUBT** Considers self separate from parents Feels dependent on parents Develops self-control and will power Struggles with a conflict between "holding on" or "letting go"	**EMERGENCE OF ORGANIZED SENSE OF SELF (9-18 MO)** Knows ways to get different types of reactions Is focused and organized while playing Initiates complex behaviors Is capable of feeling embarrassment, pride, shame, joy, empathy, anger	**Early** Attaches to transitional objects (such as a blanket) Imitates others Understands function of objects and meaning of behaviors **Late** Is egocentric Experiences separation anxiety (2 yr)
			CREATING EMOTIONAL IDEAS (18-36 MO) Uses words and gestures Participates in pretend play with others Learns to recover from anger or temper tantrums Starts associating particular functions with certain people	Loves an audience and attention Often says phrases like "me do it" and "no" Has difficulty sharing Begins to become independent and spend time alone
	3-5	**INITIATIVE AND IMAGINATION VERSUS GUILT** Displays purpose in actions Has a lively imagination Tests reality Imitates parental actions and roles Seeks new experiences that, if successful, lead to sense of initiative; needs balance between initiative and responsibility for own actions Accepts consequences of actions Makes choices and plans	**EMOTIONAL THINKING (30-48 MO)** Differentiates between real and not real Follows rules Understands relationships among behaviors, feelings, and consequences (is capable of feeling guilty) Interacts in socially appropriate ways with adults and peers	Seems optimistic and confident Asks "why" Is spontaneous Seeks other playmates Fears monsters, spiders, etc; has bad dreams (4-5 yr) Plays with imaginary playmates Tells exaggerated stories

Courtesy Jayne Shepherd. Modified from Erikson EH: *Childhood and society,* ed 2, New York, 1963, WW Norton; Greenspan, SI: *Playground politics: understanding the emotional life of your school-aged child,* Reading, Mass, 1993, Addison-Wesley; Greenspan S, Greenspan N: *First feelings: milestones in the emotional development of your baby and child,* New York, 1985, Viking Penguin.

TABLE 6-4

Psychosocial and Emotional Development—cont'd

PERIOD	AGE (YEARS)	ERIKSON	GREENSPAN	TYPICAL BEHAVIORS
MIDDLE CHILDHOOD	5-11	**INDUSTRY VERSUS INFERIORITY** Sees work as pleasurable Develops sense of responsibility and competence Learns work habits Learns to use tools Likes recognition for accomplishments Is sensitive to performance in comparison with others Tries new activities Becomes scholastically and socially competent	**THE WORLD IS MY OYSTER (5-7 YR)** Carries out self-care and self-regulatory functions with minimal assistance Enjoys relationship with parents Takes simultaneous interest wants and needs of parents, peers, and "me first" Forms relationships with peers Struggles to assert own will with peers Better handles not getting own way Better understands reasons for reality limits **THE WORLD IS OTHER KIDS (8-10 YR)** Cares about role in peer group Has best friends and regular friends Maintains nurturing relationship with parents Continues to enjoy fantasy Follows rules Orders emotions and groups them into categories Experiences competition without becoming aggressive or compliant	Early (5-7) Acts assertive and bossy; acts like a "know it all" Is critical of self Experiences night terrors Shares and takes turns Late (9-11) Desires privacy Acts with less impulsivity and more control Looks up to and focuses on being like a certain person—a "hero" ("hero worship") Becomes more competitive Expects perfection from others (11 yr)
ADOLESCENCE	12-18	**SELF-IDENTITY VERSUS ROLE CONFUSION** Has a temporal perspective Experiments with roles (parents, friends, various groups) Enters sexual relationships Shares self with others Develops ideological commitments	**THE WORLD INSIDE ME (11-12 YR)** Has a developing internal sense of right and wrong Enjoys one or a few intimate friends Takes interest in adults as role models Uses rules flexibly by understanding context Takes interest in opposite sex Has feelings of privacy about own body Has concerns about body and personality; related to puberty	Acts as if *right now* is most important thing in life Accepts and adjusts to changing body Plays to imaginary audience Believes in personal fable (of infallibility) and characterized by the phrase "It won't happen to me" Begins working Achieves emotional independence from parents

From 3 to 10 months the infant begins to learn the art of *purposeful communication*. At this stage the infant's smile is purposeful; the infant has learned that smiling causes the adults to smile back. Around 9 or 10 months the infant develops an *organized sense of self* and begins to realize the way to use behavior to get different reactions from others.[23]

EARLY CHILDHOOD

Four-year-old Phillip spends time practicing his fine motor skills. He enjoys drawing pictures and telling long, sometimes exaggerated, stories to go with his pictures. When playing with the other children in the neighborhood, Phillip tends to play with the other boys. The boys tend to play rougher games than the girls.

Physiological

The beginning of the early childhood period is ". . . marked by the development of autonomy, the beginning of expressive language, and sphincter control."[12] The rapid growth of infancy slows as children enter their second and third years. Their limbs begin to grow faster than their heads, making their bodies seem less top heavy. By 6 years the legs make up almost 45% of the body length, and the children are about 7 times their birth weight. The brain of a 5 year old is 75% of its adult weight.[14,34,36] Changes in physiological pathways give the children the sphincter control necessary for toilet training.[12]

The physiological differences between children in the early childhood stage and adults are significant. The eustachian tube is shorter and positioned more horizontally than that of adults, making children more susceptible to middle ear infections. The digestive tract is not fully mature, and the shape of the stomach is straight, resulting in frequent upset stomachs. Because of the immaturity of the retina, young children are farsighted.[12]

Sensorimotor

All of the basic components of sensorimotor development, such as vision, touch, gross motor skills, and fine motor skills, exist physiologically during the second and third years. These components are developed as the skills are refined through interactions with the environment. Balance and strength increase during the early childhood period. At age 2, toddlers walk with an increased stride length, and by 4 years their walking pattern more closely resembles that of an adult. The ability to run develops

around 3 to 4 years; by 5 or 6 years, a mature running pattern develops. Two-year-old children can climb stairs without holding on to a support; by $3\frac{1}{2}$ years, children are able to walk up and down stairs without holding on and with alternating feet.[12]

Like gross motor skills, the coordination and precision of hand and finger movements are refined with maturation and practice, especially when children enter preschool and school. At 2 years, one of children's major accomplishments is learning to draw. The first type of grasp they learn is a palmar grasp; however, during the second year, they develop the ability to hold a pencil in their hand rather than their fist. As thumb, finger, and hand precision improve enough to allow children to use a tripod grasp, their drawings progress from being scribbles to being deliberate lines and shapes. A mature, dynamic tripod grasp develops by 5 years (Figure 6-5). Three-year-old children are able to snip paper with scissors, and more mature scissor skills develop around 5 to 6 years.[11,12]

Cognitive and Language

Piaget's second phase of development, the *preoperational period*, occurs between the ages of 2 and 7 years; 2- to 4-years-olds are in the preconceptual substage of preoperational thought. The beginning of symbolic thought and strong egocentrism and the emergence of animism characterize this substage. The ability to use *symbolism* is the ability to mentally consider objects that are not pres-ent. *Egocentrism* is the inability of individuals to realize others have thoughts and feelings that may not be the same as their own. *Animism* is the act of giving inanimate objects lifelike qualities; this ability develops around age 3.[36] Children between the ages of 5 to 7 are in the *intuitive thought* substage of preoperational thought. Cognitive development, and especially language, is characterized by the use of symbolism. During this phase, children begin to engage in symbolic, or pretend, play and tend to think more logically. They are able to use words and gestures to represent real objects or events.[12]

The vocabulary of young children expands rapidly, increasing from a repertoire of 200 words at 2 years to 1500 words at 3 years. Two year olds label items and ask simple questions, whereas 3 year olds can express their thoughts and feelings in simple sentences. By age 4, children can narrate long stories, which are sometimes exaggerated. Children who are 5 or 6 are able to enunciate clearly and use their advanced language skills as a tool for learning. For example, they commonly ask questions such as, "What is this for?" "How does this work?" and "What does it mean?"[11]

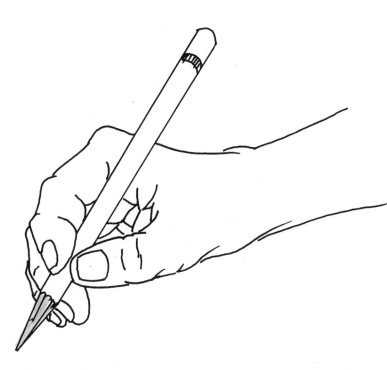

FIGURE 6-5 When using a dynamic tripod grasp, child holds pencil with thumb, index, and middle fingers. Fingers move while other joints of arm remain stable.

Psychosocial

According to Erikson, 2- to 4-year-old period of early childhood is referred to as the stage of *autonomy versus shame and doubt*. During this stage a need to be autonomous dominates children's psychosocial development; they are determined to make their own decisions and be independent. Central to this stage is the period known as the *terrible two's*, the period in which 2 year olds are trying to prove their independence. According to Erikson's theories, children begin to doubt themselves and feel ashamed if they are not given adequate opportunities for self-regulation.[10,12,17] Children between the ages of 4 to 6 are in the stage Erikson calls *initiative and imagination versus guilt*. Children show initiative in activities in which their behavior produces successful, effective results and meets with parental approval. Guilt, on the other hand, results when children assume a sense of responsibility for their own behavior. By imitating others, children learn to take responsibility for their actions and develop a sense of purpose. Gender role development is also an important period in this stage.[11,12,38]

The early childhood years comprise two of Greenspan's stages, which are called *creating emotional ideas*, and *emotional thinking*. In the stage of creating emotional ideas, 2 year olds express emotional ideas by words and gestures, engaging in pretend play, and starting to associate certain functions with certain people. In the stage of emotional thinking, 3 and 4 year olds are able to differentiate between what is real and not real, follow rules, and understand the relationship between behaviors and feelings.[23]

MIDDLE CHILDHOOD

Ten-year-old Phillip is very concerned with being accepted in his peer group—he insists on wearing the same tennis shoes as the other boys. He and his friends spend hours playing seemingly endless baseball games. They follow the rules but don't really keep score.

Physiological

Between the early childhood years and the growth spurt of adolescence, the growth rate slows. Although wide variations in growth occur in both sexes during the middle childhood years, girls and boys typically grow an average of 2 to 3 inches per year, with their legs becoming longer and trunks slimmer.[36] Girls typically grow taller than boys during this period. Facial features become more distinct and unique, partly because baby teeth have been replaced by permanent teeth. The digestive system matures, so children retain food in the digestive system longer; they eat less frequently but have increased appetites and eat in greater quantities.[12] By the age of 10, head and brain growth are 95% complete. Hearing acuity increases, and changes in the eustachian tube location decrease the risk for middle ear infections.[12,36]

Sensorimotor

Because the rate of physical development slows during middle childhood, children have the opportunity to refine their gross motor skills and become generally more adept at handling their bodies. Children tend to focus on refinement of previously learned skills. Hours of repetition leads to mastery of these skills, which creates higher self-esteem and greater acceptance from peers.[7] Increased muscle strength and endurance allow children to become more physical; their favorite activities often include running, climbing, throwing, riding a bicycle, swimming, and skating.[36] Refined fine motor skills allow children to better perform tasks such as sewing, using garden tools, and writing. The task of writing is a combination of refined grasp skills and coordinated movements that result in smooth writing strokes and smaller letters. By the age of 10 years, most children have converted from writing in print letters to writing in cursive letters.[12]

Cognitive and Language

The middle childhood years include the Piaget stage of *concrete operations*, which includes children from 7 to 11 years. This stage marks the beginning of the ability to think abstractly, or to mentally manipulate actions. For example, children are able to envision what might happen if they throw a rock across the room, but they do not actually have to throw the rock to see what is going to happen. Other characteristics of concrete operational period include the following[36]:

- Children are less self-centered.
- Children can recognize that others may have viewpoints that differ from their own.
- Children can identify similarities and differences among objects.
- Children can use simple logic to arrive at a conclusion.
- Children can simultaneously consider many aspects of a situation rather than just one aspect.
- Children realize that a substance's quantity does not change when its form does.
- Children can order objects by size, indicating an understanding of the relationships among objects.
- Children can imagine objects or pieces as parts of a whole.

Using Piaget's ideas as a basis, Kohlberg formulated schemes of moral development. During the early elementary years (between 4 and 10 years), children are in what Kohlberg calls the *preconventional level* of moral development. They make moral judgments based solely on the basis of anticipated punishment or reward. (That is, a "right," or "good," action is one that feels good and is rewarded, and a "bad" action is one that results in punishment.)[36] Between 10 and 13 years, children enter a stage called the *morality of conventional role conformity* stage. Children in this stage are eager to please others and there-

fore tend to internalize rules (by applying them to themselves) and judge their actions according to set standards. Ten and eleven year olds are concerned with meeting the expectations and following the rules of their peer group. This stage is characterized by conforming, following "the golden rule" ("Do unto others as you would have them do unto you"), and showing respect for authority and rules.[32]

During middle childhood the vocabulary of children expands, partly as a result of their focus on reading. Puns and figures of speech become meaningful, and children's jokes become based on double word meanings, slang, curse words, colloquialisms, and secret languages.[20] Communication among children during the middle childhood years has been described as *socialized communication*—conversations center around school activities, personal experiences, families and pets, sports, clothes, movies, television, comics, and "taboo" subjects (such as sex, cursing, and drinking).[32]

Psychosocial

When children begin attending elementary school, their families are no longer their sole source of security and relationships. During this period, significant social relationships are developed outside the family in the neighborhood and school. A feeling of belonging is very important to children in the middle childhood years, so they become increasingly concerned with their status among peers. They seem to have their own personal societies, separate from the adult world, that include rituals, heroes, and peer groups.[7,12,32] Peer groups usually comprise children of the same sex. Girls and boys tend to engage in their own activities with little communication between each other. During this period, children experience more pressure to conform than during any other period of development. Children struggle to simultaneously participate in group activities while balancing the group's identity with their own and establishing their role within the group.[20]

The middle childhood years include the stage Erikson named the *industry versus inferiority stage*. Erikson believed that children must learn new skills to survive in their culture; if unsuccessful, they develop a sense of inferiority.[20] During this stage the source of children's feelings of security switch from the family to the peer group as the children try to master the activities of their friends. Greenspan[22] described 8 to 10 year olds' developmental stage as *the world is other kids*. Children develop a mental picture of themselves that is based on interactions with friends, family members, and teachers. *The world inside me* stage is representative of an 11 year old's definition of self, which is based on personal characteristics rather than the peer group's perceptions. At this age, children are able to empathize and understand the feelings of others. They realize that relationships require constant, mutual adjustments, so they are able to disagree with a friend but still maintain the friendship.[22]

ADOLESCENCE

Fifteen-year-old Phillip wants to get a job working in the music store in the mall. He thinks he would be good at the job because of his extensive knowledge of popular groups and musicians. An additional benefit is that all his friends hang out at the mall.

Physiological

Adolescence is a period characterized by many dramatic physiological changes, some of which are related to the adolescent growth spurt and some to the onset of puberty. Preadolescence, characterized by little physical growth, is followed by a period of rapid growth, indicating the onset of puberty.[42] The growth spurt is triggered by neural and hormonal signals to the hypothalamus, resulting in increased production of and sensitivity to certain hormones. The onset of puberty in boys occurs between $10\frac{1}{2}$ and 16 years, with the average age being $12\frac{1}{2}$ years. The onset for girls occurs between $9\frac{1}{2}$ and 15 years, with the average age being $10\frac{1}{2}$ years. Although boys begin their growth spurt later than girls, they tend to grow more, with boys growing 8.3 inches and girls growing 7.7 inches.[15,27,42]

The onset of puberty is usually associated with the first signs of sexual development. The first visible sign of puberty in girls is breast growth, which begins around age $10\frac{1}{2}$. The average age for menarche is 12.8.[34] The onset of puberty in boys is signified by enlargement of the testes, which occurs between the ages of 10 and $13\frac{1}{2}$ years.[15] These ages are ranges; the age of the onset of puberty is *quite* variable.

Boys who mature earlier than other boys are described more positively by peers, teachers, and themselves. They tend to be the most popular, be better at sports, and begin dating more easily than boys who mature later. Boys who mature later are described as less attractive, more childish, and less masculine.[15,33,39] For girls, the scenario is reversed. Girls who mature the earliest sometimes have a poor body image and low self-esteem. They tend to confide in older adolescents and share their experiences. Girls who mature later are developing at the same age as her male peers and are likely to develop a better self-concept than the girls who mature early.[15,33,39] These differences in rates of development greatly affect adolescents' self-concept and self-esteem. To help ease these transitions, adults can educate adolescents on the following:

- Health and preparation for puberty
- Nutrition

- Issues such as smoking prevention, automobile safety, and contraception
- Developing autonomy and independence[41]

Sensorimotor

The development of gross motor skills in adolescents is directly related to the physical changes that are occurring. Increased muscle mass provides increased dynamic strength, as evidenced by better running, jumping, and throwing skills.[4] Because boys have a greater percentage of muscle mass than girls, their strength increase is greater.[7] In addition, motor coordination stops improving in girls at the age of 15 years but keeps improving in boys beyond this age. Fine motor abilities also tend to differ between the sexes. Girls show greater rates of improvement in hand-eye coordination, but overall they still do not perform as well as boys.[4,38,42]

Cognitive and Language

The development of *formal operational thought* is a hallmark of adolescence.[12] Adolescents have the ability to think about possibilities as well as realities. They can formulate hypotheses about the outcome of a certain situation, and after imagining all the possible results they can test each hypothesis to determine which one is true.[15] This process is called *hypothetico-deductive reasoning*.

Adolescents develop their moral thought in the period known as the *conventional level* of Kohlberg's stages. During this stage, adolescents approach moral problems in the context of being members of society; they want to please others by being good members of society. Adolescents follow the standards of others, conform to social conventions, support the status quo, and generally try to please others and obey the law.[33]

In high school, adolescents manipulate language; for example, they use codes, slang, and sarcasm. The use of slang during adolescence is important for establishing group membership and being accepted by peers. Adolescents also have the cognitive ability to use language for more than simple communication. For example, they can participate in debates or class discussions and argue for a position that they do not agree with; this abstract use of language is not understood by children at younger ages.[7]

Psychosocial

Egocentrism

Adolescents tend to believe that if something is of great concern to them, then it is also of great concern to others. Because adolescents believe that others have the thoughts similar to their own, they tend to be self-conscious, or *egocentric*. This egocentrism manifests itself in adolescents as an *imaginary audience*, or a perception that everyone is watching them. Another way egocentrism manifests itself in adolescents is through the *personal fable*, or the idea that they are special, have completely unique experiences, and are not subject to the natural rules governing the rest of the world. Egocentrism is the cause of much of the self-destructive behavior shown by adolescents who think that they are magically protected from harm.[33]

Identity

Erikson referred to adolescence as the *identify versus identity confusion* stage of development. The main goal during this stage is for adolescents to find or understand their identity. They work to form a new sense of self by combining past experiences with future expectations. This process allows adolescents to understand themselves in terms of who they have been and who they hope to become.[17]

The establishment of an occupational identity is a portion of the establishment of ego identity. A number of theories about occupational development exist. Ginzberg[21] outlined three periods that apply to this stage: a fantasy period, a tentative period, and a realistic period. Two of Super's[40] stages also apply to adolescents: the growth stage and the exploration stage. Adolescents explore various occupations, identify with workers in a specific occupation, discover which occupations they enjoy, and develop basic habits of working and an identity as a worker.

Peers

Peer groups support adolescents as they transition from childhood into adulthood.[12] Involvement in peer groups provides opportunities for adolescents to accomplish the following:

* Share responsibilities for their own affairs
* Experiment with new ways of handling new situations
* Learn from each other's mistakes
* Try out new roles[27]

Early adolescence (ages 12 to 14 years) is the time when children are most concerned with conforming to the values and practices of their peer group. Older adolescents are less likely to conform to a group and more likely to rely on their own independent thinking and judgment.[27]

Parents

Even though adolescents spend more time with friends, the parents still have considerable effects on them. Although adolescents seek the advice of peers on matters such as social activities, dress, and hobbies, they seek the advice of their parents on issues such as occupations, college, and money.[37]

SUMMARY

From birth through adolescence, infants and children progress through a series of stages of development. The sequences of physiological, sensorimotor, cognitive and language, and psychosocial development outlined in this chapter are typical; however, it should be noted that each individual child progresses through these sequences at a different rate. The occupational therapy practitioner should consider any physical, social, and cultural factors in the environment that may affect a client's development sequence.

References

1. Alexander R, Boehme R, Cupps B: *Normal development of functional motor skills*, Tucson, 1993, Therapy Skill Builders.
2. American Occupational Therapy Association: Uniform terminology for occupational therapy, *Am J Occup Ther* 48:1047, 1994.
3. Anisworth M: Attachment retrospect and prospect. In Parkes CM, Stevenson-Hind M, editors: *The place of attachment in human behavior*, New York, 1982, Basic Books.
4. Ausubel DP, Montemayor R, Pergrouhi S: *Theories and problems of adolescent development*, ed 2, New York, 1977, Grune & Stratton.
5. Bax M, Hart H, Jenkins SM: *Child development and child health: the preschool years*, Oxford, 1990, Blackwell Scientific.
6. Benbow M: *Neurokinesthetic approach to hand function and handwriting*, Albuquerque, 1995, Clinician's View.
7. Berger K: *The developing person through childhood and adolescence*, ed 2, New York, 1986, Worth.
8. Bly L: *Motor skills acquisition in the first year: an illustrated guide to normal development*, Tucson, 1994, Therapy Skill Builders.
9. Brazelton TB: *Neonatal behavioral assessment scale*, ed 2, Philadelphia, 1984, Lippincott.
10. Caplan F: *The first twelve months of life*, New York, 1973, Putnam.
11. Caplan T, Caplan F: *The early childhood years: the 2 to 6 year old*, New York, 1983, Putnam.
12. Case-Smith J, Shortridge SD: The developmental process: prenatal to adolescence. In Case-Smith J, Allen J, Pratt PN editors: *Occupational therapy for children*, ed 3, St Louis, 1996, Mosby.
13. Clark GF: Oral-motor and feeding issues. In Royeen CB, editor: *AOTA self study series: classroom applications for school-based practice*, Rockville, Md, 1993, American Occupational Therapy Association.
14. Dacey JS, Travers JF: *Human development across the lifespan*, Dubuque, 1996, Brown & Benchmark.
15. Dusek JB: *Adolescent development and behavior*, ed 2, Englewood Cliffs, NJ, 1991, Prentice Hall.
16. Erhardt RP: *Developmental hand dysfunction: theory, assessment, and treatment*, ed 2, Tucson, 1994, Therapy Skill Builders.
17. Erikson EH: *Childhood and society*, ed 2, New York, 1963, WW Norton.
18. Fiorentino MR: *Reflex testing methods for evaluating CNS development*, ed 2, Springfield, Ill, 1981, Charles C Thomas.

19. Fraiberg SH: *The magic years: understanding and handling the problems of early childhood*, New York, 1959, Scribner.
20. Freiberg KL: *Human development*, Massachusetts, 1979, Duxburg.
21. Ginzberg E: Toward a theory of occupational choice: a restatement, *Voc Guide Quart* 20:169, 1972.
22. Greenspan S: *Playground politics: understanding the emotional life of your school-aged child*, Reading, Mass, 1993, Addison-Wesley.
23. Greenspan S, Greenspan N: *First feelings: milestones in the emotional development of your baby and child*, New York, 1985, Viking Penguin.
24. Grunwald L: The amazing minds of infants. In Junn EN, Boyatzis CJ, editors: *Annual editions: child growth and development*, Guilford, Conn, 1995, Dushkin.
25. Haywood KM: *Life span motor development*, Champaign, Ill, 1986, Human Kinetics.
26. Hetherington EM, Parke RD: *Child psychology: a contemporary viewpoint*, New York, 1993, McGraw-Hill.
27. Kimmel DC, Weiner IB: *Adolescence: a developmental transition*, New York, 1995, John Wiley & Sons.
28. Lamb ME, Bornstein M: *Development in infancy: an introduction*, ed 2, New York, 1987, Random House.
29. Leach P: *Your baby and child*, New York, 1994, Knopf.
30. Lief NR, Fahs ME, Thomas RM: *The first three years of life*, New York, 1991, Smithmark.
31. Maier HW: *Three theories of child development*, revised ed, New York, 1965, Harper & Row.
32. Minuchin P: *The middle years of childhood*, Pacific Grove, Calif, 1977, Brooks/Cole.
33. Papaplia DE, Olds SW: *Human development*, ed 2, New York, 1992, McGraw-Hill.
34. Payne VG, Isaacs LD: *Human motor development: a lifespan approach*, ed 2, London, 1991, Mayfield.
35. Pratt PN et al: Principles and techniques of occupational therapy assessment in pediatrics. In Pratt PN, Allen, AS, editors: *Occupational therapy for children*, ed 2, St Louis, 1989, Mosby.
36. Santrock JW: *Life span development*, ed 5, Dubuque, 1995, Brown.
37. Sigelman CK, Shaffer DR: *Life span human development*, ed 2, Pacific Grove, Calif, 1995, Brooks/Cole.
38. Simon CJ, Daub MM: Human development across the life span. In Hopkins JL, Smith HD, editors: *Willard and Spackman's occupational therapy*, ed 8, Philadelphia, 1993, Lippincott.
39. Steinberg L: *Adolescence*, ed 4, New York, 1996, McGraw-Hill.
40. Super DE: *The psychology of careers*, New York, 1957, Harper & Row.
41. Vaughan VC, Litt IF: *Child and adolescent development: clinical implications*, Philadelphia, 1990, WB Saunders.
42. Watson RI, Lindgren HC: *Psychology of the child and the adolescent*, ed 4, New York, 1979, Macmillan.

Recommended Reading

Alexander R, Boehme R, Cupps B: *Normal development of functional motor skills*, Tucson, 1993, Therapy Skill Builders.

Greenspan S: *Playground politics: understanding the emotional life of your school-aged child*, Reading, Mass, 1993, Addison-Wesley.

Greenspan S, Greenspan N: *First feelings: milestones in the emotional development of your baby and child*, New York, 1985, Viking Penguin.

REVIEW *Questions*

1. What are primitive reflexes, righting reactions, equilibrium reactions, and protective extension?
2. Briefly describe the gross motor skills and fine motor skills of children at the following ages: 1 month, 6 months, 12 months, and 18 months.
3. What are the four stages of Piaget's stages of cognitive development? Give an example of a behavior that might be observed during each stage of cognitive development.

4. Why is Greenspan's stage for 2 to 7 month olds called *falling in love?* Why is Greenspan's stage for 5 to 7 year olds called *the world is my oyster?*
5. What are Erikson's five stages of development? Briefly describe each.

SUGGESTED *Activities*

1. Visit a nursery or child-care center that serves infants and toddlers. What postural reactions do you observe? Which can you elicit while playing with the infants?
2. Go to a nearby playground and watch normal children at play. Using the American Occupational Therapy Association's (AOTA's) "Uniform Terminology for Occupational Therapy"[2] as a guide, record your observations.

3. Develop a chart like the one that follows to summarize development throughout childhood:

	NEWBORN	I YEAR	4 YEARS	I0 YEARS	I5 YEARS
PHYSIOLOGICAL					
SENSORIMOTOR: GROSS MOTOR					
SENSORIMOTOR: FINE MOTOR					
COGNITIVE AND LANGUAGE					
PSYCHOSOCIAL					

7

Development of Occupational Performance Areas

JANE CLIFFORD O'BRIEN

DIANNE KOONTZ LOWMAN

JEAN W. SOLOMON

CHAPTER *Objectives*

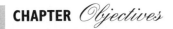

After studying this chapter, the reader will be able to accomplish the following:

- Describe the developmental sequence of oral motor control
- Identify the sequences of feeding and eating, dressing and undressing, and grooming and hygiene development
- Identify the types of food and utensils that are appropriate for infants and young children of different ages
- Identify the variables affecting a child's development of self-care skills
- Define *play* and *leisure skills*
- Describe the progression of play skills
- Explain the relevance of play to occupational therapy practice
- Identify occupational therapy professionals who have made significant contributions to the study of play
- Describe developmentally appropriate activities considered as work or productive in the context of "Uniform Terminology for Occupational Therapy"
- Explain the difference between formal and informal educational activities
- Describe age-appropriate home management activities
- Discuss care of others as it relates to humans and animals or pets
- Identify age-appropriate vocational activities

| KEY TERMS | CHAPTER OUTLINE |

Performance area

Activities of daily living

Eating

Feeding

Oral motor development

Dressing and undressing

Toilet hygiene

Grooming

Bathing and showering

Oral hygiene

Play

Leisure activities

Educational activities

Home management activities

Care of others

Vocational activities

Readiness skills

Activities of Daily Living

DEFINITION AND RATIONALE

FEEDING AND EATING SKILLS

Oral Motor Development

Infancy

Early Childhood

DRESSING AND UNDRESSING SKILLS

Infancy

Early Childhood

GROOMING AND HYGIENE

Toileting

Grooming

Bathing and Showering

Oral Hygiene

SUMMARY

Play and Leisure Activities

DEFINITION OF PLAY

OCCUPATIONAL THERAPY THEORISTS AND THEIR CONTRIBUTIONS TO PLAY

Reilly

Takata

Knox

Bundy

PLAY SKILL ACQUISITION

Infancy

Early Childhood

Middle Childhood

Adolescence

DEVELOPMENTAL RELEVANCE OF PLAY AND LEISURE

SUMMARY

Work and Productive Activities

EDUCATIONAL ACTIVITIES

HOME MANAGEMENT ACTIVITIES

CARE OF OTHERS

VOCATIONAL ACTIVITIES

READINESS SKILLS

Preschool Readiness Skills

Kindergarten Readiness Skills

Elementary School Readiness Skills

Middle Childhood and Adolescent Readiness Skills

Home Management and Care of Others Readiness Skills

Vocational Readiness Skills

SUMMARY

Chapter Summary

Occupational therapy practitioners focus on improving a child's ability to perform daily living, play and leisure, and work and productive activities. These activities occur in environmental, social, cultural, and temporal contexts. The occupational therapy practitioner evaluates a child's ability to perform in these areas by examining the performance components of each area. Knowledge of each **performance area** is therefore important to pediatric occupational therapy practice. This chapter provides a description of the performance areas within the framework of normal development.

Activities of Daily Living

DIANNE KOONTZ LOWMAN

DEFINITION AND RATIONALE

Activities of daily living (ADLs) are one of the three performance areas described in AOTA's "Uniform Terminology for Occupational Therapy."[2] The ADLs listed in Box 7-1 are the most basic tasks that children learn as they grow and mature.[35] Basic self-care skills include feeding and eating, dressing and undressing, and grooming and hygiene.[2] Because eating is a critical daily living skill essential to the child's survival, growth, health, and well-being, it falls within the occupational therapy practitioner's domain of concern.[3] A child with sufficient **eating** skills is able to actively bring food to the mouth without assistance. A child who requires **feeding** must receive assistance in the activity of eating.[3] Oral motor control relates to the child's ability to use the lips, cheeks, jaw, tongue, and palate.[37] **Oral motor development** refers to feeding, sound play, and oral exploration.[29] Feeding is an oral motor skill, but some oral motor skills, such as oral motor awareness and exploration, do not involve food at all.[14]

The normal development of oral motor skills related to eating and feeding involves the development of sucking from a nipple, coordinating the suck-swallow-breathe sequence, drinking from a cup, and munching and chewing solid foods.[12,25,26] Maturation of these skills is closely tied to the physical maturation of the infant.

FEEDING AND EATING SKILLS
Oral Motor Development

Anatomically the infant's oral mechanisms differ from those of the adult; the oral cavity of the infant appears to be filled by the tongue. The small oral cavity, coupled with sucking fat pads that stabilize the infant's cheeks, allows the infant to compress and suck on a nipple placed in the mouth. The limited mobility of the tongue results in the back and forth movement of the tongue known as *suckling*.[25,29,30] As the size ratios in the mouth change with the infant's growth, a more mature oral motor pattern emerges. By 4 to 6 months of age the area inside the infant's mouth increases as the jaw grows and the sucking fat pads decrease. These changes allow increased movement of the infant's cheeks and lips. A "true sucking" pattern develops as the infant's tongue can move up and down as well as forward and backward. Increased control of the jaw, lips, cheeks, and tongue allows the infant to move food and liquid toward the back of the mouth and prepares the infant to accept and control strained baby food.[29,31]

The full-term infant is born with reflexes that allow the infant to locate the source of food, suck, and then swallow. The infant's reflexes in relation to oral motor development follow[31]:

- *Rooting reflex:* When the infant's cheek or lips are stroked, the infant turns toward the stimulus. This reflex allows the infant to search for food and is maintained for a longer period in breast-fed infants.
- *Suck-swallow reflex:* When the infant's lips are touched, the infant's mouth opens and sucking movements begin.
- *Gag reflex:* The gag reflex protects the infant from swallowing anything that may block the airway.[29] At birth the gag reflex is highly sensitive and elicited by stimulation to the back three-fourths of the tongue. This reflex gradually moves to the back one-fourth of the tongue as the infant matures and engages in oral play.
- *Phasic bite-release reflex:* When the infant's gums are stimulated, the infant responds with a rhythmic up-

---

BOX 7-1

Activities of Daily Living

1. Grooming
2. Oral hygiene
3. Bathing and showering
4. Toilet hygiene
5. Personal device care
6. Dressing
7. Feeding and eating
8. Medication routine
9. Health maintenance
10. Socialization
11. Functional communication
12. Functional mobility
13. Community mobility
14. Emergency response
15. Sexual expression

From American Occupational Therapy Association: Uniform terminology for occupational therapy, *Am J Occup Ther* 48(11), 1994.

and-down movement of the jaw. This reflex forms the basis of munching and chewing.

- *Grasp reflex:* When a finger is pressed into the infant's palm, the infant grasps the finger. As the infant sucks, the grasp tightens, indicating a connection between sucking and the grasp reflex. Most of these early reflexive patterns begin to change or disappear between 4 and 6 months when cortical development occurs.[29,31]

Infancy

Oral skills develop concurrently and are closely related to the overall development of sensorimotor skills. Table 7-1 presents a brief overview of normal sensorimotor, oral motor, and feeding development during the first 3 years of life. Feeding initially requires that the adult provide head support and head-trunk alignment to allow the infant to coordinate the suck-swallow-breathe sequence. The infant's first suckling pattern predominates for the first 3 to 4 months of life.[12] Beginning at 4 months a "true sucking" pattern—an up-and-down tongue movement—develops as head and jaw stability appears.

At 6 months the infant has complete head control and more jaw stability allowing for better control of tongue movements. This stability allows the infant to effectively suck from a bottle and remove soft foods from a spoon.[25] At 4 to 5 months the infant demonstrates a reflexive phasic bite-release pattern when presented with a soft cracker. With practice, rhythm progresses into a munching pattern involving an up-and-down jaw movement. The munching pattern is effective with baby foods or other dissolv-

able foods.[12,25] By 7 to 8 months, some diagonal jaw movements are added to the munching pattern. Infants use their fingers to eat soft crackers and cookies.[12,25]

Around 12 months, infants enjoy and prefer eating with their fingers. Rotary chewing movements and a well-graded bite are observed. At this time, many infants transition from the bottle to the cup. While learning to drink from a cup, the infant's jaw initially continues to move in the up-and-down sucking pattern. In addition the infant bites the rim of the cup to stabilize the jaw. By 15 months the infant demonstrates some diagonal rotary movements of the tongue and jaw while chewing food. Between 15 and 18 months the infant begins to independently eat with a spoon.[12]

Early Childhood

By 24 months of age the foundation has been established for all adult eating patterns.[28] At age 2, children eat independently and eat most meats and raw vegetables (Figure 7-1). Circular rotary chewing develops between the second and third year of life and allows toddlers to eat almost all adult foods.[25,31]

By 24 months, children can hold a spoon and bring it to the mouth with the wrist supinated into the palm-up position.[29] At 30 to 36 months, children experiment with forks to stab at food. A variety of spoons are available for children learning to use utensils.[22] The size of the spoon's bowl spoon should match the size of the child's mouth. Children learning to use spoons typically use ones with shallow bowls; children must work harder

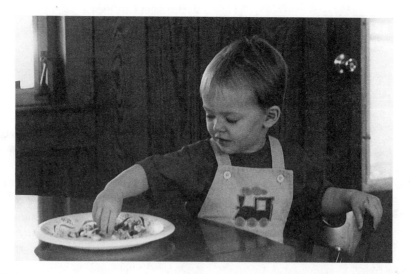

FIGURE 7-1 At age 2, children are able to sit up at the table, feed themselves, and eat almost all adult foods.

TABLE 7-1

Normal Development of Sensorimotor, Oral-Motor, and Feeding Skills

AGE	SENSORIMOTOR SKILLS	ORAL-MOTOR SKILLS	FEEDING SKILLS
BIRTH/ 37-40 WK GESTATION	Is dominated by physiological flexion Moves total body into extension or flexion Turns head side to side in prone position (a protective response) Keeps head mostly on side in supine position Tend to keep hands fisted and flexed across chest during feeding Has strong grasp reflex	Possesses strong gag reflex Possesses rooting reflex Possesses autonomic phasic bite-release pattern Sucks and suckles when hand or object comes into contact with mouth Shows minimal drooling in supine position and increased drooling in other positions	Begins bottle or breast feeding with total sucking pattern Uses mixture of suckling and sucking on bottle (dependent on head position) Possesses incomplete lip closure Is unable to release nipple
1-2 MO	Appears hypotonic as physiological flexion diminishes Practices extension and flexion Continues to gain control of head Moves elbows forward toward shoulders in prone position Possesses ATNR with head to side in supine position Experiences weakening grasp reflex Does not possess voluntary release skills	Continues to show strong gag reflex Continues to show rooting reflex Continues to show automatic phasic bite-release pattern Continues to suck and suckle when hand or object comes in contact with mouth Drools more as jaw and tongue move in wider excursions	May lose coordination of sucking-swallowing-breathing pattern with increased head movements Opens mouth and waits for food Possesses better lip closure Uses active lip movement when sucking
3-5 MO	Experiences diminishing ATNR and grasp reflex Possesses more balance between extension and flexion Has good head control (centered and upright) Brings hands to mouth constantly Supports on extended arms and props on forearms in prone position Brings hand to feet and feet to mouth in supine position Props on arms with little support in sitting position Develops tactile awareness in hands Reaches more accurately; usually with both hands Begins transfer of objects from hand to hand Does not possess controlled release skills; may use mouth to assist	Experiences diminishing rooting reflex and autonomic phasic bite-release pattern Experiences diminishing strong gag reflex at 5 months Drools less in positions with greater postural stability Uses mouth to explore objects Begins to show new oral movements in association with increased head and body control	Anticipates feeding; recognizes bottle and readies mouth for nipple Demonstrates voluntary control of mouth during bottle drinking or breast feeding Loses liquid from lip corners Is able to receive solid food from a spoon at 5 months Uses suckling during spoon feeding; gags on new textures Shows tongue reversal after spoon is removed; ejects food involuntarily

Modified from Alexander R, Boehme R, Cupps B: *Normal development of functional motor skills*, Tucson, 1993, Therapy Skill Builders; Bly L: *Motor skills acquisition in the first year: an illustrated guide to normal development*, Tucson, 1994, Therapy Skill Builders; Case-Smith J, Humphrey R: Feeding and oral motor skills. In Case-Smith J, Allen AS, Pratt PN, editors: *Occupational therapy for children*, ed 2, St Louis, 1995, Mosby; Clark GF: Oral-motor and feeding issues. In Royeen CB, editor: *AOTA self-study series: classroom applications for school-based practice*, Rockville, Md, 1993, American Occupational Therapy Association; Glass RP, Wolf LS: Feeding and oral-motor skills. In Case-Smith J, *Pediatric occupational therapy and early intervention*, Boston, 1993, Andover Medical; Lowman DK, Murphy SM: *The educator's guide to feeding children with disabilities*, Baltimore, 1999, Paul H Brookes; Lowman DK, Lane SJ: Children with feeding and nutritional problems. In Porr S, Rainville, EB, editors: *Pediatric therapy: a systems approach*, Philadelphia, 1999, FA Davis; Morris SE, Klein MD: *Pre-feeding skills: a comprehensive resource for feeding development*, Tucson, 1987, Therapy Skill Builders.
ATNR, Asymmetrical tonic neck reflex.

Continued

TABLE 7-1

Normal Development of Sensorimotor, Oral-Motor, and Feeding Skills—cont'd

AGE	SENSORIMOTOR SKILLS	ORAL-MOTOR SKILLS	FEEDING SKILLS
6 MO	Has total head control Shifts weight and reaches with one hand in prone position Begins shifting weight in quadruped position Transfers objects from hand to hand in supine position Reaches with one hand while supporting with other in sitting position Reaches to be picked up Begins to use thumb in grasp Begins to hold objects in one hand Shows visual interest in small things	No longer has rooting reflex or autonomic phasic bite-release pattern Experiences decrease in strength of gag reflex Maintains lip closure longer in supine, prone, and sitting positions Drools when babbling, reaching, and teething; drools less during feeding	Sucks from bottle or breast with no liquid loss and long sequences of coordinated suck-swallow-breathing Suckles liquid from a cup with liquid loss Coughs and chokes when drinking too much liquid from cup Moves upper lip down to scrape food from spoon and uses suckling with some sucking to move food back Gags on new textures Opens mouth when spoon approaches Uses phasic up-and-down jaw movements, suckling, or sucking when presented with solids Moves tongue laterally when solids placed on side biting surfaces Begins finger feeding Plays with spoon
7-9 MO	Shifts weight and reaches in quadruped position Creeps Develops extension, flexion, and rotation; expands movement options in sitting position May pull to stand and hold on to support Reaches with supination Uses index finger to poke Develops voluntary release skills	Experiences diminishing gag reflex; becomes more similar to an adult protective gag reflex Uses facial expressions to convey likes and dislikes Uses mouth in combination with visual examination and hand manipulation to investigate new objects Bites on fingers and objects to reduce teething discomfort Produces more coordinated jaw, tongue, and lip movements in supine, prone, sitting, and standing positions; rarely drools except when teething	Suckles liquid in cup; loses liquid when cup is removed Takes fewer sucks and suckles before pulling away from cup to breathe Independently holds bottle Feeds self cracker using fingers Holds jaw closed on soft solids to break off pieces Uses variable up-and-down movement while chewing; moves tongue laterally and jaw diagonally when solids placed on biting surfaces Assists with cup and spoon feeding

Modified from Alexander R, Boehme R, Cupps B: *Normal development of functional motor skills*, Tucson, 1993, Therapy Skill Builders; Bly L: *Motor skills acquisition in the first year: an illustrated guide to normal development*, Tucson, 1994, Therapy Skill Builders; Case-Smith J, Humphrey R: Feeding and oral motor skills. In Case-Smith J, Allen AS, Pratt PN, editors: *Occupational therapy for children*, ed 2, St Louis, 1995, Mosby; Clark GF: Oral-motor and feeding issues. In Royeen CB, editor: *AOTA self-study series: classroom applications for school-based practice*, Rockville, Md, 1993, American Occupational Therapy Association; Glass RP, Wolf LS: Feeding and oral-motor skills. In Case-Smith J, *Pediatric occupational therapy and early intervention*, Boston, 1993, Andover Medical; Lowman DK, Murphy SM: *The educator's guide to feeding children with disabilities*, Baltimore, 1999, Paul H Brookes; Lowman DK, Lane SJ: Children with feeding and nutritional problems. In Porr S, Rainville EB, editors: *Pediatric therapy: a systems approach*, Philadelphia, 1999, FA Davis; Morris SE, Klein MD: *Pre-feeding skills: a comprehensive resource for feeding development*, Tucson, 1987, Therapy Skill Builders.

TABLE 7-1

Normal Development of Sensorimotor, Oral-Motor, and Feeding Skills—cont'd

AGE	SENSORIMOTOR SKILLS	ORAL-MOTOR SKILLS	FEEDING SKILLS
10-12 MO	Creeps with good coordination Cruises holding on to support with one hand Stands independently Learns to walk independently Uses superior pincer grasp with finger tip and thumb Smoothly releases large objects	Produces more coordinated jaw, tongue, and lip movements when sitting, standing, and creeping on hands and knees; rarely drools except when teething	Easily closes lips on spoon; uses upper and lower lips to remove food from spoon Uses controlled, sustained biting motion on soft cookies or crackers Chews with mixture of up-and-down and diagonal rotary movements Feeds self independently using fingers Likes to feed self but needs assistance with using spoon; inverts spoon before putting in mouth
13-18 MO	Walks alone Learns to go up and down stairs Has more precise grasp and release	Moves upper and lower lips By 15-18 months, has excellent coordination of sucking, swallowing, and breathing	Uses an up-and-down sucking pattern to obtain liquid from a cup Shows well-coordinated rotary chewing movements by 18 months Has well controlled and sustained biting movements Practices self-feeding; becomes neater Holds cup and puts cup down without spilling liquid
19-24 MO	Demonstrates equilibrium reactions while standing and walking Runs with more narrow base of support	Uses up-and-down tongue movements and tip elevation Develops internal jaw stabilization Swallows with easy lip closure	Efficiently drinks from cup Has well graded and sustained bite
24-36 MO	Jumps in place* Pedals tricycle* Scribbles* Snips with scissors*	Uses tongue humping rather than tongue protrusion to initiate swallow	Possesses circular rotary jaw movements* Closes lips while chewing* Holds cup in one hand* Handles spoon more accurately* Uses fingers to fill spoon* Begins to drink from straws*

*From this point on, skills learned during the first 24 months are further refined.

TABLE 7-2

Developmental Sequence for Self-Care Skills

AGE (YEARS)	DRESSING AND UNDRESSING SKILLS	GROOMING AND HYGIENE
1	Cooperates in dressing (for example, holds foot up for shoe or sock, holds arm out for sleeve) Pushes arms through sleeves and legs through pants	Cooperates during hand washing and drying Has regular bowel movements
1½	Takes off loose clothing (such as mittens, hat, socks, and shoes) Partially pulls shirt over head Unties shoes or takes off hat as an act of undressing Unfastens clothing zippers with large pull tabs Puts on hat	Allows teeth to be brushed Pays attention to acts of eliminating Indicates discomfort from soiled points Begins to sit on potty when placed there and supervised (for a short time)
2	Removes unfastened coat Purposefully removes shoes (if laces are untied) Helps pull down pants Finds armholes in over-the-head shirt	Attempts to brush teeth in imitation of adults Washes own hands with assistance Shows interest in washing self in bathtub Urinates regularly
2½	Removes pull-down pants or shorts with elastic waist Removes simple clothing (such as open shirt or jacket) Assists in putting on socks Puts on front-button type coat or shirt Unbuttons large buttons	Dries hands Wipes nose if given a tissue and prompted to do so Has daytime control of bowel and bladder; experiences occasional accidents Usually indicates need to go to toilet; rarely has bowel accidents
3	Puts on over-the-head shirt with some assistance Puts on shoes without fastening (may be on wrong feet) Puts on socks with some difficulty positioning heel Independently pulls down pants or shorts Zip and unzips coat zipper without separating or inserting zipper Needs assistance to remove over-the-head shirt Buttons large front buttons	Washes own hands Uses toothbrush with assistance Gets drink from fountain or faucet with no assistance Uses toilet independently but needs help wiping after bowel movements

Modified from Case-Smith J: Self-care strategies for children with developmental deficits. In Christiansen C, editor: *Ways of living: self-care strategies for special needs*, Bethesda, 1994, AOTA; Coley IL: *Pediatric assessment of self-care activities*, St Louis, 1978, Mosby; Cook RE, Tessier A, Klein MD: *Adapting early childhood curricula for children in inclusive settings*, Columbus, 1996, Merrill; Johnson-Martin NM, Attermeier SM, Hacke B: *The Carolina curriculum for preschoolers with special needs*, Baltimore, 1990, Paul H Brookes; Johnson-Martin NM et al: *The Carolina curriculum for infants and toddlers with special needs*, ed 2, Baltimore, 1990, Paul H Brookes; Klein MD: *Pre-dressing skills: skill starters for self-help development, revised*. Tucson, 1983, Communication Skill Builders; Orelove, FP, Sobsey, D: *Educating children with multiple disabilities: a transdisciplinary approach*, ed 3, Baltimore, 1996, Paul H Brookes; Shepherd J, Procter SA, Coley IL: Self-care and adaptations for independent living. In Case-Smith J, Allen JA, Pratt PN, editors: *Occupational therapy for children*, ed 2, St Louis, 1996, Mosby.

to eat food from spoons with deeper bowls. Child-size spoons and forks are easier for children to hold and manipulate and bowls and plates with raised edges also are easier for children to scoop against.[22,29]

By 24 months, toddlers also can efficiently drink from cups. Children may begin drinking through straws between 2 and 3 years, especially if they have been exposed early to the use of straws. Given the variety of silly, long, short, and decorated straws available, children are happy to independently use their own straws.[22] By 30 to 36 months, children try to serve themselves liquids and family-style servings of food.[29]

TABLE 7-2

Developmental Sequence for Self-Care Skills—cont'd

AGE (YEARS)	DRESSING AND UNDRESSING SKILLS	GROOMING AND HYGIENE
3½	Usually finds front of clothing Snaps or hooks clothing in front Unzips front zipper on coat or jacket, separating zipper Puts on mittens Buttons series of three or four buttons Unbuckles belt or shoe Puts on boots Dresses with supervision (needs help with front and back)	Pours well from small pitcher Spreads soft butter with knife Seldom has toileting accidents; may need help with difficult clothing
4	Removes pullover garment independently Buckles belt or shoe Zips coat zipper, inserting zipper Puts on pull-down pants or shorts Puts on socks with appropriate heel placement Puts on shoes with assistance in tying laces Consistently knows front and back of clothing	Washes and dries hands and face without assistance Brushes teeth with supervision Washes and dries self after bath with supervision Cares for self at toilet (may need help with wiping after bowel movement)
4½	Puts belt in loops	Runs brush or comb through hair Tears toilet tissue and flushes toilet after use
5	Puts on pullover shirt correctly each time Ties and unties knots Laces shoes Dresses unsupervised	Scrubs fingernails with brush with coaching Brushes and combs hair with supervision Cuts soft foods with knife Blows nose independently when prompted Wipes self after bowel movements
5½	Closes back zipper	Performs toileting activities, including flushing toilet, independently
6	Ties bow knot Ties hood strings Buttons back buttons Snaps back snaps Selects clothing that is appropriate for weather conditions and specific activities	Brushes and rinses teeth independently

DRESSING AND UNDRESSING SKILLS

Dressing and undressing also are essential basic self-care skills learned in infancy and early childhood.[2] *Dressing* includes selecting clothing and accessories appropriate for the weather and occasion, putting clothes on sequentially, and fastening and adjusting clothing and shoes.[2] Young children develop independent dressing skills at various ages according to the family's cultural expectations for self-dressing and the types of clothing worn, opportunities for practice, and the child's motivation for independence.[10] Dressing skills require coordinated movements of almost every body part.[32] Typically the development of independent dressing skills occurs at age 4 to 5 years.[10,20,36] Table 7-2 lists the general sequence of dressing and undressing skills.

Infancy

During the first year of development, the infant is established in the daily routines and begins to cooperate in dressing activities.[16] The infant learns to remove loose-fitting clothing, such as hats, mittens, and socks. By age 1 the infant has achieved many of the motor skills needed for the development of dressing skills. They can separate movements so that the arms or legs can move separately from the trunk, have begun to stabilize with one hand the action of the other, and can adjust their posture during reaching.[21] Infants have the necessary control to push arms and legs through sleeves and pants or play at pulling off a hat.[21]

Early Childhood

By age 2, refined balance and equilibrium reactions provide children with the necessary motor skills to raise their arms to pull shirts over their heads. They can move their hands behind them to attempt to put their arms into the sleeves of a button-front shirt. By 3 years, children are more aware of details and can find arm and leg holes easily. By 4 years, children recognize correct and incorrect sides; as fine motor skills progress they can also use buckles, zippers, and laces. By 5 years, all skills of balance, equilibrium, and fine motor coordination are refined enough to allow children to dress themselves unsupervised.[16,21] Figure 7-2 shows children putting on their boots before going outdoors.

GROOMING AND HYGIENE

Grooming and hygiene are important self-care skills which tend to develop following eating and dressing skills. (See Table 7-2 for the general sequence of grooming and hygiene skills.) The cultural expectations and social routines of the family determine when independence in grooming and hygiene is achieved.[36] **Toilet hygiene** involves clothing management, maintaining toileting position, transferring to and from toileting, and cleaning the body. **Grooming** involves washing, drying, combing, and brushing hair. **Bathing and showering** involves soaping, rinsing, and drying the body. In early childhood, **oral hygiene** involves brushing teeth.[2]

Toileting

Physiologically, voluntary control of urination do not usually occur until between 2 and 3 years of age. Independent toileting is a developmental milestone with wide variation among children. During infancy the infant gradually develops regularity in bowel movement and urination. The infant also may indicate when diapers are wet or soiled and even sit on the toilet when placed. Toilet training typically is not introduced until

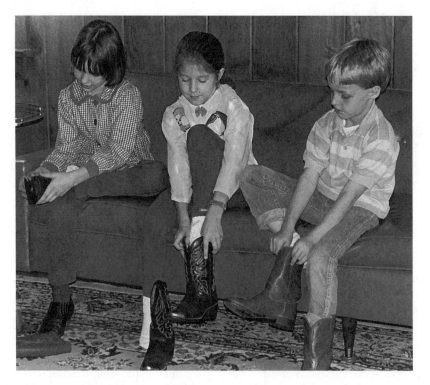

FIGURE 7-2 By age 5, children are able to dress themselves without adult supervision. They show adequate strength, balance, equilibrium, and fine motor coordination.

the child remains dry for 1 or more hours at a time, shows signs of a full bladder or need to toilet, and is at least 2½ years old.[32] Daytime bowel and bladder control is usually attained between 2½ and 3 years, although the child still may need assistance with difficult clothing or fasteners.[16] Nighttime bladder control may not be attained until 5 or 6 years of age. During the day, 5 year olds can anticipate immediate toilet needs and completely care for themselves while toileting, including wiping and flushing the toilet.[16]

Grooming

Face washing, hand washing, and hair care are typical grooming skills learned in early childhood. The infant cooperates in hand washing. By age 2, children can wash their hands but need assistance turning on water and getting soap. By age 4, children wash their hands and face unsupervised. With supervision and coaching, 5 year olds can scrub fingernails with a brush and comb hair.[16]

Bathing and Showering

Around age 2, children begin to show interest in bathing by assisting in washing while in the bathtub. Because bathing is a pleasurable activity for most children and parents, learning to wash self themselves begins in the context of play.[12] Typically, most children are able to wash and dry themselves with supervision by age 4. It is not until age 8 years that most children can independently prepare the bath or shower water, wash, and dry themselves.[36]

Oral Hygiene

Before age 2, infants allow their parents to brush their teeth. Two year olds imitate parents who are brushing their teeth. Children continue to brush their own teeth with supervision until the age of 5 or 6 years.[36] At that time, refinement of skill in the use of tools enables children to independently complete all steps of caring for their teeth, including preparing, brushing, and rinsing teeth.[12]

SUMMARY

The ADLs of feeding and eating, dressing and undressing, and grooming and hygiene are the most basic tasks learned by children as they grow and mature. The specific age at which young children develop independent self-care skills varies according to the family's cultural expectations, opportunities for practice, and the child's motivation for independence. Occupational therapy practitioners are in an excellent position to teach parents and teachers ways to facilitate the development of self-care skills in children.

Play and Leisure Activities

JANE CLIFFORD O'BRIEN

Play is the occupation of childhood. Through play, children learn cognitive, social-emotional, motor, and language skills.[4,5,15,33,35] In adulthood, play often takes the form of **leisure activities,** which are activities that are not associated with time-consuming duties and responsibilities.[2] During play and leisure activities, people refine skills, relax, reflect, and engage in creative activity.

Children must have certain skills to engage in play. Occupational therapy practitioners evaluate the play of children to determine ways to facilitate play and enable children to play at their highest potentials. In this way, occupational therapy practitioners assist children in gaining skills for adulthood.

DEFINITION OF PLAY

Scholars have struggled for centuries to define *play.** Play has been viewed as (1) a method to release surplus energy, (2) a link in the evolutionary change from animal to human being (recapitulation theory), (3) a method to practice survival skills, and (4) an attitude or mood.[27,32] More recent theories have asserted that play provides the stimulation needed to satisfy a physiological need for optimal arousal.[33]

Theorists describe play in terms of the development of cognitive, emotional, social, language, and motor skills.[4,5,15,33,35] These theorists propose that play develops as children learn necessary skills. For example, Piaget proposed that children's play developed from sensorimotor (practice) play to symbolic play to games with rules as the child acquires cognitive skills.[35] Table 7-3

---

*References 6, 7, 13, 15, 18, 19, 33-35.

TABLE 7-3

Piaget's Stages of Play

AGE (YEARS)	STAGE
0-2	**Sensorimotor:** Practices games, exploratory behaviors, reflexive behaviors, repetition
2-6	**Symbolic:** Uses imaginary objects, pretend play
6-10	**Games with rules:** Participates in team sports, activities with flexible rules, goals

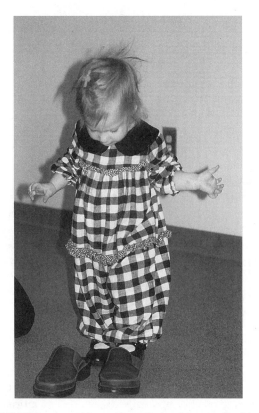

FIGURE 7-3   A toddler enjoys playing "dress-up" with her mother's shoes, a typical activity for an 18 month old.

describes Piaget's stages of play. McCune-Nicolich proposed that children engage in more make-believe play as their language skills develop.[35] See Table 7-4 for a description of the progression of symbolic or make-believe play. Figure 7-3 shows an 18-month-old toddler playing "dress-up" with her mother's shoes. Early theorists such as Erikson and Freud believed that children work out emotional conflicts in play.[35] Psychoanalysts also theorized they could use play to evaluate these conflicts.

Developmental theorists describe the changes in play in terms of motor skill progression.[5,23,33] In doing so, they divide play into the categories of functional (sensorimotor), constructive (manipulative), dramatic (pretend), and games with rules.[33] Parten identified the social aspects of play as progressing from solitary to parallel to group play.[33] Figure 7-4 shows two children engaging in cooperative play.

Play encompasses a variety of skills and occupies much of the child's day. Thus occupational therapy practitioners have a firm understanding of its complexities. AOTA's "Uniform Terminology for Occupational Therapy" defines *play* or *leisure activities* as ". . . intrinsically motivating activities for amusement, relaxation, spontaneous enjoyment or self-expression."[2]

Occupational therapy practitioners view play as a performance area in addition to ADLs and work and productive activities. As such, occupational therapy practitioners work with children to facilitate and remediate

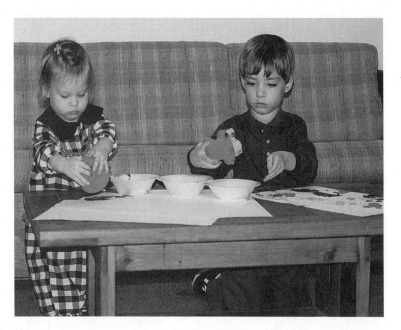

FIGURE 7-4   Children sharing their paints as they create their pictures. They are absorbed in the play process.

TABLE 7-4

Symbolic Play

AGE (MONTHS)	PLAY CHARACTERISTICS
12	Play directed towards self
	Imitation of patty-cake and other movements
	Simple pretend play directed toward self (eating, sleeping)
	Imitation of familiar actions
18-24	Roleplaying with objects (such as feeding a doll)
	Use of nonrealistic objects in pretend
24-36	Engagement in multistep scenarios (such as giving doll a bath, dressing the doll, and putting the doll to bed)
36-48	Use of language in play
	Advance plans and development of stories
	Acting out sequences with miniatures
48	Imaginary play
	Role-playing entire scenarios
	Creation of stories with "pretend" characters

play skills. The following occupational therapy theorists have made significant contributions to the study of play in occupational therapy practice.

OCCUPATIONAL THERAPY THEORISTS AND THEIR CONTRIBUTIONS TO PLAY

Reilly

Mary Reilly, a noted occupational therapist and researcher, described play as a progression through three stages: exploratory behaviors, competency, and achievement.[34] *Exploratory behaviors* are intrinsically motivated behaviors engaged in for their own sake.[34] Infants engage in exploratory behaviors that focus on sensory experiences.[34] The second stage of development, *competency*, occurs when children search for challenges, novelty, and experimentation. Children in this stage often want to do everything alone and "their way."[34] This stage is often present in early and middle childhood. The *achievement* stage of play emphasizes performance standards (such as winning) and competition. Children at this stage of development take more risks in their play.

Takata

Occupational therapist Nancy Takata developed the *Play History* to provide occupational therapy practitioners with a format for obtaining information about a child's play.[34] The interview format helps describe a child's play skills. Occupational therapy practitioners with a solid knowl-

edge of typical play patterns can use this information to design treatment.

Knox

The *Knox Preschool Play Scale* (PPS) was constructed by occupational therapist Susan Knox and is based on the work of Piagetian cognitive stages and Parten's social stages.[33] The Knox PPS divides play into four domains: space management, material management, imitation, and participation. The scale provides age equivalents for each domain and an overall play age. This scale is easy to administer and provides information on the motor skill requirements for play.

Bundy

Professor and occupational therapist Anita Bundy designed the *Test of Playfulness* (ToP) to objectively measure playfulness.[7,8] Bundy found that a child's attitude about and approach to activities (that is, playfulness) provides valuable information to occupational therapy practitioners. Some children who do not possess the skills for play may still be playful. Other children have the skills but do not appear to be having fun.

The ToP examines the context in which children perform play activities.[7,8] For example, two 4-year-old boys playing "Godzilla" may engage in rough-and-tumble "fighting." Because the context of the fighting is play, the children are not being mean-spirited or hurtful. They are clearly playing and not fighting.

TABLE 7-5

Toys and Play Activities for Various Ages

AGE (YEARS)	TOYS AND ACTIVITIES
0-1	**Manipulative, sensory:** rattles, musical sounds, bells, swings, soft toys, boxes, pots and pans, wooden spoons, books,
1-2	**Movement, manipulative, sensory:** push-pull toys, balls, pop-beads, pop-up toys, toy phones, musical books, noisy toys, ride-on toys, trucks, cause and effect toys
2-4	**Pretend play, movement, manipulative, sensory:** dolls, trucks, action figures, playdough, markers, water play, balls, blocks, Legos, books, dress-up toys, hats, shoes, clothes, tricycles
4-6	**Pretend play, craft activities, movement:** swings, gyms, bicycles, scooters, ball games, beads, painting, play dough, arts and crafts, dolls, cooking, group games (for example, follow-the-leader, tag, red rover)
6-8	**Pretend play, craft activities, movement:** gymnastic play, jumping rope, coordinated games (for example, keep-away with ball), arts and crafts, wood kits, model airplanes, painting, drawing, skating, bike riding, swimming
8-10	**Movement, group games, manipulative:** basketball, baseball, soccer, bike riding, skateboarding, tennis, swimming, volleyball, arts and crafts requiring more skill, cooking, collecting
10 and up	**Movement, games that challenge, skilled manipulative resulting in products:** competitive sports, strenuous activities, sewing, knitting, woodworking, bowling, walking, going to the beach, flying kites, boating, camping, reading

PLAY SKILL ACQUISITION

Children acquire play skills as they mature and develop. Play affords opportunities for a child to develop. For example, a child needs balance and coordination to ride a bike. At the same time, riding the bike improves the child's balance and coordination. A variety of play opportunities are important for development. Table 7-5 provides an outline of toys and play activities suitable for different age groups.

Infancy

Infants explore the environment and learn through their senses.[5,24] They enjoy visual, tactile, auditory and movement sensations.[6] Toys with bells and noise encourage infants to explore the environment.[23] Play should focus on enhancing the infant's capabilities while furnishing new opportunities for exploration. Occupational therapy practitioners and caregivers must allow infants to repeat activities until they have mastered them.[5,34] Infant play encourages body awareness. Infants typically explore their hands and feet spontaneously. Playing games such as pat-a-cake help them understand that their bodies are fun as does face-to-face play with an adult.[4,5,14] Peek-a-boo is a favorite game at this age. Enjoyable toys encourage mobility, elicit actions, increase motor skills, and facilitate natural creativity.

Parents and caregivers establish bonds with infants by playing comfortably with them. Adults must respond to the cues of the infant. Cues that indicate stress include crying, hiccups, gaze aversion, yawning, finger splaying, and tantrums.[6,27] If infants cry or show signs of stress, they should be comforted and the type of play should be changed. Occupational therapy practitioners should remember that play is fun.

Early Childhood

Continued exploration and the development of friendships accentuate childhood play.[6,24] Play provides children with opportunities to learn negotiation, problem-solving, and communication skills. Figure 7-5 shows children challenging their skills in play. Play also develops and refines motor skills.[6,15,24] Adults should be cautious about intervening too quickly during play. Children need opportunities to work out differences among themselves.

Children enjoy manipulative play, imitation, games, and social play with other children of the same sex.[6] They enjoy dramatic and rough-and-tumble play.[6,35] Role-playing scenarios that facilitate dramatic play stimulates a child's imagination, creativity, and problem-solving abilities.

Middle Childhood

Middle childhood is a time of refinement of skills, such as speed, dexterity, strength, and endurance. Children become more competent in play activities. They enjoy games with rules and competition. Childhood is a time

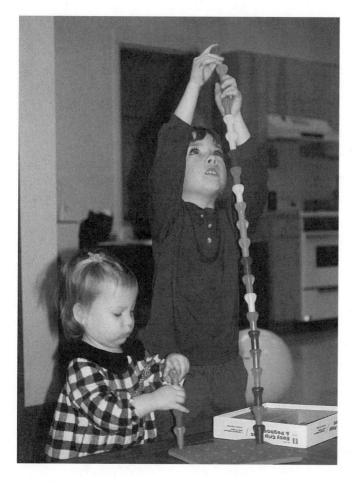

FIGURE 7-5 Children challenge their motor, social, and cognitive skills during play. These children must use their fine motor skills to build a tower.

for children to experiment with many play activities. Some activities are easy whereas other activities are difficult. Children should be encouraged to play, have fun, and realize everyone has different talents. This is all part of growing up and finding their identities.

Adolescence

Adolescents are in search of independence.[6,24] Parents need to facilitate socially appropriate play and leisure activities. Adolescents enjoy activities in which they can participate with peers.[6,24] They may wish to participate in school or community clubs. Practitioners and parents need to listen carefully to adolescents to help them discover their goals and talents. At this stage of development, play is beneficial in the establishment of independence.

DEVELOPMENTAL RELEVANCE OF PLAY AND LEISURE

Play is important in each stage of development. It provides children with opportunities to develop motor, social-emotional, cognitive, and language skills. (The appendix ["Play Analysis Guide"] at the end of this chapter provides a guide to the observation of play.) Play allows children to interact with others, challenge themselves, and learn their strengths and weaknesses; therefore play contributes to quality of life. Play and leisure remain important throughout a person's life. People engage in play or leisure activities because they enjoy them and are motivated intrinsically to participate in them.[9]

SUMMARY

Play and leisure activities are crucial components of child development for the acquisition of skills children will use in adulthood. Play and leisure activities provide the foundation for problem solving, skill development, social interactions, and negotiating.

Occupational therapy practitioners can be key players in teaching parents, teachers, and peers ways to play and be playful with children who have special needs. Occupational therapy practitioners have the skills required to assist children and families in developing play skills so that children may reach their potential.

Work and Productive Activities

JEAN W. SOLOMON

Work and productive activities are one of the three occupational performance areas described in AOTA's "Uniform Terminology for Occupational Therapy." Work and productive activities are purposeful activities for self-development, social contribution, and livelihood.[2] *Work* is defined as any physical or mental activity that is directed toward production or the accomplishment of something.[1] *Productive* is defined as something that yields a useful result.[1] The outcome of work and productive activity results in a product or an accomplishment.

EDUCATIONAL ACTIVITIES

Educational activities are the opportunities that facilitate learning for children and adolescents.[36] Educational activities can be formal or informal. Formal educational activities are structured and may be mandated by public law for specific age groups. These activities are provided in settings such as preschool programs, day-care, public schools, or Sunday school classes. Informal educational activities are less structured and occur in a variety of settings. Examples of informal activities in which younger children engage include playing school with an older sibling or playing a shopping game with peers. Figure 7-6 shows children engaged in "playing school," a typical informal educational activity. Adolescents frequently study together, creating opportunities for informal learning.

HOME MANAGEMENT ACTIVITIES

Home management activities are tasks that are necessary to obtain and maintain personal and household possessions.[2] Temporal and environmental performance contexts significantly influence a child or adolescent's participation in home management tasks. Children's ages and physical, social, and cultural environments determine their roles in this domain. Children and adolescents may have chores that they are expected to complete on a regular schedule. Examples of chores include making the bed, setting the dinner table, and cutting the grass. Some children and adolescents have the incentive of a monetary allowance to complete the assigned chores. Others do not have a monetary incentive but are still expected to assist in the maintenance of their households.

CARE OF OTHERS

Care of others refers to the physical upkeep and nurturing of pets or other human beings.[2] As with household management, care of others is also significantly influenced by performance contexts. In large families, older siblings may be required to assist their parents in the care of younger siblings. A child living on a farm may assist with

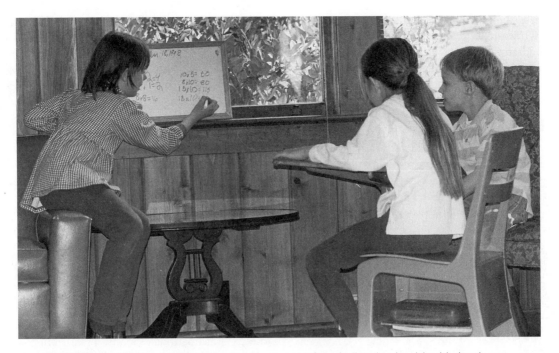

FIGURE 7-6 Children enjoy "playing school," a typical informal educational activity. Notice the students attending to the teacher.

feeding and caring for the farm animals. A child who living in an urban area may walk the family dog several times a day in the park.

VOCATIONAL ACTIVITIES

Vocational activities are work-related activities that typically have a monetary incentive or salary. Like educational activities, vocational activities can be formal or informal. Formal vocational activities are jobs. Public laws determine the age at which a person may hold a job. Informal vocational activities include neighborhood lemonade stands and cutting a neighbor's grass for a fee. Figure 7-7 shows a child "selling" cookies to a friend. Like home management and care of others, vocational activities in which a child or adolescent might participate are significantly influenced by performance contexts for that individual.

READINESS SKILLS

Readiness skills are those performance abilities that are necessary to effectively engage in educational, home management, care of others, and vocational activities. *Readiness* is a stage of preparedness for "what comes next."[17,36] Different readiness skills are necessary for different tasks. Readiness skills must be considered within the temporal and environmental contexts of AOTA's "Uniform Terminology for Occupational Therapy." The chronological age of the child or adolescent directly relates to the necessary readiness skills. For example, different readiness skills are expected of a kindergarten student and a high school student. Social, cultural, and physical environments also influence expectations of readiness.

Readiness skills necessary for successful participation in formal educational activities vary according to performance contexts. This section discusses educational readiness skills for children enrolled in preschool programs, kindergarten, and elementary school.

Preschool Readiness Skills

Children entering preschool programs need certain readiness skills, which include independence in toileting with minimal assistance with fasteners, independence in self-feeding, and cooperative play behavior. Children attending a preschool program also are expected to understand rules and schedules. They need to exhibit the beginning of behavioral and emotional maturity (that is, controlling tempers and mood swings).

Kindergarten Readiness Skills

The child attending kindergarten is expected to have the readiness skills of a typical preschooler with additional preacademic and academic skills. The child must be able to sit quietly while listening to a story and should have adequate fine motor skills for coloring and manipulating

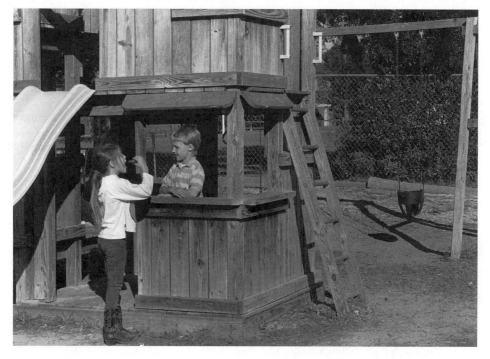

FIGURE 7-7   A young boy sells cookies to his friend, an informal vocational activity.

small objects.[11,17] They must possess gross motor skills such as running, hopping, and jumping, and they are expected to recognize letters and numbers.

Elementary School Readiness Skills

Children attending elementary school are expected to have greater independence and skill in the occupational performance areas and components than younger children. Independence in the bathroom and cafeteria is necessary. In addition to independence in eating, children in elementary school are expected to carry their lunch trays and to assist in cleaning the table at the end of a meal. Children must remain in their classroom chairs for extended periods of time. The ability to remain "on task" and attend to work while seated is termed *in-seat behavior*.

Expectations of reading, writing, spelling, and math skills increase with grade level. The child attending elementary school should have adequate perceptual and motor skills to participate in games and organized sports.

Middle Childhood and Adolescent Readiness Skills

Educational readiness skills for middle childhood and adolescence build on the competencies gained during the preceding periods. Appropriate social skills and manners are expected, and increased skill in creative thinking, problem solving, and the development of ideas is required. Expressive writing is learned during this period. During middle childhood, children and adolescents also begin to seek their independence. They question authority figures but must learn to work with them effectively in educational settings.

Home Management and Care of Others Readiness Skills

Readiness skills also are necessary for successful participation in home management and care of others activities. Specific readiness skills are relative to particular tasks. Activity analysis (breaking an activity into steps) can determine the readiness skills needed to perform a specific task. For example, making a bed requires the coordination of the two sides of the body, sequencing skills, and a pad-to-pad pinch. Setting the dinner table requires sequencing, balance, and dexterity while carrying and placing plates and silverware. The different readiness skills necessary to care for others can be illustrated by comparing the requirements for caring for a pet and baby-sitting a sibling. These two tasks obviously require different abilities. (See Chapters 12 and 13 for additional information on activity analysis.)

Vocational Readiness Skills

Readiness skills for formal and informal vocational activities are as varied as those required for home management and care for others. They also depend greatly on performance contexts. To successfully engage in formal vocational activities, skills such as promptness, appropriate dress, and effective communication with peers and supervisors are important. Activity analysis is beneficial when considering appropriate formal and informal vocational activities.

SUMMARY

Work and productive activities are one of the three performance areas described in AOTA's "Uniform Terminology for Occupational Therapy." Activities include educational, home management, care of others, and vocational activities. Readiness skills also develop during childhood and can differ according to each child's age and the task being performed. Although all children and adolescents participate in educational tasks, great variability exists in the ways they participate in home management activities, care for others, and participate in vocational activities.

Chapter Summary

Occupational therapy practitioners should have a firm knowledge of the occupational performance areas of daily living, play and leisure, and work and productive activities to effectively work with children and their families. Occupational therapy practitioners also should use knowledge of performance contexts in which the activity occurs because these contexts can influence the activity and the success of the child. Finally, the ability to analyze each of the performance areas through activity analysis is essential while working with children and adolescents.

References

1. *American Heritage Dictionary*, ed 3, New York, 1996, Houghton Mifflin.
2. American Occupational Therapy Association: Uniform terminology for occupational therapy, *Am J Occup Ther* 48(11):1047, 1994.
3. Avery-Smith W: Eating dysfunction positions paper, *Am J Occup Ther* 50(10):846, 1996.
4. Axline VM: Play therapy procedures and results. In Schaefer C, editor: *The therapeutic use of play*, New York, 1976, Jason Aronson.
5. Bantz DL, Siktberg L: Teaching families to evaluate age-appropriate toys, *J Pediatr Health Care* 7(3):111, 1993.
6. Berger KS: *The developing person through the lifespan*, ed 3, New York, 1994, Worth.
7. Bundy AC: Assessment of play and leisure: delineation of the problem, *Am J Occup Ther* 47:217, 1993.

8. Bundy AC: Play and playfulness: What to look for. In Parham LD, Fazio LS, editors: *Play in occupational therapy for children*, St Louis, 1997, Mosby.

9. Bundy AC: Play theory and sensory integration. In Fisher AG, Murray EA, Bundy AC, editors: *Sensory integration: theory and practice*, Philadelphia, 1991, FA Davis.

10. Case-Smith J: Self-care strategies for children with developmental deficits. In Christiansen C, editor: *Ways of living: Self-care strategies for special needs*, Bethesda, Md, 1994, American Occupational Therapy Association.

11. Case-Smith J, Allen JA, Pratt PN, editors: *Occupational therapy for children*, ed 3, St Louis, 1996, Mosby.

12. Case-Smith J, Humphrey R: Feeding and oral motor skills. In Case-Smith J, Allen JA, Pratt PN, editors: *Occupational therapy for children*, ed 3, St Louis, 1996, Mosby.

13. Cass JE: *The significance of children's play*, London, 1971, Batsford.

14. Clark GF: Oral-motor and feeding issues. In Royeen CB, editor: *AOTA self-study series: classroom applications for school-based practice*, Rockville, Md, 1993, American Occupational Therapy Association.

15. Cohen D: *The development of play*, New York, 1987, New York University Press.

16. Coley IL: *Pediatric assessment of self-care activities*, St Louis, 1978, Mosby.

17. ERIC Clearinghouse on Elementary and Early Childhood Education, University of Illinois at Urbana-Champaign, Children's Research Center. http://www.npin.org/respar/tests/learning/kinrea.htm/.

18. Florey L: Development through play. In Schaefer C, editor: *The therapeutic use of play*, New York, 1976, Jason Aronson.

19. Greenstein DB: It's child's play. In Galvin J, Sherer M, editors: *Evaluating, selecting, and using appropriate assistive technology*, Gaithersburg, Md, 1996, Aspen.

20. Johnson-Martin NM et al: *The Carolina curriculum for infants and toddlers with special needs*, ed 2, Baltimore, 1990, Paul H Brookes.

21. Klein MD: *Pre-dressing skills: skill starters for self-help development*, rev ed, Tucson, 1983, Communication Skills Builders.

22. Klein MD, Delaney TA: *Feeding and nutrition for the child with special needs: handouts for parents*, Tucson, 1994, Therapy Skill Builders.

23. Linder TW, editor: *Transdiscipinary play based assessment*, Baltimore, 1990, Paul H Brookes.

24. Llorens LA: *Application of a developmental theory for health and rehabilitation*, Rockville, Md, 1976, American Occupational Therapy Association.

25. Lowman DK, Lane SJ: Children with feeding and nutritional problems. In Porr S, Rainville EB, editors: *Pediatric therapy: a systems approach*, Philadelphia, 1999, FA Davis.

26. Lowman DK, Murphy SM: *The educator's guide to feeding children with disabilities*, Baltimore, 1999, Paul H Brookes.

27. Marfo K, editor: *Parent-child interaction and developmental disabilities*, New York, 1988, Praeger.

28. Millar S: *The psychology of play*, New York, 1974, Aronson.

29. Morris SE, Klein MD: *Pre-feeding skills: a comprehensive resource for feeding development*, Tucson, 1987, Therapy Skill Builders.

30. Murphy SM, Caretto C: Anatomy of the oral and respiratory structures made easy. In Lowman DK, Murphy SM, editors: *The educator's guide to feeding children with disabilities*, Baltimore, 1999, Paul H Brookes.

31. Murphy SM, Caretto C: Oral-motor considerations for feeding. In Lowman DK, Murphy SM, editors: *The educator's guide to feeding children with disabilities*, Baltimore, 1999, Paul H Brookes.

32. Orelove FP, Sobsey D: *Educating children with multiple disabilities: a transdisciplinary approach*, ed 3, Baltimore, 1996, Paul H Brookes.

33. Parham LD, Primeau L: Play and occupational therapy. In Parham LD, Fazio LS, editors: *Play in occupational therapy for children*, St Louis, 1997, Mosby.

34. Reilly M, editor: *Play as exploratory learning: studies in curiosity behavior*, Beverly Hills, 1974, Sage.

35. Rubin K, Fein GG, Vandenberg B: Play. In Mussen PH, editor: *Handbook of child psychology*, ed 4, New York, 1983, Wiley.

36. Shepherd J, Procter SA, Coley IL: Self-care and adaptations for independent living. In Case-Smith J, Allen JA, Pratt PN, editors: *Occupational therapy for children*, ed 2, St Louis, 1996, Mosby.

37. Wolf LS, Glass RP: *Feeding and swallowing disorders in infancy: assessment and management*, Tucson, 1992, Therapy Skill Builders.

REVIEW *Questions*

1. Describe the developmental sequence of oral motor control, feeding, and eating skills.
2. Which foods and utensils are appropriate for children at various ages?
3. List the developmental sequences of dressing and undressing, toilet hygiene, grooming, bathing and showering, and oral hygiene.
4. Provide examples describing the progression of play skills.
5. Which terms describe play?
6. Describe the contributions of Reilly, Takata, Knox, and Bundy to the study of play in occupational therapy.
7. What is the difference between formal and informal work and productive activities? Give an example of each.
8. List the readiness skills expected for a child entering kindergarten. Why are these skills important?

SUGGESTED *Activities*

1. In a small group, list and discuss examples of how different cultural expectations might affect the development of self-care skills.
2. Visit a local child-care center.
   a. Observe preschool children of different ages eating lunch. What similarities and differences do you notice?
   b. Note all the different ways you see children putting on their coats.
   c. Visit the 2-year-old class. How many children are in diapers? How many are toilet trained?
3. Participate in play with an infant, child, and adolescent. Describe the way their play differed.
4. Watch a child playing for 15 minutes. Describe the way Reilly, Knox, Takata, and Bundy would describe the child's play.
5. Describe your favorite play activities as a child, adolescent, and adult. Record the setting, materials, group members, and feelings. Share your activities with classmates. How are the activities the same? Different?
6. In a small group, discuss your recollection of your formal education. In what ways do your stories differ and at what age?
7. Make a log of the home management, care of others, and vocational activities that you remember engaging in as a child and adolescent. Compare logs with classmates.

CHAPTER 7 APPENDIX

Play Analysis Guide

NAME OF CHILD: DATE OF EVALUATION:

DATE OF BIRTH:

CHILD'S AGE:

   I. **Describe the physical setting.**
      Who was present?
  II. **Describe the activities performed by the child.**
     A. *Gross Motor*
        Balance:
        Coordination:
        Motor Planning:
        Sequencing:
        Endurance:
        Mobility:
        Quality of Movement:
        Overall Skill:
     B. *Fine Motor*
        Manipulation of Objects:
        Grip:
        Strength:
        Overall Effectiveness:
     C. *Social*
        Participation:
        Negotiating:
        Peer Interactions:
        Sharing:
     D. *Imitative*
        Creativity:
        Novelty:
        Use of Toys:
     E. *Language*
        Expression:
        Communication:
        Imagination:
     F. *Attitude*
        Approach:
        Affect:
        Spontaneity:
        Teasing:
        Mischief:
 III. **Describe the adult supervision. Did it facilitate or inhibit play?**
 IV. **Other**

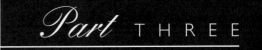

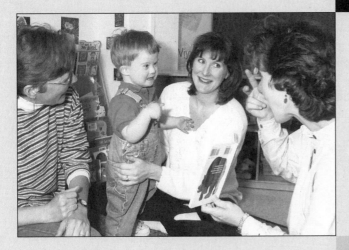

Pediatric Disorders

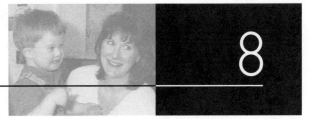

Cerebral Palsy

JOYCE A. WANDEL

After studying this chapter, the reader will be able to accomplish the following:

- Describe the various types of movement disorders labeled *cerebral palsy*
- Identify and describe the impaired components of normal postural control and movement in children with cerebral palsy
- Explain the ways normal and impaired muscle tone influence human movement abilities
- Recognize the differences among motor development, motor learning, and motor control
- Identify the certified occupational therapy assistant's role in the assessment, treatment, and management of individuals with cerebral palsy
- Identify team members involved in the provision of services to children with cerebral palsy

KEY TERMS | CHAPTER OUTLINE

DEFINITION, DESCRIPTION, AND INCIDENCE

Jeremy, a 12-year-old boy, acquired **cerebral palsy** *at birth when the placenta that connected him to his mother's uterine wall became prematurely dislodged during his delivery. He was without sufficient oxygen for several minutes. As a result of this anoxia (lack of oxygen), Jeremy experienced damage to the parts of his brain that control movement. Jeremy developed cerebral palsy affecting all of the muscles in his body, including those that he uses for eating, breathing, and focusing his vision. At age 12, Jeremy has yet to learn to stand or walk independently. He relies on others to assist him with all activities of daily living (ADLs) and attends a school that can accommodate students with physical handicaps. For mobility, Jeremy uses an electric wheelchair that he controls through a switch he activates by tilting his head. Because he cannot easily coordinate his speaking and breathing muscles, his speech is very difficult to understand. Jeremy is now learning to use switches to operate a computer for communication and school work.*

Origin

Cerebral palsy, first described by English physician William Little in 1843,[4] is a general term used to describe a variety of postural control and movement disorders that result from a lesion or damage to one or more parts of the central nervous system. These lesions occur in areas responsible for controlling the quality and quantity of skilled movement (Box 8-1). Cerebral palsy occurs when sensory, perceptual, and motor areas of the central nervous system cannot accurately relay and integrate essential information that the brain needs to correctly plan and direct the skilled, efficient movements used in everyday interactions with the environment. The lesion or damage causes impairment in muscle activity in part or all of the body. The muscles shorten and lengthen in uncoordinated, inefficient ways and are unable to work together to create smooth, effective motion. This type of muscle activity is referred to as *impaired coactivation.*

Progression of Disordered Movement Development

Children with cerebral palsy demonstrate difficulty achieving and maintaining normal postures while lying down, sitting, and standing because of impaired muscle coactivation. They also develop abnormal movement compensations, movements, and body postures that evolve as they try to function within their environments. Over time, such movement compensations create barriers to a child's ongoing motor skill develop-ment. Instead of freely moving and exploring the world, as does the child with a normally developing sensori-motor system, children with cerebral palsy may rely on early automatic reflex movement patterns as their primary means of mobility.

Normally developing infants demonstrate an asymmetrical tonic neck reflex between ages 1 month and 4 months.[11] As infants turn their heads to one side, the upper extremity on that side extends outward. This early automatic behavior lays the groundwork for the child's future independent ability to visually regard the hand and engage in coordinated eye-hand activities (Figure 8-1).

BOX 8-1

Definition of Cerebral Palsy

Cerebral palsy is a disorder of motor functioning caused by a permanent, nonprogressive brain defect or lesion present at or shortly after birth. It causes atypical muscle movements and can affect the muscles controlling breathing, speech, and eye movement.

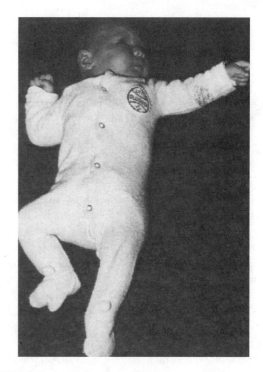

FIGURE 8-1 Normal infant exhibiting asymmetrical tonic neck reflex. (From Case-Smith J, Allen AS, Pratt PN: *Occupational therapy for children,* ed 3, St Louis, 1996, Mosby.)

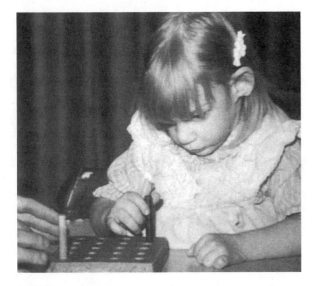

FIGURE 8-2 A child with hemiplegia and spasticity in her left arm and leg. Note the fisting of her left hand as she places the peg into the pegboard with her right hand. (From Case-Smith J, Allen AS, Pratt PN: *Occupational therapy for children,* ed 3, St Louis, 1996, Mosby.)

CLINICAL *Pearl*

In the normally developing infant, automatic reflex movement patterns are never obligatory. Therefore normal infants may not always exhibit the motor responses of the asymmetrical tonic reflexes when their heads are turned to the side.

Children with cerebral palsy continue to rely on this automatic movement pattern because they are unable to direct their muscles to move successfully in other patterns. The pattern becomes repetitive and fixed (Figure 8-2). The repetition of the pattern prevents these children from gaining independent voluntary control of their own movements. The use of **primitive reflex patterns** limits the children's access to participation in meaningful activities. The combination of impaired muscle coactivation and the use of reflexively controlled postures may also lead to future contractures in the muscle, tendon, and ligamentous tissues, causing the tissues to become permanently shortened. Deformities of bones and alterations of typical shape or alignment also may occur.[6]

The nervous system damage that causes cerebral palsy can occur before or during birth or before a child's second year, the time when myelination of the child's sensory and motor tracts and central nervous system structures occurs rapidly.[3] Cerebral palsy is described as nonprogressive, nonhereditary, and noncontagious. As a nonprogressive condition the original defect or lesion occurring in the

BOX 8-2

Risk Factors Associated with the Development of Cerebral Palsy

PRENATAL
- Genetic abnormalities
- Maternal health factors (chronic stress, malnutrition)
- Teratogenic agents (drugs, chemical exposure, radiation)

PERINATAL
- Prenatal conditions (for example, toxemia secondary to maternal diabetes)
- Premature detachment of the placenta
- Medical problems associated with prematurity (for example, compromised respiration, cardiovascular dysfunctions)
- Multiple births

POSTNATAL
- Degenerative disorders (for example, Tay-Sachs disease)
- Infections (for example, meningitis, encephalitis)
- Alcohol or drug intoxication transferred while breastfeeding
- Malnutrition
- Trauma
- Anoxia

central nervous system typically does not worsen or change over time. However, because the lesion has occurred in immature brain structures, the progression of the child's motor development may appear to change. Normal nervous system maturation shifts control of voluntary movement toward increasingly higher and more complex areas of the brain. The child with cerebral palsy exhibits some changes in movement ability that result from the expected progression of motor development skills, but these changes tend to be delayed relative to age and often show much less variety than those seen in the normal child.

Frequency and Causes

Cerebral palsy is diagnosed in 500,000 to 700,000 or 0.05% of Americans, and approximately 1,500 babies are born with cerebral palsy in the United States each year.[9] Unfortunately, the exact cause frequently cannot be determined, but known contributing risk factors may be prenatal, perinatal, or postnatal. Prenatal factors may include genetic abnormalities or maternal health factors such as stress, malnutrition, exposure to damaging drugs, and pregnancy-induced hypertension. Some gestational conditions of the mother, such as diabetes, may cause perinatal risks to the child as well. Perinatally, children born very prematurely with low birth weights demonstrate an increased risk for cerebral palsy. Medical problems associated with premature births may directly or indirectly damage the developing sensorimotor areas of the central nervous system. In particular, respiratory disorders can cause the premature newborn to experience *anoxia,* an acute lack of oxygen needed for cells to function and survive. Typical postnatal, child-centered conditions that may result in significant damage to the developing central nervous system may be malnutrition and anoxia but can also stem from infection, trauma, or exposure to environmental toxins. Research also suggests a link between multiple births and an increased risk for cerebral palsy (Box 8-2).[8,13]

POSTURE, POSTURAL CONTROL, AND MOVEMENT

To understand the functional movement problems that develop in children with cerebral palsy, the occupational therapy practitioner must be familiar with the ways people normally control their bodies and execute skilled movements. The term *posture* describes the alignment of the body's parts in relation to each other and the environment. The ability to develop a large repertoire of postures and change postures easily during an activity depends on the integration of several automatic, involuntary movement actions referred to as the **postural mechanism.** (See Chapter 6 for a more extensive discussion on the components of normal movement.) The normal postural mechanism includes several key components[14]:

- Normal muscle tone
- Normal postural tone
- Developmental integration of early, primitive reflex movement patterns
- Emergence of righting, equilibrium, and protective extension reactions
- Intentional voluntary movements

Disruption in the normal postural mechanism is a key cause for the movement problems that are seen in cerebral palsy.

Righting, Equilibrium, and Protective Reactions

The functions that aid individuals in maintaining or regaining posture are **righting reactions** and **equilibrium reactions,** often referred to as *balance reactions.* These functions can be thought of as static or dynamic. When

people are sitting and not engaged in any activity, they are using static balance. When they bend to pick up an object on the floor, they use dynamic balance to right themselves. *Righting* means to bring the body back into "normal" skeletal alignment[16] using only the necessary muscle groups. When righting and equilibrium reactions are not sufficient to regain an upright posture quickly and safely, individuals use another reflexive reactions called **protective extension reactions.** When people fall, they frequently use this reaction, automatically reaching outward from their bodies to catch themselves or break the fall.

CLINICAL *Pearl*

Frequently, children who have cerebral palsy have delayed or absent protective extension responses. These children may move cautiously for fear of falling or, because of their impaired balance, may be at risk for physical injury when moving.

When movement abilities develop normally, children experience and practice many different movements and positions as they work toward mastery of an upright, two-legged stance. Postural stability and the ability to reestablish it through righting and balance reactions evolve developmentally through experimentation and experiences in a variety and combination of positions (for example, prone, supine, sitting, kneeling, standing). As children refine their control of specific postures through developmental progression, they gain the stable background needed for the infinite variety of skilled, voluntary movements used for environmental interactions. For example, when a person reaches across the dinner table to pass a serving dish, that person must remain stable in the chair while going through several hand and arm motions to lift the dish, move it across the table, and then carefully release it to the person waiting for the dish. Such a task requires the use of the muscles of the trunk and pelvic girdle areas as stabilizers; that is, these areas must do more "holding" as the upper extremity and shoulder girdle muscles perform most of the visible movements. In addition to the different types of muscle activity used for this task, the person must also rely on quick-responding righting and equilibrium reactions and visual perception to remain seated in the chair. The person passing the dish will probably lean to the left or right or forward. In this instance, just as in every executed movement, the leaning or moving from the center of gravity requires shifting of the body's weight. Each time a person shifts weight, righting and equilibrium reactions are used to counterbalance the weight shifts during the movements and help regain an upright posture with body parts correctly realigned. Vision, hearing, and other sensory information also provide perceptual information about whether the person is moving just the right distance when reaching and whether that person is upright in the context of the immediate surroundings.

Muscle Tone

Children's ability to perform sequential movements is supported by the ability of their muscles to maintain the correct amount of tension and elasticity during the movements; the neurophysiological state of the muscle is referred to as **muscle tone.** Best described as a state of continuous mild contraction in the muscle, muscle tone is determined largely by two factors. First, muscle tone is most influenced by gravity. The muscle must have enough tone to move against gravity in a smooth, coordinated motion. Second, emotions and mental state, including levels of alertness, fatigue, and excitement, influence muscle tone. Normal muscle tone develops along a continuum, with some variability among the normal population.

The muscles' qualities of contractility and elasticity are necessary for an accurate response to the stimuli changes experienced during movement, an event referred to as *coactivation*. In the previous example a greater degree of force resistance is required for the initial lifting of the serving dish than is required for its actual movement toward a person. For a person to carefully lower the dish without dropping it again requires more force resistance. Although muscle strength is important for the movement of muscles against an outside force (weight) or gravity, normal muscle tone also is essential. Tone allows the muscles to adapt readily to the changing sensory stimuli resulting from the positional changes of the dish in relation to the arm. The total movement appears smooth and coordinated because normal muscle tone can be sustained in all muscles including the muscle groups that contract to initiate movement at joints (agonists) and those that simultaneously relax to allow movement at joints (antagonists). When agonist muscle groups initiate the lifting of the dish, the gradual relaxation and elongation of the opposing antagonist muscle group result in a smooth, directed movement. When the dish is held still for several seconds, the agonist and antagonist muscle groups work with equal force. Cocontraction occurs, resulting in postural stabilization; each muscle group has just the right amount of muscle tone needed for the muscle contractions to keep the joint stable while not in motion. Individuals with intact sensorimotor functioning can perform an infinite number and variety of movements; all require points of postural stability or fixation to provide the stable background for skilled, active movements.

Common Problems of Motor Development in Children with Cerebral Palsy

1. Abnormal muscle tone
   - Hypertonicity: rigid, high tone
   - Hypotonicity: flaccid, floppy, very low tone
   - Fluctuating: rigid, floppy, rigid, floppy, and so on
2. Persistence of primitive reflex patterns interfering with voluntary movements
3. Poorly developed normal movement patterns, including balance reactions
4. Distorted body awareness and body scheme because of inaccurate sensory information
5. Joint hypermobility
   - Reduced limb stability
   - Use of postural compensations
6. Muscle weakness
7. Reduced skill development and refinement of movement
8. Decreased exploration of the environment

Children with cerebral palsy experience disorder in the central nervous system functions that regulate postural control, righting, and equilibrium and muscle tone. A certified occupational therapy assistant (COTA) who is planning therapeutic interventions for children with cerebral palsy must possess an understanding of the ways postural control and motor skills develop. This knowledge is imperative for planning functional therapeutic activities that are appropriate for the child's age and physical abilities (Box 8-3).

POSTURAL DEVELOPMENT AND MOTOR CONTROL

As newborns grow, they are continually developing and refining postural control. As with motor skills the characteristics of posture vary with age. In the past 20 years, much research has been devoted to the understanding of motor control so that practitioners may provide effective neurological rehabilitation to persons with cerebral palsy and other neurological disorders. Motor control theory is complex, and detailed explanations are beyond the scope of this text. However, the COTA should recognize the two main schools of thought on motor control. This knowledge can guide the occupational therapy practitioner in seeking information that can contribute to implementing effective therapeutic approaches. The theories can be grouped into two models of motor control: the traditional reflex-hierarchical models and the more recent systems models.[7,16]

Reflex-Hierarchical Models

Reflex-hierarchical models propose that purposeful movement is initiated only when the individual experiences a need to move. When the desire to move is stimulated, the person searches long-term memory for a pattern of movement that will accomplish the desired task. The stored movement patterns that the person has practiced the most are most likely to be used again because they are more embedded in memory. The person prepares to execute the movement, incorporating additional information from the environment to make the movements meet the demands of the task. The previous example of lifting and passing a serving dish can help illustrate this model. From the general experience of lifting and moving objects, an individual can recall from long-term memory the necessary movement patterns. The individual also needs to collect some information from the environment such as the approximate size and weight of the dish. This information helps the individual determine whether both hands are required for the task and what type of grasp should be used to lift and hold on to the dish. Sensory feedback determines whether the individual's movement efforts have been successful (that is, have met the task demands). With continual repetition, these movement patterns can develop into motor skills. Reflex-hierarchical models support the idea that motor learning optimally occurs when a person engages in repetition of the same task during frequent, regular practice, and breaking down a task into small parts is the most effective way to learn the entire task.[10]

According to reflex models, many children with cerebral palsy use the tonic reflexes controlled by the lower levels of the central nervous system for managing most of their movement. These movement patterns are "hard-wired" into the human nervous system and do not depend on the application of learned patterns for performing tasks. Children with cerebral palsy lack the ability to independently learn to control movement from higher-level brain centers. Their abnormal postural mechanisms and disordered muscle tones cause them to repeatedly use and store in memory those movement patterns that are governed predominantly by the early tonic reflex patterns.

Systems Models

Systems approaches to understanding motor behavior propose that postural control is greatly influenced by an individual's many volitional or functional daily tasks and activities. The sitting posture needed for a person to put on shoes while sitting on a bed is quite different from the posture needed when a person is strapped into the seat of an airplane. Systems models purport that posture and movement must be flexible and adaptable so that a person can perform a wide range of daily activities. Reflex models state that control of posture and movement is the outcome or product of a process, but systems models postulate that posture is anticipatory to the initiation of movement. Postural adjustments actually precede movements; they prepare the body to counterbalance the weight shifts that are caused by the movement activity. In this way, less balance disturbance occurs. For example, a person catches two balls, one of which is a small tennis ball and the other a large, heavy medicine ball. Before catching either ball, that person has seen the balls, used visual perception to make decisions about their sizes and weights, and assumed an appropriate postural stance. This anticipatory process is called *feed forward*. According to the systems approach, feed forward actions require that posture be highly variable and subject to being affected by all the factors motivating the person to choose to catch the balls. No one right way to execute movement exists; rather, movement is strongly influenced by many variables. This model contrasts with reflex models that state motor development follows a steplike progression, starting with the primitive reflexes and progressing to voluntary movement control through the higher brain centers. The research of the systems theorists has shown that motor activity is most often initiated by the interaction of sensory, perceptual, environmental, and other factors leading to task-focused, goal-directed movement. One other concept from the systems model research has important therapeutic implications for the treatment of children with cerebral palsy or other neurologically based disorders. Postural control and movement are at their greatest levels of efficiency, flexibility, and adaptability after randomized practice and repetition.[7,16] Children in elementary school have many opportunities to practice learning to print their names so that the letters will be neatly aligned and a small, equal size. Although children practice printing in school during class, they are also practicing any time they spontaneously write their names during typical childhood activities and games. Over time, this repeated motor pattern develops into a skill; children can adapt the postures and movements used in the activity to fit several different tasks. They can write their names at the top of school papers while seated at their desks or at the bottom of pictures they are drawing while stretched out on the floor. By repeating this task in many different contexts, children gain the skill of motor problem solving. The systems models suggest that children with cerebral palsy need to be challenged with meaningful activities giving them opportunities to solve motor problems and practice their motor strategies in a variety of environments. (See Chapter 15 for additional information related to motor control and motor learning.)

CLASSIFICATION AND DISTRIBUTION

Cerebral palsy can be classified according to the location of the lesion in the central nervous system. For example, a lesion in the motor cortex typically causes increased, or hypertonic, muscle tone during flexor and extensor co-contraction. This increased tone produces **spasticity;** as a movement is initiated, excessive muscle tone builds up and then rapidly releases, triggering a hyperactive stretch reflex in the muscle. It may show up at the beginning, middle, or end of a movement range, but the result is poor control of voluntary movement and little ability to regulate force of movement. A basal ganglia lesion produces a state of widely fluctuating tone called **athetosis.** In athetosis, tone rapidly shifts from normal or hypertonic to unusually low or hypotonic. Movement is very unsteady and appears purposeless and uncontrollable. The person may appear to be swiping at an object or writhing.

CLINICAL *Pearl*

Children with athetosis are often very bright. They also tend to appear physically asymmetrical because they are unable coordinate the movements of both sides the body and show significant muscle tightness and a fixed posture on one side of the body. These children assume the fixed, static posture on one side of the body for stability while using the limbs on the opposite body side for purposeful actions. For example, a child with athetosis may stabilize the right arm between crossed legs while reaching with the left arm.

Ataxia is a less common tone abnormality. Children with ataxia also show tonal shifts but to a lesser degree than those with athetosis. These children can be more successful in directing voluntary movements but appear clumsy and may shake involuntarily. They have much difficulty with balance, coordination, and maintenance of a stable alignment of the head, trunk, shoulders, and pelvis.[15]

CLINICAL *Pearl*

The child who has ataxia may use visual fixation to maintain balance while moving toward an object.

Children with cerebral palsy often show combinations of tone problems. Children with spastic cerebral palsy move their extremities with abrupt hypertonic motions

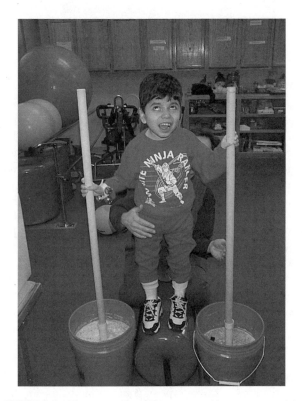

FIGURE 8-3   The occupational therapy practitioner uses specialized positioning and handling techniques to improve the child's ability to act on the environment.

but also may exhibit marked hypotonicity in their trunk muscles. Medical and allied health practitioners commonly use two ways to describe each child's movement control problems. One is by the type of movement disorder, which is characterized by the predominant muscle tone observed, and the other is by distribution, which identifies the body parts most affected by the child's movement control problems (Figure 8-3). The three most common distribution patterns are **quadriplegia,** involving all four extremities; **diplegia,** involving predominantly the lower half of the body; and **hemiplegia,** involving one side of the body (see Figure 8-2).

CLINICAL *Pearl*

Children who have moderate to severe spastic diplegia have functional limitations in both arms and the lower extremities.

Monoplegia and triplegia, which involve one and three extremities, respectively, are more rare. In addition to these categories of characteristic tone and topographical distribution, the disorder may also be diagnosed as mild, moderate, or severe. Each level suggests a degree of muscle tone abnormality, types of abnormal reflex activity, potential for functional activity, and typical associated problems. Knowledge of the degree of muscle tone abnormality and a child's cognitive, sensory, and perceptual status can help the occupational therapy practitioner establish realistic and practical therapeutic goals and interventions. A child with mild involvement and normal cognition has greater potential to succeed at gaining new motor skills. A child with severe motor involvement and impaired cognition may benefit more from assistive technologies that compensate for absence of motor skills.

FUNCTIONAL IMPLICATIONS AND ASSOCIATED PROBLEMS
Muscle and Bone Tissue Changes

A host of associated disabilities, health, and social problems can be caused by cerebral palsy and influence each person's functional potential. The disorder is nonprogressive in terms of lesion changes in the central nervous system, but over time the resulting postural disorder may cause muscle tissue contractures, bone deformities, and joint dislocation or misalignment. These changes further limit functional movement and if they are severe, the child may become highly dependent on others for all ADLs. As the child ages, the potential for painful arthritis in misaligned joints increases. Individuals who are unable to assume more than a few positions or independently shift their weight also risk skin breakdown because their body weight is often concentrated over a few joints for prolonged time periods.

Cognition and Language Impairments

More than 60% of children with cerebral palsy have cognitive and language impairments. The severity of deficits can range from mild to severe; as many as 30% of individuals with cerebral palsy possess significant communication impairments.[2] Cognitive and linguistic competency can play a significant role in a child's ability to benefit from therapeutic and educational interventions. Children with normal or near-normal cognition can consciously generate problem-solving strategies to perform some functional movement activities that are automatic for most people.

CLINICAL *Pearl*

Because approximately 40% of children with cerebral palsy have normal or above normal intelligence, the occupational therapy practitioner should not assume that a child is cognitively delayed based on physical appearance or lack of motor control.

Sensory Problems

Sensory problems are also present in individuals with cerebral palsy. Visual impairments such as blindness, uncoordinated eye movements, or eye muscle weakness affect as many as 50% of children with cerebral palsy; auditory reception and processing deficits impact 25%.[2] Additional sensory problems include hypersensitivity or overreacting to touch, textures, and changes in head position, causing some children to become visibly upset when handled or moved by others. Children with multiple sensory processing problems have more difficulty understanding their environments. Some children's tactile sensation problems are also linked to abnormal oral movement patterns. Many children dislike certain food textures and may have problems coordinating their chewing, sucking, and swallowing movements. Children with severe problems in this area may be surgically fitted with a gastrostomy tube for feedings. Occupational therapy practitioners must consider a child's sensory limitations and strengths when setting therapeutic goals. The practitioner should consider each child individually to determine which sensory experiences are likely to improve the child's occupational performance abilities.

CLINICAL *Pearl*

The occupational therapy practitioner working with children who have cerebral palsy should offer these children opportunities for a variety of sensory experiences. However, the practitioner should not force sensory experiences that a child finds aversive.

Physical and Behavioral Manifestations

Additional problems can include seizures and other medical conditions not directly related to the child's movement disorder. Abnormal postures and weak muscle activity may compromise cardiac and respiratory functions and prevent these systems from working efficiently. The resulting low endurance and fatigue can influence the child's capacity for activity. The occupational therapy practitioner monitors each child's physical endurance and may plan therapeutic goals to increase strength and endurance.

Behavioral problems and social delays are not unusual. Children with cerebral palsy may become accustomed to receiving assistance from others, and problems such as "learned helplessness" may prevent these children from attempting developmental challenges needed for continued growth and mastery of skills. The inability to manage social and peer interactions can lead to social isolation, social immaturity, and a repertoire of undesirable social behaviors. The occupational therapy practitioner often can assist families and work collaboratively with the child's educational team (which can include teachers, consultants, and administrators) to suggest strategies to enhance the child's social development.

OTR AND COTA ROLES

The registered occupational therapist (OTR) and COTA collaborate to provide services. The individual needs of the child and family and the child's chronological age shape each step in the assessment and intervention process. In infancy and early childhood, occupational therapy practitioners focus on family care and management issues such as feeding and bathing, mobility around the home, and family participation. During the early school years the OTR and COTA assist the child with classroom participation, self-care skills, peer socialization, leisure and vocational readiness, and educational and community mobility. For the adolescent with cerebral palsy, occupational therapy services can focus on engagement in work or other productive activities, development of independent living skills, sexual identification and sexual expression, and mobility in the community at large.

Assessment

The OTR and COTA collaboratively assess each individual's needs. Together, they evaluate performance areas, components, and contexts listed in the "Uniform Terminology for Occupational Therapy."[1] The OTR may use one or several standardized tests requiring specialized administration and interpretation skills that can provide the team with specific information about reflex development, sensorimotor functioning, motor skills, and developmental skill levels in the "Uniform Terminology for Occupational Therapy" occupational performance areas. The experienced, trained COTA may assist in the administration of some tests. Observation is a crucial part of the assessment process because many children with cerebral palsy cannot easily follow the directions of standardized tests because of their impaired motor skills. Both practitioners can observe the child's functional abilities at home and in school and leisure activities. Observation of function and dysfunction in the "Uniform Terminology for Occupational Therapy" performance components provides the practitioner with data on the child's muscle tone, reflex activity, gross and fine motor skills, sensory systems, cognition, perception, and psychosocial development. The COTA may be the practitioner who sees the child regularly, whereas the OTR may rely on the COTA to bring this information to their supervision sessions to plan the most effective occupational therapy intervention. Early assessment is most desirable whenever possible. The earlier the patterns of postural abnormality are recognized, the earlier interventions can be planned to facilitate developmental progress, which minimizes the risk of serious deformities and development of undesirable behaviors.

Assessment data create a "picture" of the child's functioning and indicates the child's strengths and weaknesses. The OTR and COTA use this information to formulate goals to match the child's needs and developmental abilities or potential. Examples include increasing a child's ability to participate in a classroom writing activity or teaching family members to reduce the child's hypertonicity so that they can bathe or feed their child. Goals for the adolescent might address accessing public transportation or learning ways to perform homemaking skills. Thorough occupational therapy assessment data are essential when working as part of a service delivery team. Classroom teachers may rely on the occupational therapy practitioner's expertise to assist in the establishment and implementation of educational goals. Vocational skills trainers need to know the student's physical performance abilities and attitudes toward new tasks. Families may use occupational therapy input to select recreational activities for their child.

Intervention

Nathan, a 10-year-old boy with cerebral palsy, wanted to participate in a special "Day at the Beach" activity with his classmates. Plans included mixing tropical fruit drinks for refreshments. The COTA treating Nathan had already helped him acquire the skills needed to activate a switch-operated computer in his classroom. The COTA then obtained another switch and electronic interface device and attached them to a standard kitchen blender. With the press of a switch, Nathan was able to blend tropical fruit drinks for his classmates.

Individuals with cerebral palsy who receive occupational therapy services can experience a sense of empowerment and control when they successfully perform meaningful occupations, be it in the self-care, work, or leisure domain. Occupational therapy practitioners develop and implement interventions to promote functional performance within each individual's capacities. Through training and consultation, they also assist caregivers and educators in the provision of interventions that facilitate and support the child's occupational performance. Intervention strategies include positioning and handling. (See Chapter 17 for thorough coverage of this topic.) The occupational therapy practitioner determines the variety of postures a child can assume, maintain, achieve independently or with physical assistance. Optimal positions are determined for ADLs. Upright sitting positions are needed for most classroom activities, while a relaxed, semireclined position may be optimal for assisted bathing. Practitioners also can select and recommend positioning equipment such as chairs, supine or prone standers, and side-lyers that supports the child during functional activities with the best possible postural alignment, control, and stability. Handling techniques such as slow rocking, slow stroking, imposed rotational movement patterns, and bouncing are used to influence the child's muscle tone, activity level, and ability for independent movement. Techniques such as weight bearing and weight shifting can promote postural alignment and independent movement.[12] A stiff, hypertonic child fixed in a strong extensor posture can be positioned in a wheelchair easily after the practitioner has slowly and alternately rotated the child's shoulders in a forward and back motion. Handling relaxes this child's tone throughout the body (see Figure 8-3). Each joint can move more easily and the child can then be placed in the wheelchair with good postural alignment and comfort. Positioning and handling methods are especially important for those individuals with cerebral palsy who are most unable to move independently. These methods also help a child work toward achievement of performance area goals such as increased independence in dressing, feeding, playing, or doing school work. Most handling techniques are based on specialized treatment approaches such as the neurodevelopmental treatment described in Chapter 15.[12] An occupational therapy practitioner can learn these treatments in special training programs or under the direction of a skilled therapist. The COTA can implement positioning recommendations, teach them to caregivers, and use handling methods to improve the child's functional performance by following the instructions of the OTR.

Persons with cerebral palsy can achieve greater independence in daily living tasks with assistive and adaptive devices. (See Chapters 13 and 16, respectively, for more information on occupational performance areas and assistive technologies.) The COTA may recommend adapted utensils for the child with limited grasp abilities, suggest a large weighted pen to aid a student with tremors, or attach a large zipper pull on a child's coat for a self-dressing activity. The COTA consults with the OTR to determine the safest and most appropriate devices to match each child's abilities. This task is particularly important in the selection of feeding equipment that can influence safe swallowing. The COTA should become familiar with a number of assistive device vendors so that equipment recommendations can be offered for all appropriate occupational performance areas and budget considerations. With a little creative thinking a COTA often can fabricate assistive devices from inexpensive materials. Inexpensive PVC plastic pipe from a hardware store can be assembled to make an inverted U-shaped frame with sus-

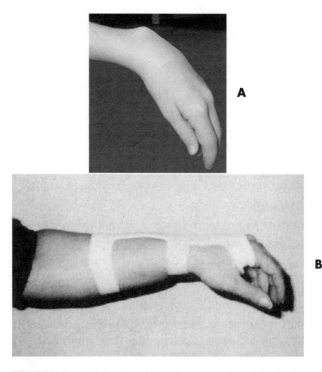

FIGURE 8-4 **A,** Unsplinted hand is postured inefficiently for function. **B,** Orthotic device that helps keep bones and joints in good alignment and increases child's ability to use hand.

pended toys to be placed in front of a child. For children with limited reaching and grasping abilities, this could be the right way to help them engage in a meaningful play activity.

Many children with cerebral palsy may benefit from a custom-designed *orthotic device*, a bracing system designed to control, correct, or compensate for bone deformities (Figure 8-4). Occupational therapy practitioners can design these to accomplish a variety of goals. A COTA may make a resting orthotic hand splint to decrease or prevent further deformity in a child whose muscle tone abnormalities are causing ulnar deviation. The OTR may design an upper extremity orthotic to stabilize wrist and elbow joints so that a student may successfully use a keyboard-typing device at school. Therapists occasionally may help family and school team members solve self-injurious behavior problems by designing appliances to prevent children from biting or otherwise injuring themselves. A COTA who fabricates orthotic devices should have good knowledge of and experience in splinting and work under the supervision of an OTR to devise safe and appropriate wearing schedules while instructing caregivers. The COTA may be required to monitor the application, use, and safety of the fabricated orthosis.

COTAs assist clients who have cerebral palsy in a variety of settings. Intervention programs can occur in the family home, the child's school setting, or in a hospital. In each setting the COTA is part of an interdisciplinary treatment team whose goal is to maximize the health, functional capacities, and quality of life for the child. As an occupational specialist the COTA combines knowledge and skill to help each child accomplish purposeful and meaningful daily living tasks within the home, school setting, and community.

CASE *Study*

Missy is a 6-year-old girl. During her birth, she experienced a prolonged period of anoxia that resulted in spastic diplegia. Missy has moderate hypertonia throughout her lower extremities and mild tone problems in her upper extremities that cause difficulties with fine motor and in-hand manipulation tasks such as drawing, writing, and brushing her teeth. Missy demonstrates good balance reactions from her middle trunk area upward but easily loses her balance when seated on a chair without armrests. She frequently topples over when she tries to bend to retrieve something dropped on the floor. Missy is a bright, happy child of normal intelligence and good vision and hearing abilities. From ages 3 to 6, Missy attended a special preschool and kindergarten program where she received occupational and physical therapy services. Physical therapy practitioners worked with Missy to develop functional mobility skills. Missy now ambulates independently with a wheeled walker, can lower and raise herself to and from the floor level using an environmental support, and can transfer on and off a preschool-size toilet. Occupational therapist practitioners helped Missy increase her independence in dressing with the use of Velcro closures and zipper pulls, and they used therapeutic handling and strengthening techniques to improve Missy's manipulation skills with drawing materials and pencils. Because Missy has been so successful in learning self-management skills, her parents and the special education team believe that she is ready to enroll in the regular first-grade classroom of her local elementary school.

Occupational therapy consultation services are recommended to assist in Missy's successful school transition. Before Missy starts school, the COTA and OTR participate in a team staffing meeting. Missy's parents, her new first-grade teacher, the school's physical education teacher, and the school principal also attend the meeting. The team members decide that the occupational therapy team will consult with the classroom teacher to address Missy's seating needs and make sure she can participate in the typical first-grade activities. The school district OTR reviews the occupational therapy documentation from Missy's previous practitioners and then schedules a classroom visit for herself

and the COTA, Mike, during the first week of school. During their visit they note that the classroom desks are too high for Missy. Missy cannot maintain a stable, upright posture on a desk chair and loses her balance whenever she leans sideways. Missy also has difficulty keeping her papers firmly on the desk surface when writing and drawing. The OTR and Mike note two other problems. Because of Missy's lack of developed balance reactions in her lower body, she is unable to remove or put on her coat while standing in the coat room area with the other children. At snack time Missy has difficulty opening her cardboard juice cartons. The teacher also tells Mike that each student is expected to have a daily job, and she would like assistance in selecting one for Missy.

The OTR and Mike review Missy's functional motor skills and tone problems. They note that Missy sits in a regular chair with her hips rolled back, her knees and toes pointing inward, and her upper body bent forward because of her lack of postural control and stability in her pelvic area and lower extremities. The OTR instructs Mike to locate a smaller chair with arms for Missy and discusses with him ways to determine a good functional seating position.

The following week the COTA, Mike, and Missy's teacher locate a chair with armrests that provides Missy with good stability. Her feet are flat on the floor and her hips fit back on the seat with a 90-degree bend. Mike places a piece of Dycem, a nonskid rubbery material, on the seat to provide Missy with additional stability so that she can shift her weight and lean somewhat without significant loss of balance. A desk of suitable height is found, and nonslip grips are placed under the desk feet so that Missy can reach a standing position easily by pushing on the desk. Mike recommends using removable sticky putty to help Missy keep her papers in place, and he finds a small bench that can be positioned against the wall in the coat room. Missy can easily manage her coat by sitting on the bench and leaning against the wall. The teacher has learned that Missy enjoys exploring the building but has fewer opportunities to do so than her classmates because she needs additional travel time with her walker. The teacher believes Missy would like the job of taking the daily attendance report to the school office but is not certain how Missy could accomplish this. Mike suggests strapping an attractive bicycle basket of Missy's choice to her walker. The basket also can be handy for transporting other classroom materials. To solve Missy's snack time drink problem, Mike chooses a small piece of brightly colored splinting material and fashions a ring with an inch-long, pencil-like protrusion for Missy's middle finger. Missy can slide on the ring with the protrusion pointing down from her palm and then use the force of her open hand to punch a hole in the juice carton. The basket and the ring enable Missy to be as independent as the other children at snack time. Mike remembers that repeated practice of skills in a variety of situations and environments can increase a person's independent motor skill ability. He contacts Missy's mother who agrees that Missy can use her ring to manage her drinks at home. After speaking with Mike, the physical education teacher places a bench against a wall in the area where the children change into their gym shoes. Missy now can don and doff her Velcro-closure gym shoes independently.

SUMMARY

Cerebral palsy is a term that encompasses a number of postural control and movement disorders resulting from damage to some areas of the central nervous system controlling movement and balance. Common problems associated with cerebral palsy include limitations in movement options, delays in occupational skill development, muscle tone abnormalities that cause secondary problems such as contractures, and bone or joint deformities. Cerebral palsy can involve total or partial areas of the body, and many individuals with cerebral palsy experience a number of associated disorders such as impaired vision, hearing, and communication; below normal cognition; and seizures.

COTAs can play a vital role in helping children who have cerebral palsy increase their ability to function independently and expand their repertoire of occupational performance roles. Grounded with an understanding of movement control and skill development, COTAs can apply their knowledge of positioning and handling methods to improve an individual's abilities to interact with the environment. COTAs can recommend and instruct in the use of assistive devices and specialized equipment to enable children with cerebral palsy to engage in purposeful activities matching their occupational roles and interests. With guidance from the OTR, COTAs can help children during therapy by using techniques to develop postural control, righting and equilibrium reactions, and controlled movement against gravity. Individual therapy plans incorporate therapeutic interventions that correspond to each child's unique developmental skills and occupational needs. COTAs offer service in many environmental contexts and find creative ways for each child to engage in meaningful activities at home, at school, and in their community.

References

1. American Occupational Therapy Association: Uniform terminology for occupational therapy, *Am J Occup Ther* 48:1047, 1994.
2. Batshaw M, Perret Y: *Children with disabilities: a medical primer*, ed 3, Baltimore, 1992, Brookes.
3. Cech D, Martin S: *Functional movement development across the life span*, Philadelphia, 1995, Saunders.
4. Connecticut Children's Medical Center: What's new in cerebral palsy, *Pediatric Ortho Update* 2:2, 1990.
5. Copeland M, Kimmel J: *Evaluation and management of infants and young children with developmental disabilities*, Baltimore, 1989, Brookes.
6. Gordon C, Schanzenbacher K, Case-Smith J, Carrasco R: Diagnostic problems in pediatrics. In Case-Smith J, Allen A, Pratt P, editors: *Occupational therapy for children*, ed 3, St Louis, 1996, Mosby.
7. Horak F: Assumptions underlying motor control for neurologic rehabilitation. In Contemporary management of motor control problems: proceedings of the II step conference, *Found Phys Ther*, 1991.
8. Kuban O, Leviton A: Cerebral palsy, *New Eng J Med* 330(3):188, 1993.
9. Levy S: The developmental disabilities. In Kurtz L, Dowrick P, Levy S, Batshaw M, editors: *Handbook of developmental disabilities*, Gaithersburg, Md, 1993, Aspen.
10. Mathiowetz V, Haugen JB: Evaluation of motor behavior: traditional and contemporary views. In Trombly CA, editor: *Occupational therapy for physical dysfunction*, Baltimore, 1995, Williams & Wilkins.
11. Scherzer A, Tscharnuter I: *Early diagnosis and therapy in cerebral palsy*, New York, 1982, Marcel Dekker.
12. Schoen S, Anderson J: Neurodevelopmental treatment frame of reference. In Kramer P, Hinojosa J, editors: *Frames of reference for pediatric occupational therapy*, Baltimore, 1993, Williams & Wilkins.
13. Stanley F, Blair E: Cerebral palsy. In Pless I, editor: *The epidemiology of childhood disorders*, New York, 1994, Oxford University Press,
14. Solomon JW: Evaluation of motor control. In Early MB, editor: *Physical dysfunction practice skills for the occupational therapy assistant*, St Louis, 1998, Mosby.
15. Sugden D, Keogh J: *Problems in movement skill development*, Columbia, SC, 1990, University of South Carolina Press.
16. Vansant A: Motor control and motor learning. In Cech D, Martin S, editors: *Functional movement development across the life span*, Philadelphia, 1995, Saunders.

REVIEW *Questions*

1. Cerebral palsy can be classified by type or distribution over body areas. What are these classifications?
2. How does a COTA incorporate knowledge of motor control theories into treatment approaches for cerebral palsy?
3. What is the postural mechanism, and how is it disrupted in children with cerebral palsy?
4. Describe ways COTAs facilitate function for very young children, school-age children, and adolescents.
5. Name several physical or psychological conditions that frequently occur in children with cerebral palsy.
6. Using "Uniform Terminology for Occupational Therapy," identify Missy's (see the Case Study) occupational performance areas and occupational performance components that were addressed by the COTA.
7. Explain the importance of structured observation in the assessment of children with cerebral palsy.
8. Differentiate between a contracture and a deformity. Explain the therapeutic interventions the COTA can offer for these problems.

SUGGESTED *Activities*

1. Explore several therapeutic equipment catalogs and identify seating and positioning systems used for children with cerebral palsy.
2. Challenge your own balance reactions in several positions. For example, try sitting on the edge of a table with your feet off the floor. Notice the way your head leads your body toward regaining an upright position. Which muscle groups are needed to make this happen?
3. Walk across a room and observe the way weight shifting occurs with each step you take.
4. Sit in a chair at a table. Try assuming a posture in which your hips are rolled back in the chair seat and your legs are extended straight in front of you with your toes pointed inward. Now try to complete a writing task on the table. Notice which tasks take most of your attention and energy.
5. Visit the Internet web site for United Cerebral Palsy at *http://www.ucpa.com*. Explore information resources that can be helpful to a COTA.

9

Mental Retardation

DONNA NEWMAN

CHAPTER *Objectives*

After studying this chapter, the reader will be able to accomplish the following:

- Identify possible causes of mental retardation
- Explain the difference in levels of severity of mental retardation
- Identify functional consequences for each level of severity of mental retardation
- Identify the amount of support needed for each level of severity of mental retardation
- Explain the roles of the registered occupational therapists and certified occupational therapy assistants in assessments of and interventions with children who have mental retardation

| KEY TERMS | CHAPTER OUTLINE |

A child with mental retardation has below average intellectual functioning that causes developmental delays and functional impairments. Functional impairments can include impairments in social, motor, language, academic, and activities of daily living (ADLs) skills. The child may have physical disabilities as well as intellectual difficulties depending on the causes of the mental retardation. In less severe cases the child's deficits may not be noticeable until school age.

DEFINITION

Mental retardation is a developmental disorder that is characterized by significantly subaverage intellectual functioning as well as deficits in two or more skill areas. These skill areas can include ADL, communication, social, academic, leisure, and homemaking skills as well as other skills that are required to attain and maintain independence. Mental retardation is the most common of the developmental disorders; some studies state that it affects 2% to 3% of the population. By definition, mental retardation must manifest itself before the child is 18 years of age.[2]

MEASUREMENT

One of the initial signs of mental retardation is a significant delay in children's motor and cognitive development. Although their learning speed may be slower than children who do not have mental retardation, children with mental retardation are capable of learning. The amount of material these children are capable of learning depends on the severity of their mental retardation. The level of severity is determined using several factors: results of intelligence testing, adaptive functioning, and mental age.

Intelligence Testing

Intelligence is determined using standardized tests that measure the underlying abilities of the child and help predict how well the child will do in school and society in the future. The tests are scored on a scale of 0 to 145, with the average score generally being 100. Individuals who score below 70 to 75 are generally categorized as having mental retardation. (See "Intelligence Quotient" in this chapter for an extended explanation of intelligence testing.)

Adaptive Functioning

Adaptive functioning skills include all of the skills that are necessary for ADL independence, such as dressing, grooming, mobility, social, and communication skills.

Children's functioning in the various areas is compared to the normal development level for their chronological age.

Mental Age

Mental age is another term that is used to describe a child's functional level. Mental age is the age at which an average child is able to perform a certain task. For example, a child who is 5 years old but only performs tasks that an average 3 year old performs would have a mental age of 3.[7] Mental age is usually determined according to a child's performance on certain standardized tests. These tests ensure that each child is given the same opportunities and tasks so that their performance can be equitably compared to the chronological age standard.

ETIOLOGY AND INCIDENCE

As many as 5% of all infants of live births have major birth defects and various forms of physical disabilities.[4] The causes of mental retardation are varied and numerous, ranging from birth defects and genetic disorders to complications during birth and problems in infancy. Some causes of mental retardation are determined when children are older, whereas a large percentage are never known. Physicians frequently categorize causes based on when they occur; prenatal causes occur before birth, perinatal causes occur at birth, and postnatal causes occur after birth.

Prenatal Causes

Genetic

Each human cell contains pairs of chromosomes. On these chromosomes are genes, which contain deoxyribonucleic acid (DNA). DNA is the material that contains the unique physical and genetic plan for each individual. The store of DNA information on each of the genes is called the *genetic code*. Each human cell contains 23 pairs of chromosomes. The first 22 pairs are called *autosomes*, and the twenty-third pair is the *sex chromosomes*, the chromosomes that determine the sex of the individual. During reproduction, half of the chromosomes come from the mother, and half come from the father. The new resulting cell should have 23 pairs of chromosomes, or 46 chromosomes total.

In some cases, too many or too few chromosomes are present (for example, 47 instead of 46), or an abnormal gene negatively affects the developing fetus. Although some genetic disorders are inherited, others are caused by errors in cell division. Two examples of genetic conditions associated with mental retardation are Down syndrome and Fragile X syndrome. Down syndrome is called *trisomy 21* because individuals with the condition have three

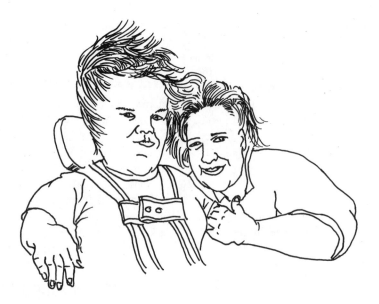

FIGURE 9-1 Adult with disproportionately sized head caused by unshunted hydrocephalus.

copies of chromosome 21 instead of a pair. Individuals with Fragile X syndrome have an abnormal, or "fragile," X chromosome that has a weak area. (See Chapter 11 for additional information about genetic disorders.)

Acquired

Acquired causes of mental retardation are environmental factors known as *teratogens*. A teratogen is any physical or chemical substance that may cause physical or developmental complications in the fetus.[4] Teratogens can include prescription medications, alcohol, or illegal drugs consumed by the mother, maternal infections, and other toxins (which are discussed later in the chapter). The effects of teratogens on the fetus range from congenital anomalies (defects) to mental retardation. Exposure to teratogens does not always result in fetal damage. The type of agent, amount of exposure, and point at which exposure occurred during embryonic and fetal development all play important roles. Exposure to teratogens during the first 12 weeks of pregnancy can be the most dangerous because it is during this time that the fetal brain, spinal cord, most internal organs, and limbs develop. (See Chapter 11 for further discussion of acquired causes.)

Perinatal Causes

Anoxia or hypoxia at birth

Anoxia is a total lack of oxygen in a specific area of the body[8]; *hypoxia* is a decreased amount of oxygen.[8] When either condition occurs in the brain, mental retardation can develop, with its severity depending on the location and size of the area deprived of oxygen, the amount of time the area was without oxygen, and metabolic changes that have taken place in the body as a result of cell death in that area. During labor, numerous circumstances can lead to anoxia or hypoxia. Examples include the mother's pelvis being too small (resulting in bleeding around the brain as the baby attempts to pass through the birth canal), the umbilical cord being compressed, or the infant presenting buttocks first instead of head first.

Prematurity

A premature infant is one who is born before completion of the thirty-seventh week of gestation.[8] Numerous maternal factors can cause prematurity, such as poor nutrition, lack of prenatal care, toxemia, multiple fetuses, a weak cervix, numerous previous births, and being an adolescent.[5] Although prematurity does not necessarily mean mental retardation will develop, some complications caused by prematurity can result in mental retardation. For example, prematurity can cause *respiratory distress syndrome (RDS)*, which is a condition in which the premature infant's lungs are not yet producing *surfactant*, a chemical on the surface of the lungs that helps keep them from collapsing. Another complication of prematurity that can occur is *apnea*, a condition in which the infant stops breathing; apnea can last from seconds to minutes. Prematurity can also cause *hydrocephalus*, a condition in which the cerebrospinal fluid accumulates in the brain and can cause the head to grow disproportionately large (Figure 9-1). The extent of the infant's prematurity and associated complications affect the severity of the mental impairment (if any develops).

Postnatal Causes

Infections

Numerous infections can cause brain damage and resulting mental retardation in infants and children. One such infection is *viral meningitis*, a condition in which a virus attacks the protective covering around the brain and spinal cord, known as the *meninges*.[5] Several different viruses cause meningitis, including the chicken pox virus. Meningitis in small children and infants can cause permanent brain damage that leads to mental retardation, the severity of which depends on the amount of brain damage received. Viruses can also cause *encephalitis*, or inflammation of the brain. Encephalitis can be caused by a single virus or by complications of chicken pox, rabies, measles, influenza, and other diseases.[8] Again, the severity of any resulting mental retardation varies depending on the areas and amount of the brain that have been damaged.

Traumas

Any severe traumatic injury of the brain has the potential to cause brain damage and subsequent mental impairment. Automobile accidents are the most common form of head injuries, especially in cases in which the child is not restrained by a seat belt.[7] Head injuries are also caused by falls, bicycle accidents, pedestrian-automobile accidents, near-drowning accidents, and physical abuse.

Toxins

Toxins are poisonous substances and cause particular problems when ingested.[8] Because infants and small children often place objects and substances in their mouths, certain common household substances can pose serious and life-threatening problems. For example, older homes often have lead-based paint on the walls. Inhaling, licking, or eating paint chips can lead to lead poisoning, which can build up during several months and cause barely noticeable developmental problems. Once diagnosed, lead poisoning can be treated, but residual, permanent damage may exist, depending on the severity of the poisoning. Other common household toxins include mercury from thermometers and cleaning agents such as ammonia and bleach. (See Chapter 11 for information on environmentally induced disorders.)

CLASSIFICATIONS

Intelligence Quotient

In previous years the most common way to diagnose and classify mental retardation was by using intelligence quotient (**IQ**) testing. IQ tests are administered by a qualified psychologist and have two components: motor and verbal. Some of the more common IQ tests used are the WISC-R, Kaufman, and Stanford-Binet tests. The challenge of administering an IQ test, especially to children with more severe disabilities, is that the test is difficult to

TABLE 9-1

Categories of Mental Retardation Based on IQ Scores

IQ RANGE	MENTAL RETARDATION CATEGORY
55 to 69	Mild
40 to 54	Moderate
25 to 39	Severe
Less than 25	Profound

From Case-Smith J: *Pediatric occupational therapy and early intervention*, Stoneham, Mass, 1993, Butterworth-Heinemann.

TABLE 9-2

Categories of Mental Retardation Based on Needed Levels of Support

LEVEL	SUPPORT NEEDED
Intermittent	Needs support in special circumstances only
Limited	Needs certain supports or assistance in specific (but not all) occupational performance areas (for example, financial support or time-limited support, such as vocational training) on a regular basis
Extensive	Needs support in all occupational performance areas on a regular basis
Pervasive	Needs constant support in all areas of life

From Smith R: *Children with mental retardation: a parent's guide*, Bethesda, Md, 1993, Woodbine House.

completely adapt. If a child is physically unable to perform in a certain area, the score is lowered. The test categorizes mental retardation based on particular scores[3] (Table 9-1).

Functional Ability

Although IQ testing still occurs, the American Association on Mental Retardation (AAMR) has created a new system for classifying mental retardation that is based on IQ *and* each individual's strengths and weaknesses.[7] This new system recognizes that individuals who score the same on an IQ test can have widely varying capabilities and performance levels. The new classification has four **levels of support** that are based on the amount of support the individual needs to function in the environment (Table 9-2).

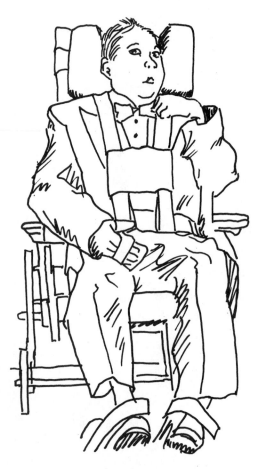

FIGURE 9-2 Adolescent with multiple disabilities and mental retardation.

Multiple Disabilities

Numerous children who have mental retardation also have additional disabilities. The more severe the mental retardation, the greater the chance of physical deficits being present. These deficits can include visual impairments, hearing loss, muscle tone problems, sensory disorders, and seizures (see Chapters 11 and 15). Treating children with multiple disabilities can be more challenging than treating children with one disability, but they still have the potential to make progress (Figure 9-2).

CLINICAL *Pearl*

While working with children who have multiple disabilities, do not underestimate their abilities; they may surprise you.

FUNCTIONAL ABILITIES

The functional abilities of a child with mental retardation varies greatly depending on the severity of the mental retardation and presence of additional deficits. The following descriptions of **levels of severity** gives a general idea of the capabilities of individuals in each category of mental retardation.

CLINICAL *Pearl*

The parents or primary caregivers of a child who has mental retardation may have invaluable information concerning their child's functional abilities.

Mild Mental Retardation

*Carrie is 25 years old today. As the staff and residents of the DeHay House sing "Happy Birthday," Carrie smiles and laughs. Carrie moved into the DeHay House group home and began going to the local sheltered workshop 4 years ago. She moved into an apartment behind the group home last year. Carrie now has a job at a day-care center within walking distance of her apartment. Carrie's primary responsibilities at the day-care center are kitchen duties; however, she also plays with the children and reads them stories. Occasionally, Carrie does not recognize and cannot pronounce certain words that are in the stories she reads to the children. The older children and day-care staff are always willing to help Carrie by explaining the words to her. Carrie is always on time and works very hard at the day-care center. Carrie is a person who has **mild mental retardation.***

Individuals with mild mental retardation have IQs of 55 to 69 and usually require an intermittent level of support. Children in this category may not seem significantly different than other children until they attempt to attain higher levels of cognitive skills. These individuals usually master academic skills ranging from the third to the seventh grade; however, it takes them longer than average students to attain the skills. Academic skills they are capable of attaining include reading at the fourth- or fifth-grade level, writing simple letters or lists such as grocery lists, and performing simple mathematical functions such as multiplication and division. As adults, their social, vocational, and self-help skills are usually sufficient enough to allow them to partially or completely support themselves financially, and they can therefore live independently or in a minimally supervised setting in the community.

Moderate Mental Retardation

Kelly is 7 years old. She attends her neighborhood school and is enrolled in a self-contained classroom for children who have mental disabilities. Kelly is nonverbal but able to indicate her needs by pointing to pictures on a simple communication board. She is a very picky eater. Her teacher has requested that Kelly be evaluated by an occupational therapist.

After the initial evaluation, a registered occupational therapist (OTR) recommends that Kelly be placed on a home and classroom program to decrease her oral sensitivity. The family and classroom staff are instructed in specific techniques designed to decrease Kelly's tactile defensiveness (that is, difficulty processing tactile sensory information) in the face and mouth areas. The OTR monitors Kelly's progress once every 2 weeks. Within 3 months, Kelly has begun eating a variety of foods at school and home. Kelly is a child who has **moderate mental retardation.**

Individuals who have moderate mental retardation have an IQ of 40 to 54 and usually need limited support. At a young age, it may be more noticeable that these children are experiencing developmental delays. They are likely to have deficits in academic, communication, and social skills. With special education, individuals who have moderate mental retardation are usually able to attain the skills of a second-grade student, which include the following:

- Writing name in cursive
- Reading simple texts
- Understanding written numbers and quantities (for example, being able to select three apples from a pile of apples)
- Understanding basic concepts of money

Adolescents and adults may require some supervision to complete ADLs and independent ADLs (IADLs). These individuals can do some meaningful work in sheltered workshops or community-supported employment settings. Numerous adults with moderate mental retardation live successfully in group homes or other supervised living arrangements.

Severe Mental Retardation

Thomas is a short, chubby little boy. He is able to walk and feed himself independently. Thomas is on a toileting schedule at home and school. Thomas is 9 years old and not able to talk, recognize colors, or purposefully use a crayon. Thomas has **severe mental retardation.**

Individuals with severe mental retardation have an IQ of 25 to 39 and usually need extensive support. Because many children with retardation also have additional disabilities, their functional independence depends greatly on their physical limitations. Basic self-care skills such as feeding and assisting in hygiene tasks may be learned because these activities are habitual. Wants and needs can be communicated verbally or nonverbally using communication boards and various other technologies. As adolescents and adults, individuals with severe mental retardation may be successful in supervised prevocational training activities. They are unable to live independently and require extensive supervision and support. It is unlikely that these individuals will achieve any particular academic grade level in school because tasks such as reading and writing are extremely difficult for them.

Profound Mental Retardation

Danielle is a frail little girl. She is unable to sit or stand because she has poor head and trunk control. She depends on others for all self-care needs including eating, toileting, and dressing. Danielle has **profound mental retardation.**

An IQ of less than 25 classifies individuals as having profound mental retardation and typically means that they need a pervasive level of support. Because of the numerous physical disabilities that may accompany profound mental retardation, these individuals often have difficulty making developmental progress.

Depending on the extent of their physical limitations, individuals with profound mental retardation may learn to communicate and perform basic self-care activities such as hygiene and grooming tasks. Extensive help is required for all other ADL skills, and maximum support is needed in living arrangements.

CLINICAL *Pearl*

Children who have profound mental retardation have preferences for certain people, toys, and food and typically have a sense of humor. The occupational therapy practitioner should try to respect their preferences and find their sense of humor.

FUNCTIONAL IMPLICATIONS

The previous section provided a basic idea of the way individuals in each category function; this section focuses on the specific implications of mental retardation in each of the following areas: cognitive development, motor development, language development, sensory abilities, and behavioral issues.

Cognitive Development

Cognitive development can be affected in several ways:

- Slower learning ability
- Shorter attention span
- Difficulty with problem solving and critical thinking
- Difficulty generalizing information and mastering abstract thinking
- Difficulty storing and retrieving information

As mentioned previously, children with more severe mental retardation generally have more severe and numerous cognitive deficits. Techniques for treatment need to be altered according to their cognitive abilities. For example, children with short attention spans can be treated in shorter sessions, and children who have problems with abstract thinking can be taught practical skills.

Motor Development

Motor development in children with mental retardation vary greatly, especially in children with other physical deficits; they may have problems with muscle tone, such as hypotonicity, spasticity, or athetosis, that greatly affect and sometimes prevent motor development. Children with mental retardation often reach major physical milestones later than usual, and often when they finally master a particular motor skill, they appear awkward or uncoordinated. Children with mental retardation *must* have intervention early to promote the development of motor skills. If intervention does not occur early enough, these children may never completely attain needed motor skills.

Language Development

Speech and language problems are frequently associated with mental retardation. Some are caused by physical problems that inhibit speech, such as low mouth muscle tone that causes unclear articulation and difficulties taking deep breaths or speaking loudly. Other problems are caused by cognitive difficulties; for example, a shorter memory and attention span could make recalling and retrieving words difficult, whereas difficulties with abstract thinking could make mentally grasping certain concepts a challenge. As with physical milestones, it can take longer for children with mental retardation to reach speech and language milestones. The severity of a child's speech and language deficits depends on the severity of the child's mental retardation, presence of physical disabilities, age at which speech intervention was received, and degree of support and encouragement the child receives at home.

Sensory Abilities

Children with mental retardation may have problems processing various sensory stimuli. One such problem is difficulty processing the sensation of touch, which is referred to as *tactile defensiveness*. Children with tactile defensiveness dislike being touched on certain areas of their body or avoid contact with certain textures. Children who have *oral hypersensitivity* may have feeding difficulties; they may dislike certain flavors or textures or have an oral reaction that causes them to bite down on the feeding utensil when food is placed in their mouth. Both of these situations can lead to nutritional problems and other medical complications, such as impaired skin integrity and dehydration.

Another example of sensitivity to particular sensations is having an exaggerated reaction (startle reaction) in response to loud noises or other certain sounds. Children with mental retardation may also have sensory problems relating to body movement and muscle coordination, which lead to further motor deficits.

Behavioral Issues

As with most other skills, children with mental retardation attain their social skills later than other children, so

TABLE 9-3

Behavior Difficulties Associated with Mental Retardation

BEHAVIOR	EXAMPLES
Hyperactivity	Being impulsive and excessively active
Aggressiveness	Hitting, kicking, throwing tantrums
Distractibility	Having difficulty paying attention
Excessive shyness	Not maintaining eye contact Not speaking in the presence of strangers

these children often appear to be misbehaving or behaving inappropriately more than their peers. However, just as exceptions are made for the behavior of toddlers and preschool children, exceptions must also be made for children with mental retardation. For example, a 5-year-old child with mental retardation may act like a preschooler, but this is because this child's mental age is not that of a typical 5 year old; this must be taken into consideration before labeling a child's behavior as a problem.

Numerous behavior difficulties are associated with mental retardation, including hyperactivity (impassivity and excessive activity that result in difficulty functioning in social situations), aggressiveness (such as hitting, kicking, and throwing tantrums), excessive shyness, and distractibility (difficulty paying attention to one task because of distractions) (Table 9-3). Each of these behaviors can cause problems in the school and home settings. They may also interfere with children's relationships with peers and the attainment of social skills. Studies have shown that children with certain types of mental retardation are prone to hyperactivity problems; among such children are those with certain types of cerebral palsy or Fragile X syndrome.[7]

OTR AND COTA ROLES

Assessment

The evaluation of individuals with mental retardation varies according to their chronological, developmental, and motor ages; the severity of their mental retardation; the presence of multiple disabilities; and the setting in which occupational therapy services are provided. The majority of the assessment is done by the OTR and focuses on sensorimotor performance components, ADL performance areas, play and work and productive skills, and overall developmental skills.[6] Age-appropriate standardized tests may be used by the OTR during the evaluation process. The COTA may administer specified standardized tests after the establishment of service competency and at the discretion of the supervising OTR.

An interview of the child's parents or primary caregivers is essential to the evaluation process. The interview, which is conducted by an occupational therapy practitioner, is a tool that is used to gain useful information for the treatment planning process. Effective interviews can reveal information relevant to support systems for the child and information about the parents' or caregivers' expectations and goals for the child.

The typical settings of care for infants and young children with mental retardation include home, preschool or day-care, and outpatient settings. The level of service provided by the occupational therapy practitioner depends on a variety of issues, including funding sources, the severity of mental retardation, the coexistence of multiple disabilities, the availability of home and community resources, and other services that are being provided. Evaluation of infants and young children typically include an assessment of their neuromusculoskeletal and sensorimotor statuses and ADL and play skills. The OTR is primarily responsible for evaluating the neuromusculoskeletal and sensorimotor statuses; the COTA assists the OTR in assessing ADL and play skills. (See the Case Study at the end of this chapter for an example of the occupational therapy process that is used to assess and treat a young child with mild mental retardation and cerebral palsy.)

All services that are provided for a child with mental retardation who is attending public school must be educationally relevant and a part of the individualized education plan (IEP) (see Chapter 4). The definition of *educationally relevant* changes depending on the severity of the mental retardation and the coexistence of multiple disabilities.

The occupational therapy services provided for older adolescents and young adults with mental retardation (at all levels of severity) are usually consultative or monitoring services. Types of occupational therapy services for older adolescents and young adults may include the following:

- Modifying activities to allow independence in a sheltered workshop (for example, creating jigs [devices for guiding an activity] or other adaptations)
- Monitoring adaptive equipment used in a workshop, the home, or a group home
- Prescribing and monitoring exercise programs
- Monitoring the use of orthotic devices and splints
- Recommending behavior management programs
- Modifying or recommending adaptive equipment for leisure-time activities
- Intervention

Intervention

Occupational therapy intervention for a child with mental retardation varies greatly depending on the level of severity of the retardation, the presence of physical disabilities, and the amount of support family members or caregivers can provide. Sensorimotor techniques can be used to address developmental delays, motor dysfunction, and difficulties with sensory processing. (See Chapter 15 for a discussion of sensorimotor approaches to treating these deficits.) Behavioral approaches such as using a "time out" (placing the child in a quiet area away from the activity and other children) or backward chaining (having the child perform the last step of a task to receive reinforcement, then the last two steps for reinforcement, and so on) can be used to address behavioral issues (see Chapter 13). Augmentative communication systems and environmental controls can be used to facilitate communication and allow children to interact with their environments. (See Chapter 16 for additional examples of assistive technology.) Because of the varying degrees of existing disabilities and possibility of the presence of multiple disabilities, no one specific intervention plan works for all children with mental retardation. The OTR typically sets up the initial intervention plan, sometimes using significant input from the COTA (especially if the COTA assisted with portions of the evaluation). The COTA can carry out and make appropriate changes to the treatment plan and make recommendations for discharge plans under the supervision of the OTR.

CASE *Study*

Paul, 4-year-old child with mild mental retardation, also has a medical diagnosis of spastic quadriplegia cerebral palsy. Paul receives home-based services through the statewide early intervention program, WEECARE. Paul does not demonstrate significant cognitive delays. He plays appropriately with toys and is able to use tools such as a spoon and crayon correctly. He is receiving speech therapy services once each week to improve his articulation. He is seen by a physical therapist once each week to improve his balance and ability to walk using a posterior walker and bilateral ankle-foot orthoses (AFOs). He has recently been evaluated to determine whether he would benefit from occupational therapy services.

The initial occupational therapy evaluation was performed in Paul's home. His parents and the early interventionist who works with Paul on a weekly basis were present during the initial visit. Jeannie, the OTR, assessed Paul's sensory processing skills, range of motion (ROM) in his extremities and trunk, muscle tone, postural control, and motor skills. Amy, the COTA, interviewed the parents. At the end of the visit, Amy scheduled an appointment to complete the initial evaluation. Amy assessed Paul's play and ADL skills during her next visit. Jeannie and Amy met to discuss the results of the initial evaluation and an intervention plan.

Results of Initial Occupational Therapy Evaluation

Sensory processing

Paul demonstrates tactile defensiveness in his hands and around his mouth. He avoids holding soft toys such as stuffed animals. He prefers to eat crunchy foods such as potato chips or crackers.

Range of motion

Paul has full passive range of motion (PROM) in both of his arms. Active range of motion (AROM) is limited in his shoulders, elbows, forearms, and wrists bilaterally. Paul has difficulty reaching above his head. He is not able to completely straighten his elbows (lacking 15 degrees to complete full extension) in either weightbearing or nonweightbearing positions. Paul is unable to turn his palms up into full supination while using a spoon for self-feeding. He has difficulty extending his wrists while holding a crayon or other objects and tools. Paul uses a palmer grasp to hold a spoon or crayon.

Paul demonstrates full PROM in his trunk and legs. AROM is slightly decreased.

Muscle tone

Paul demonstrates increased flexor tone or spasticity in both of his arms. He has increased extensor tone in his trunk and legs. His legs are more affected than his arms. Paul's abdominal muscles are weak.

Postural control

Paul demonstrates associated reactions in his hands and mouth while performing fine motor activities. Although protective extensive responses are present in his arms, they are slow. He has good head control and fair trunk control.

Motor skills

Paul is able to sit independently and crawl on the floor. He is able to stand with support while wearing his AFOs. He has a freedom stander and posterior walker.

Paul prefers using his left hand for most fine motor activities. He is able to hold a crayon while engaging in prewriting tasks (that is, tasks that are performed before true writing skills are developed, such as scribbling). Paul uses a palmer grasp to hold tools. His abnormal muscle tone interferes with his ability to make smooth and coordinated arm movements.

Activities of daily living

Paul is on a toileting schedule and rarely has accidents. He adjusts his arm and leg positions to assist his caregivers with putting on and taking off his clothing. He is able to finger feed independently. Paul is also able to feed himself using a spoon but is slow and messy. Paul can independently use a "sippy cup."

Play skills

Paul engages in exploratory play activities according to his motor abilities. He enjoys manipulating toy trucks and blocks. Paul is creative during play and crashes the cars into the blocks. Paul enjoys playing but becomes frustrated by his limited mobility. He cries when toys go too far out of his reach.

The OTR and COTA recommended that Paul receive weekly occupational therapy services. The treatment plan was developed based on the initial occupational therapy evaluation and the family's priorities. The long-term goals follow:

Improve sensory processing in hands and around mouth.
Increase AROM in both arms so that it is within functional limits.
Improve functional grasp and pinch patterns.
Increase age-appropriate ADL independence.

The OTR and COTA collaborated on establishing short-term objectives (STOs) for each long-term goal. The short-term objectives are as follows:

1. Improve sensory processing in both arms and around the mouth.
   - STO #1: For three consecutive therapy sessions, Paul will play with a variety of soft toys and objects 3 out of 4 times that he plays with objects.
   - STO #2: Paul will tolerate a variety of textured foods during meal time 50% of the time.
2. Improve AROM in both arms.
   - STO #1: Paul will reach for toys and objects above his head with full elbow extension 3 out of 4 trials for five consecutive therapy sessions.
   - STO #2: Paul will actively supinate his forearm through 50% of the range while self-feeding 100% of the time.
3. Improve functional grasp and pinch patterns.
   - STO #1: Paul will isolate his index finger from the other digits for pointing 100% of the time.
   - STO #2: Paul will use his index and middle fingers and thumb to grasp small objects 3 out of 4 trials for three consecutive therapy sessions.

4. Increase age-appropriate ADL independence.
   - STO #1: Paul will independently take off a pull-over shirt 100% of the time.
   - STO #2: Paul will put on a pullover shirt with minimal assistance 3 out of 4 trials for three consecutive therapy sessions.

The OTR and COTA agreed that the COTA would see Paul on a weekly basis, and the OTR would perform a supervisory visit once monthly. Because of Paul's age, it was agreed that occupational therapy sessions would consist of 45 minutes of direct service and 15 minutes of consultation with the family and early interventionist.

SUMMARY

The causes of mental retardation are numerous and varied and sometimes preventable. Many children who have mental retardation also have various physical disabilities and behavioral problems. The four levels of mental retardation are defined by a child's IQ and functional level of support. The occupational therapy practitioner should treat all children as individuals, with various abilities and needs despite their level of retardation. Intervention varies depending on the degree of the mental retardation, the presence of physical disabilities, and available family support.

References

1. American Association on Mental Retardation: *Mental retardation: definition, classification and system of supports*, ed 9, Washington, DC, 1992, The Association.
2. American Psychiatric Association: *Diagnostic and statistical manual of mental disorders (DSM IV)*, ed 4, Washington, DC, 1994, The Association.
3. Case-Smith J: *Pediatric occupational therapy and early intervention*, Stoneham, Mass, 1993, Butterworth-Heinemann.
4. Case-Smith J, Pratt P, Allen A: *Occupational therapy for children*, ed 3, St Louis, 1996, Mosby.
5. Mader S: *Understanding human anatomy and physiology*, ed 3, Dubuque, Iowa, 1997, William C Brown.
6. Neistadt M, Crepeau E: *Willard & Spackman's occupational therapy*, ed 9, Philadelphia, 1998, Lippincott-Raven.
7. Smith R: *Children with mental retardation: a parent's guide*, Bethesda, Md, 1993, Woodbine House.
8. *Taber's cyclopedic medical dictionary*, ed 17, Philadelphia, 1993, FA Davis.

REVIEW *Questions*

1. Explain the different ways of diagnosing and categorizing mental retardation.
2. Explain the reason it is important to treat a child with mental retardation as an individual instead of as a "category."
3. Explain the way multiple disabilities can affect a child with mental retardation.
4. Explain the reason it is better to diagnose mental retardation based on functional level than IQ score.
5. Describe the roles of the OTR and COTA in treating mental retardation.

SUGGESTED *Activities*

1. Volunteer at a facility that specializes in working with children who have severe disabilities.
2. Attend a Down syndrome support group to learn about the challenges faced by the families and caregivers of individuals with the syndrome.
3. Volunteer your time in a school system or early intervention program. Ask to see a sample individual family's service plan (IFSP) and IEP.
4. Volunteer to babysit or provide respite care for a child who has mental retardation.

10

Psychosocial Disorders

SUSAN D. STOCKMASTER

CHAPTER *Objectives*

After studying this chapter, the reader will be able to accomplish the following:

- Describe signs and symptoms of mental disorders seen in children and adolescents
- Describe the impact of mental disorders on occupational performance in children and adolescents
- Identify appropriate evaluation methods for this population and describe the role of the occupational therapy practitioner in evaluation
- Identify appropriate goals and intervention techniques for this population

KEY TERMS

CHAPTER OUTLINE

T ommy is a 13-year-old adolescent who is being discharged from a local psychiatric hospital. He has been an inpatient for the past 2 weeks for evaluation and treatment of his mental status. Tommy was admitted to the hospital by his mother and stepfather following an outburst at home during which he threatened both his parents with a butcher knife. This afternoon Tommy and his family will meet with the psychiatrist from the hospital, his school psychologist, and a community mental health worker to plan for his discharge.

Children and adolescents with psychiatric disorders have difficulty managing their feelings, thoughts, and behaviors. It is estimated that more than 7.5 million children and adolescents in the United States have psychiatric disorders.[10] The American Psychiatric Association's preferred term for a disorder that affects feelings, thoughts, and behaviors is **mental disorder,** which is defined as the following:

> An illness with psychological or behavioral manifestations or impairments in functioning caused by a social, psychological, genetic, physical/chemical, or biological disturbance. The disorder is not limited to relations between the person and society. The illness is characterized by symptoms or impairment in functioning.[4]

Mental disorders in children and adolescents include many of the same disorders seen in adults, including mood disorders (for example, major depressive disorder and schizophrenia), anxiety disorders (for example, obsessive-compulsive disorder), and substance-related disorders.

Children and adolescents with mental disorders receive intervention services in a variety of settings including psychiatric units in acute care hospitals, independent psychiatric hospitals, day treatment centers, community mental health and settings, and public schools.

The mental disorders discussed in this chapter are those that begin in childhood or adolescence or occur predominantly in children and adolescents. General categories of disorders covered in this chapter include disruptive behavior disorders, anxiety disorders, eating disorders, tic disorders, mood disorders, and substance-related disorders. This chapter presents disorders specific to children and adolescents in each category, provides information on the impact of these disorders on occupational functioning, and makes recommendations for occupational therapy assessment and intervention.

DISRUPTIVE BEHAVIOR DISORDERS

According to the Diagnostic and Statistical Manual of Mental Disorders IV,[4] **disruptive behavior disorders** are characterized by socially disruptive behavior that is often more distressing to others than to the individual with the disorder. Attention deficit hyperactivity disorder (see Chapter 11), conduct disorder, and oppositional defiant disorder are the most frequently encountered disruptive behavior disorders.

Conduct Disorder

Peter is an 11-year-old boy who has difficulty getting along with the other children in his class and neighborhood. Both children and adults consider him a bully. At school he was caught stealing money from his teacher's desk. Many neighbors have become concerned about his aggressive behavior toward their pets. Peter is doing poorly in the fifth grade. Next week a parent conference will be held to discuss Peter's aggressive behavior and poor school performance.

Longstanding behaviors that violate the rights of others and the rules of society are the predominant features of conduct disorder. Children and adolescents with this disorder often display the following behaviors:

- Physical aggression toward other people or animals
- Participation in mugging, purse-snatching, shoplifting, or burglary
- Truancy (absence from school without permission)
- Running away from home

Additionally, these major symptoms may be accompanied by the use of addictive substances, recklessness, and temper outbursts. Individuals with conduct disorder lack concern for others and lack feelings of guilt or remorse. Left untreated, a significant number of those suffering from conduct disorder will develop antisocial personality disorder as adults and may commit serious crimes including rape, physical assault and battery, and homicide.[4]

Despite an image of toughness, conduct disorder is often accompanied by poor self-esteem and symptoms of anxiety, depression, and suicidal thoughts. School performance is typically impaired, especially verbal and reading skills, and is complicated by truancy and suspension (restriction from school for a specific period of time) for behavioral problems.[6] Learning disorders and other academic difficulties can often catalyze the development of disruptive behavior disorders.

Oppositional Defiant Disorder

LaTonya is a 13-year-old seventh-grade student. She has always been a somewhat difficult child, and lately she seems to argue constantly with her parents and younger sister and lose her temper over seemingly trivial issues. She refuses to obey her parents' rules and has started deliberately violating *her curfew. She lies to her parents about her activities and companions. When confronted by her parents about her behavior, LaTonya blames her friends for her actions, saying that they would not let her come home on time even though she wanted to leave.*

The primary symptoms of oppositional defiant disorder are negative, hostile, and defiant behaviors that are more severe than normal developmental behavioral fluctuations.[4] Unlike conduct disorder, individuals with this disorder do not seriously violate the rights and ignore the feelings of others. Children and adolescents with oppositional defiant disorder often display outbursts of temper, argue with adults, and defy adult requests and rules. These children may seem angry and resentful of rules, become easily annoyed, and blame others for their mistakes. The normal "difficult" periods of childhood and adolescence should not be confused with this disorder.[4]

Children and adolescents with oppositional defiant disorder do not display the severe impairments in functioning seen in conduct disorder. They rarely engage in activities that cause physical harm to others and as a rule do not engage in criminal activity. They may have difficulty in school because of their oppositional behavior toward teachers and stormy relationships with family and peers because of their defiance of rules, outbursts of temper, and tendency to blame others for their actions.[6] Oppositional defiant disorder often is the visible manifestation of underlying childhood depression or an inability to effectively cope with anger and other uncomfortable feelings.

CLINICAL *Pearl*

The occupational therapy practitioner working with children and adolescents with disruptive behavior disorders must possess a thorough knowledge of normal developmental behavioral fluctuations to recognize abnormal behavioral patterns.

ANXIETY DISORDERS

Anxiety disorders are characterized by anxiety and avoidance of situations causing anxiety.[4] Children and adolescents can suffer from a variety of anxiety disorders that are also found in adults, such as obsessive-compulsive disorder and posttraumatic stress disorder. This chapter examines separation anxiety disorder, which is usually limited to children and adolescents.

Separation Anxiety Disorder

Sally is a 3-year-old girl who stays at home with her mother. Throughout the day, Sally constantly follows her mother while she tries to clean the house. She will not take a nap or fall asleep at night unless her mother lies next to her. Her mother has tried leaving Sally at "Mother's Day Out," a church-sponsored day-care program available twice a week. The one time Sally's mother left her at the church program, Sally cried hysterically and became physically ill; she complained of a headache and began vomiting. The caretakers could not calm Sally and contacted her mother. Sally calmed down a few minutes after her mother returned.

Separation anxiety disorder is characterized by extreme anxiety when a youth anticipates or is separated from home or an individual to whom the youth is most attached, usually a parental figure. Children and adolescents with this disorder may experience extreme anxiety when traveling away from home or to unfamiliar areas, refuse to visit or sleep over at the homes of friends, or refuse to participate in events that require overnight stays, such as summer camp. These individuals often cling to the adults to whom they are most attached and may actually follow them around the home. Physical symptoms including headaches, stomachaches, nausea, and vomiting may occur with separation and even the anticipation of separation. In extreme cases, students may refuse to attend school or participate in social and recreational age-appropriate activities.[4]

Separation anxiety disorder generally resolves or decreases in severity as the child or adolescent ages. However, while the illness is present, school performance and social development can be significantly impaired. The child's refusal to attend school or misery while at school can result in poor academic performance. The child's refusal to spend time away from the adult to whom the child is most attached also can limit normal interpersonal development.[6]

TIC DISORDERS

Tic disorders are involuntary, recurrent motor movements or vocalizations. Common motor tics include eye blinking, neck jerking, coughing, shoulder shrugging, facial grimacing, foot stamping, touching of objects, and grooming behaviors. Vocal tics include throat clearing, grunting, sniffing, snorting, barking, the repetition of obscene words (*coprolalia*), and the repetition of others' words (*echolalia*). Tics often increase in stressful situations and decrease during sleep or absorbing activities such as computer games.[4] Tourette's syndrome is the most common tic disorder for which treatment is sought.

Tourette's Syndrome

Brian is a 7-year-old third grader. Recently he has started to jerk his neck to the side and make strange faces. He also has started making barking and grunting noises. These behaviors have occurred intermittently throughout the day for the past 3 weeks. Brian's parents and teacher seem to be annoyed by these behaviors and his classmates and friends have started to avoid him. Brian is embarrassed but is unable to control the movements and noises. His school performance is suffering because the jerks and noises distract him. Brian's teacher has scheduled a conference to discuss these behaviors with Brian and his parents.

Tourette's syndrome is a genetic condition in which both motor and vocal tics occur frequently and daily. Symptoms of attention deficit hyperactivity disorder and learning disabilities (see Chapter 11) also may be present.[4] These tics typically affect all areas of occupational performance to some degree. School work, activities of daily living (ADL) tasks, and leisure activities are disrupted by the motor and vocal tics, and children and adolescents with this disorder are often avoided by adults as well as peers because of the bizarre nature of the tics.[6] Tourette's syndrome is chronic although most cases improve during adolescence and early adulthood.[4]

EATING DISORDERS

Eating disorders involve a disturbance in eating behaviors and occur primarily in adolescents and young adults.[4] Eating disorders are extremely serious because of the resulting physical problems and can be fatal if left untreated. The most common eating disorders are anorexia nervosa and bulimia nervosa. An individual may have symptoms of one or both disorders simultaneously. Because anorexia nervosa and bulimia nervosa share many symptoms, they are discussed together in this section.

Anorexia Nervosa and Bulimia Nervosa

Jennifer is a 16-year-old junior in high school. She is a bright, well-behaved student who always makes good grades and is a cheerleader. During the past 6 months her parents have become worried about her health. They have noticed that Jennifer picks at her food during meals and looks thin even in the baggy clothes she has been wearing to hide her body. Despite her apparent weight loss, Jennifer thinks she looks fat when she looks at herself in the mirror. She has been taking laxatives every day and does aerobic exercise for at least 3 hours in addition to her daily cheerleading practice. Jennifer has not menstruated in over 4 months.

Her friends also have become concerned about her. Recently they heard her vomiting in the school bathroom immediately after lunch. Sometimes Jennifer buys cake and ice cream and hides it in the basement at home. When she knows everyone is asleep, she sneaks down to the basement and eats the food rapidly, cramming the food into her mouth in big bites. Immediately after she has eaten all the cake and ice cream she can hold, Jennifer goes to the bathroom and makes herself vomit to get rid of the food.

Anorexia nervosa is characterized by an intense fear of gaining weight or becoming fat, even when the individual is less than the normal weight for age and height. Adolescents with this disorder are preoccupied with body size. Their body image is distorted, and they see themselves as overweight in all or some body parts, regardless of how thin they become. Vigorous, lengthy exercise sessions are common, and laxatives, diuretics, and purging (self-induced vomiting) may be used to control weight. Individuals with this disorder are often preoccupied with food and enjoy preparing elaborate meals for others although they eat little of the food they prepare.[4] Food consumption for an entire day may consist of as little as an apple and several diet colas. When confronted by parents or concerned friends, they deny or minimize the severity of the problem and resist treatment efforts.

Anorexia nervosa can lead to significant medical problems because of malnutrition, ceased menstruation, hypothermia (decreased body temperature), and cardiovascular impairments such as bradycardia, hypotension, and arrhythmias. Renal function can be impaired and electrolyte imbalance may occur. Repeated vomiting of stomach acid with food can cause dental erosion. Osteoporosis may result from the insufficient intake of calcium and estrogen-containing foods. Approximately 10% of those with anorexia nervosa die from starvation or an electrolyte imbalance.[4]

Bulimia nervosa shares many characteristics with anorexia nervosa but is less severe. The primary symptom of bulimia nervosa is binge eating episodes followed by purging episodes. A binge is a period of time in which a significantly larger than normal amount of food is consumed, usually very rapidly. Individuals with this disorder feel unable to control their eating during binges. As noted above, purging is self-induced vomiting. As with anorexia nervosa, individuals with bulimia nervosa are preoccupied with body shape and weight and often use strict dieting, vigorous and extensive exercise, and laxatives and diuretics to control their weight. Physical complications are similar to but less severe than those seen in anorexia nervosa, and death from bulimia nervosa is rare.[4]

Generally, individuals with eating disorders perform well in school and work settings. ADL functioning is intact except for eating; the individual may be obsessed with food. Social function is often impaired because of the individual's preoccupation with weight and fear of rejection. Additionally, most individuals with eating disorders have low self-esteem caused in part by a view of themselves as overweight and feelings of ineffective weight control. Their senses of worth are externalized and based on others' judgment of their values and appearances. Leisure time may be spent obsessing about food or weight, and the individuals may avoid leisure situations that involve food for fear of discovery.[6]

CLINICAL *Pearl*

When conducting cooking and eating activities with clients who have eating disorders, the occupational therapy practitioner must be aware of the potential for the child or adolescent to hide or purge the food. Special attention should be paid to a client who uses or requests to use the restroom during or shortly after eating.

MOOD DISORDERS

Mood disorders are characterized by a disturbance in mood. The Diagnostic and Statistical Manual of Mental Disorders (DSM-IV) defines mood as "a pervasive and sustained emotion that colors the perception of the world."[4] Mood disorders include conditions in which the mood can be either dysphoric (unpleasant) with sad, anxious, or irritable feelings, or elevated (overly pleasant) with an exaggerated sense of well being that may be described as "on top of the world."[4] This category includes manic episodes, depressive episodes, bipolar disorder, and major depressive disorder.

Major depressive disorder tends to be viewed as a disorder of adults and the elderly. It may be difficult to imagine children and adolescents as depressed, but experts recognize that depression is frequently found in this age group although the symptoms may differ from those of adults and may be camouflaged as anger or behavior problems. Symptoms of major depressive disorder often accompany the other disorders discussed in this chapter and can result in suicidal behavior if left untreated.

Major Depressive Disorder

Wendy is a 10-year-old student in the fifth grade whose parents have recently separated. She lives with her mother and 12-year-old brother. She is usually a good student and a pleasant, well-behaved child, but lately she has been irritable and cranky at home and at school. She also has been picking fights with her older brother. Her grades have dropped significantly over the past several weeks. Wendy has stopped spending time with her friends at school. After school, instead of playing with the other children in the neighborhood, she comes home, goes to her bedroom, and goes to sleep. Her mother has noticed that she eats very little at meals and has stopped asking for snacks between meals. She has stopped reading and playing computer games, activities she previously enjoyed, and has given her brother many of her favorite computer games. She complains of headaches, stomachaches, and constant fatigue. For the past few days, she has been making statements to her brother such as "I won't be around to bother you much longer," and "Pretty soon you can have all my things."

Major depressive disorder can be manifested in feelings of sadness or irritability, anhedonia (loss of interest in previously enjoyed activities), significant weight change (gain, loss, or failure to gain weight normally), inability to sleep or excessive sleeping, restlessness, fatigue, feelings of worthlessness, difficulty with concentration, and suicidal thoughts. Somatic complaints such as headaches and stomachaches are common in children with major depressive disorder.[4]

Depending on the severity of the disorder, occupational performance can be severely impaired in all areas. Difficulty with concentration and loss of energy causes academic performance to decline. The child or adolescent with major depressive disorder may neglect basic activities of daily living (ADLs) as a result of apathy and fatigue. The child or adolescent loses interest and stops participating in previously enjoyed leisure activities. Group leisure activities are avoided because of social isolation.[6] Isolation and social withdrawal impairs social development.[4]

Suicidal behavior can occur in severe cases of major depressive disorder. Suicide is the third leading cause of death for 15 to 19 year olds and the fourth leading cause of death among the 10- to 14-year-old age group.[1] Signs that a child or adolescent is suicidal are often the same as those for a major depressive disorder. The individual expressing suicidal thoughts or exhibiting these symptoms must receive professional psychiatric help immediately and must be closely monitored to prevent suicidal behavior. Children or adolescents who engage in self-mutilating behavior or appear to suddenly recover from depression are of special concern. In psychiatric terminology, sudden, unexplained improvement is known as *flight into health* and can signify that the final decision to end one's life has been made. Box 10-1 contains a list of suicidal risk signals.

BOX 10-1

Suicidal Risk Signals

If you can answer "Yes" to any of the following questions about a young person, you may have identified a suicidal individual. Professional help must be sought.

Yes   **No**

☐   ☐   *Depression:* Does this person appear sad, irritable, or worthless? Is this person exhibiting symptoms of depression? Symptoms of depression include insomnia, anorexia, withdrawal from others, decreased ability to concentrate, and fatigue. Depression can be concealed by substance abuse, aggressive behavior, and risk-taking behavior.

☐   ☐   *Preoccupation with death and dying:* Has this person been writing poems, stories, or songs about death and suicide?

☐   ☐   *Talking about suicide:* Has this person been expressing a desire to die, making suicidal threats, or joking about suicide?

☐   ☐   *Hopelessness about the future:* Can this person tell you about plans for the next week or next month? Has this person been "putting affairs in order?" Has this person been giving away prized possessions or writing a will?

☐   ☐   *Changes in life situation:* Have there been any major recent changes such as death of a parent, separation or divorce of parents, school problems, or boyfriend or girlfriend problems?

☐   ☐   *Previous suicide attempts:* Has this person ever attempted to commit suicide?

☐   ☐   *Lack of support from family and friends:* Has this person expressed feeling unloved or unwanted?

☐   ☐   *Excessive use of drugs or alcohol:* Has this person begun or increased use of substances?

☐   ☐   *Risk-taking behavior:* Does this person engage in dangerous behavior such as driving too fast or walking in the middle of the road rather than on the sidewalk?

Modified from Hafen BQ, Frandsen KJ: *Youth suicide: depression and loneliness,* Evergreen, Col, 1984, Cordillera; Hermes P: *A time to listen: preventing youth suicide,* San Diego, 1987, Harcourt Brace Jovanovich.

CLINICAL *Pearl*

If signs of self-mutilating behavior or a flight into health is observed, the occupational therapy practitioner should immediately report the behavior to a supervisor or an appropriate team member such as a nurse, psychologist, or mental health counselor. The behavior also should be documented as soon as possible after it is observed. The child or adolescent must not be left unattended.

SUBSTANCE-RELATED DISORDERS

Substance-related disorders as defined by the DSM-IV include several categories of disorders resulting from misuse of drugs, toxins, or medications. The terms substance abuse and dependence are often used interchangeably; however, the terms refer to two different levels of substance misuse. *Substance abuse* is a pattern in which use of substances results in adverse consequences, such as consumption of alcohol while driving or tardiness for school because of hangovers. *Substance dependence* is a more serious disorder; hospitalization is frequently need to help the individual stop using the substance. Substance dependence is a pattern of continued substance use despite serious cognitive, behavior, and physiological symptoms. According to the DSM-IV, the following seven characteristics indicate substance dependence disorder:

1. The development of tolerance (the need to use larger amounts of the substance to obtain the desired results)
2. Unpleasant withdrawal symptoms if use of the substance is decreased or stopped
3. Use of the substance in increasing amounts or for increasingly longer periods of time
4. A desire to stop or failed attempts to stop using the substance
5. Excessive time spent in getting, using, and recovering from the substance
6. Neglect of occupational performance role responsibilities
7. Continued use despite the presence of problems caused by the substance

Although an individual may have all or most of the symptoms listed, at least three of the seven symptoms must be present for a diagnosis of substance dependence to be made.[4]

Another frequently used term that refers to substance misuse is *addiction*, defined as an "intense physiological and psychological craving for a drug."[16] As can be inferred from the characteristics of the disorder, the terms *dependence* and *addiction* are essentially synonymous.

Substance abuse and dependence in adolescents has shown significant growth in the 1990s. The Institute for Social Research at the University of Michigan in conjunction with the National Institute on Drug Abuse conducts an annual survey on tobacco, alcohol, and drug use by eighth-, tenth-, and twelfth-grade students. Results of the 1995 survey of approximately 50,000 students indicate increased use of all substances by this population.[1] According to a 1995 study of 74,000 Minnesota high school students, 13.8% of ninth-grade and 22.7% of twelfth-grade students met the criteria for substance abuse while 8.2% of ninth-grade and 10.5% of twelfth-grade students met the criteria for substance dependence as defined by the DSM-IV.[12]

Substances leading to abuse and dependence include alcohol, amphetamines (uppers), cannabis (marijuana), cocaine, hallucinogens (for example, LSD), opioids (for example, heroin) phencyclamines (for example, PCP, angel dust), sedatives, hypnotics, anxiolytics (for example, Valium, Librium), and inhalants (for example, nitrous oxide, acetone). Although young people may misuse all the listed substances, a thorough discussion of each substance is beyond the scope of this chapter. Inhalant dependence has been selected for discussion to illustrate substance-related disorders.

Inhalant Dependence

Michael is a 15-year-old high school student who has been hospitalized in an adolescent chemical dependency unit. In the weeks before the hospitalization, Michael's parents noticed behavior changes such as appearing "spaced out" and silly at dinner. In the past, Michael has received average grades at school, but he failed two subjects during the last term. He used to play basketball with several neighborhood boys in his driveway after school and on the weekends, but for the past several weeks has spent a lot of time in the garage with two friends of whom his parents do not approve. Although he receives a generous allowance each week, he no longer seems to have money. His mother found a paper bag and several cans of gold spray paint hidden at the back of a storage cabinet in the garage.

Data acquired in 1993 from the Monitoring for the Future survey indicated alarming information about the use of inhalants: one in nine eighth-grade students admitted to having used inhalants at least once.[17] Inhaling toxic substance is called *huffing* or *sniffing* by users. Substances commonly inhaled include gasoline, fingernail polish remover, glue, paint thinner, spray paint, dry erase and permanent markers, correction fluids, and aerosol can propellants. Fluid inhalants (for example, gasoline and paint thinner) are often used with a cloth soaked in the substance that is held over the mouth and nose during inhalation. Substances in aerosol form are frequently sprayed into a paper or plastic bag, which is then held over the mouth and nose during inhalation. The use of inhalants results in rapid absorption of the substance into the blood stream and creates an almost immediate intense "high." Psychotic experiences including auditory, visual, and tactile hallucinations (sensory perceptions incompatible with reality, such as the feeling of insects crawling beneath the skin) and delusions (beliefs incompatible with reality, such as users believing they are being poisoned by their parents) may occur. Furthermore, chronic use of inhalants can cause anxiety, depression, and permanent respiratory, heart, kidney, liver, and brain damage. In chronic users, death can result from cardiac or respiratory damage.[4]

Regardless of the substance, dependence can lead to significant impairment in all areas of occupational performance. Young people with substance dependence disorders often spend much time procuring, using, and recovering from the substance; therefore ADLs may be neglected. Decreased attendance and performance in school or work may be a consequence of dependence. In severe cases of dependence on some substances (for example, inhalants), permanent cognitive deficits may occur. Additionally, the adolescent may be suspended if caught using the substance at school. Previous leisure interests are typically replaced by activities that revolve around use of the substance, such as dropping out of school activities and spending more time partying. Socially, the adolescent may stop spending time with friends who do not use substances and will develop relationships with those peers who abuse substances.

CLINICAL *Pearl*

The occupational therapy practitioner should avoid treatment activities requiring materials that may be inhaled, such as permanent markers, when working with children and adolescents with inhalant dependence disorders. The occupational therapy practitioner must be aware of any possible inhalant materials in the occupational therapy treatment setting.

IMPACT ON OCCUPATIONAL PERFORMANCE

The term *occupational performance* describes the individual's overall participation in activities required to function in daily life. According to AOTA's "Uniform Terminology for Occupational Therapy," occupational performance comprises three major performance areas: ADLs, work, and play or leisure.[3] ADLs include bathing, grooming, dressing, eating, and other tasks engaged in for the purpose of maintaining the self or environment. Work includes the activities through which individuals provide for their welfare. School and household chores are the predominant work activities for children and adolescents. Additionally, some adolescents hold part-time jobs. Play includes activities engaged in for pleasure or self-expression. Play is the predominant activity of young children. Each performance area requires specific skills that include sensorimotor, cognitive, and psychosocial skills.

Successful participation in occupational performance activities and mental health are interdependent. A mentally healthy child or adolescent is able to successfully participate in occupational performance areas, and this successful performance gives the child a sense of competence and confidence that contributes to good mental health. Conversely, impaired occupational performance can intensify an existing dysfunction.

All disorders discussed in this chapter result in some degree of impairment in occupational performance. General symptoms produced by the disorders include decreased energy, social withdrawal, decreased self-esteem, impaired academic performance, anxiety, and physical complaints or conditions. These symptoms may affect ADL performance, work (school and chores), and play and leisure skills. Table 10-1 describes the impact of each disorder discussed in this chapter on occupational performance areas. The impact of these disorders on social skills also is included in this table, because the ability to relate to others is affected in some manner by mental disorders. Social skills are not considered a major performance area by "Uniform Terminology for Occupational Therapy"; they

TABLE 10-1

Impact of Selected Mental Disorders on Occupational Performance

PSYCHOSOCIAL DISORDER	ACTIVITIES OF DAILY LIVING FUNCTIONING	SCHOOL AND WORK FUNCTIONING	PLAY AND LEISURE FUNCTIONING	SOCIAL FUNCTIONING
DISRUPTIVE BEHAVIOR DISORDERS **Conduct Disorder**	Generally, these skills are not impaired; however, risky behavior (such as use of illegal substances and promiscuity) may result in neglect of ADLs.	School or work performance is impaired by the child or adolescent's refusal to follow rules, behavioral problems, inattentiveness, truancy, or suspension.	Individuals with this disorder tend to engage in reckless activities such as using illegal drugs and joining gangs rather than the usual age-appropriate leisure activities. Additionally, the individual with this disorder may become physically aggressive or bully others during games or sports activities.	Aggressive behavior toward others, destruction of other's property, deceitfulness, and lack of remorse or guilt may impair the development of social skills.
Oppositional Defiant Disorder	The disorder usually results in impairment in this area only if the child or adolescent refuses to comply with authority figures' requests and directions.	The child or adolescent's negative or stubborn behavior or refusal to follow rules and instructions impair school or work performance.	Play and leisure activities are impaired by the tendency to defy rules of games and sports. Solitary leisure activities may not be affected.	Social skills are impaired. Children and adolescents with this disorder frequently annoy others by being argumentative, losing their temper, and blaming others for their own mistakes. Both adults and peers may avoid the individual.

Continued

TABLE 10-1

Impact of Selected Mental Disorders on Occupational Performance—cont'd

PSYCHOSOCIAL DISORDER	ACTIVITIES OF DAILY LIVING FUNCTIONING	SCHOOL AND WORK FUNCTIONING	PLAY AND LEISURE FUNCTIONING	SOCIAL FUNCTIONING
ANXIETY DISORDERS **Separation Anxiety Disorder**	These skills are impaired only if an activity involves separation from the individual to whom the child or adolescent is attached, such as going to the store alone.	Concentration and attention span in school may be severely affected by the child or adolescent's despair at separation from the individual to whom they are attached and by physical symptoms. In extreme cases, the child or adolescent may refuse to attend school.	Leisure and play activities are impaired if the activity occurs away from the person to whom the child or adolescent is attached. Leisure and play activities within the home or with the object of attachment present are usually not impaired.	Social development is impaired if the social activity occurs away from the person to whom they are attached. The child may refuse to attend events such as birthday parties, camping trips, or pajama parties unless the person to whom the child is attached is also present. Social activities in the home or with the object of attachment present are usually not impaired.
EATING DISORDERS **Anorexia Nervosa and Bulimia Nervosa**	Skills are generally not affected with the exceptions of food preparation and eating. The individual with an eating disorder does not consume adequate nutrition and may obsess about food.	Work and school performance are not affected unless the individual's preoccupation with food disturbs concentration. In extreme cases, hospitalization is required, resulting in absence from work or school.	Leisure and play skills are often impaired, as the individual with an eating disorder will use any available time for exercise.	The individual with an eating disorder often avoids social contact for fear of having the disorder discovered by others or because of poor self-esteem and self confidence. Additionally, social events involving food (such as going to a restaurant with friends) may be avoided.
TIC DISORDERS **Tourette's Syndrome**	Motor tics may interfere with performance of ADLs. Motor and vocal tics may interfere with ADLs that require public activities, such as shopping.	Tics may interfere with the ability to concentrate on school or work tasks. Additionally, the tics may be disruptive to others making concentration difficult. The adolescent may have difficulty finding employment in a setting with other people because of the bizarre nature of some tics.	Leisure activities with others may be impaired because of avoidance by others. Motor tics may interfere with physical leisure activities. Leisure activities that are engrossing and performed alone are often unimpaired; in fact, the tics may decrease or disappear during these activities.	The child or adolescent with a tic disorder is often avoided by both adults and children because of the bizarre and disruptive nature of many tics. Additionally, the sufferer is often embarrassed to be seen by others and thus is socially withdrawn.

TABLE 10-1

Impact of Selected Mental Disorders on Occupational Performance—cont'd

PSYCHOSOCIAL DISORDER	ACTIVITIES OF DAILY LIVING FUNCTIONING	SCHOOL AND WORK FUNCTIONING	PLAY AND LEISURE FUNCTIONING	SOCIAL FUNCTIONING
MOOD DISORDERS **Major** **Depressive** **Disorder**	Decreased energy and apathy impair the child or adolescent's participation in ADLs. Sleep and appetite disturbances also affect this area. In severe cases, personal hygiene and grooming are performed only with encouragement and supervision.	Symptoms of this disorder include decreased energy and concentration. Both symptoms impair the individual's performance on academic activities, chores, and work tasks.	The child or adolescent with this disorder typically suffers from anhedonia and stops engaging in previously enjoyable activities, such as toys or games.	Decreased socialization is a typical feature of this disorder. The child or adolescent with this disorder withdraws from others and appears disinterested in social interaction.
SUBSTANCE-RELATED DISORDERS	ADLs may be neglected because of the time spent getting, using, and recovering from substances. Use of substances may result in apathy about hygiene and appearance. Excessive use of substances can result in neglect of proper nutrition. Large amounts of money may be spent buying substances.	School and work performance is impaired. Tardiness, absences, and neglect of school or work assignments and homework may occur. Suspension may result if the individual is caught using substances at school or work. In severe chronic cases, permanent cognitive impairment may result.	Activities with individuals who do not use substances are often replaced by those associated with the substance use. The individual may drop out of school or neighborhood sports and spend time "hanging out" or partying. In severe cases, the individual will spend all leisure time in substance-related activities.	Interaction with both adults and peers may be impaired. The young person with this disorder may withdraw from family and peers, and develop friendships with other substance-using peers.

are considered skills needed for successful participation in the major performance areas. Regardless, a discussion of the impact of mental disorders on occupational performance would not be complete without this inclusion.

DATA GATHERING AND EVALUATION

Evaluation provides a starting point from which to develop the treatment plan for any dysfunction. According to Early, "The main purpose of evaluation in psychiatric occupational therapy is to find out what things the client needs or wants to be able to do, and whether or not the client can do them."[8] The registered occupational therapist (OTR) and the certified occupational therapy assistant (COTA) have related roles in evaluation of the child or adolescent with a mental disorder. The OTR has the

ultimate responsibility for the treatment planning process, which includes gathering and interpreting the evaluation information. The OTR determines specific areas of evaluation and specific assessment methods and tools. Once service competency is established, specific aspects of the information gathering process may be assigned to the COTA, including review of records, interviews, observations, and structured assessments. Information collection should focus on occupational performance and the individual's daily roles. ADLs are evaluated to determine the specific areas impaired by the disorder; for the child or adolescent these areas include bathing, dressing, grooming, and eating. Educational and vocational skills are evaluated to identify specific areas of deficit in school, chores, or work skills (if appropriate), such as concentration and attention span, ability to follow instructions, rate of work, and neatness of work. Leisure skills are evaluated to identify the individual's participation in play and fun activities, which are essential for a healthy balance of occupations. The child or adolescent's social skills should be evaluated to determine ability to express feelings and relate to others appropriately. Because decreased self-esteem is a common symptom of most disorders discussed in this chapter, the occupational therapy practitioner must address the child or adolescent's self-esteem during the evaluation process.

Many methods can be used to gather information about the child or adolescent's current level of functioning. The COTA may be assigned the task of reviewing the client's records. Inpatient and outpatient settings typically maintain medical records that can provide information about the client's age, sex, academic level and performance, family situation, cultural background, diagnosis, medical history, psychiatric history, medications, and current symptoms. In the school setting, educational records are reviewed for pertinent information.

Interviews with the child or adolescent and family members can provide information about the individual's home environment, performance of self-care tasks, relationships with family members, and participation in leisure activities. Other members of the treatment team also may provide valuable insight into the child or adolescent's occupational performance. For example, in an inpatient setting, nursing staff members can identify the client's specific problems with ADLs. In the school setting, teachers will be able to identify specific problems that interfere with learning and academic performance.

Observation is one of the most important evaluation tools of the occupational therapy practitioner. Much can be learned about specific deficits in occupational performance by observing the individual's activities. ADLs, work, and social skills can be assessed through observation. For example, by observing the child or adolescent during a classroom activity, the occupational therapy practitioner may be able to identify specific problems in concentration, attention span, work skills (such as neatness and rate of completion), and behavioral deficits that interfere with learning. Observation of the child or adolescent during recess will provide information about social skills including the amount and appropriateness of interactions with peers and participation in available leisure activities. A structured observation opportunity may be designed as part of the evaluation process. The child or adolescent may be asked to perform a specific activity (such as stringing beads to make a bracelet) while the COTA observes the performance for strengths and deficits in behavior, interactions, and work skills.

Structured evaluation tools may be used to assess occupational performance of children and adolescents. Specific occupational therapy assessments for use with this population are limited, but many occupational therapy departments have developed facility-specific assessments by modifying and combining available tools to meet the needs of the specific setting and client population.

Structured assessment tools for the assessment of self-esteem in the child or adolescent include the Piers-Harris Children's Self-Concept Scale. This instrument was developed to assess the ways children and adolescents ages 8 to 18 feel about themselves. The assessment consists of an 80-item, self-report questionnaire that addresses the child or adolescent's self-perception in the areas of behavior, intelligence and academic performance, appearance and personal traits, anxiety, popularity, and happiness. The test is available in paper or computer version and is inexpensive, easy to administer, and can be conducted by paraprofessionals (including COTAs) in either individual or group settings. A high score on the assessment indicates a positive self-evaluation and a low score indicates a negative self-evaluation.[15] This assessment can provide a good indication of the impact of the mental disorder on the child or adolescent's self-esteem.

The adolescent role assessment was developed by an OTR to assist occupational therapy practitioners in the identification of developmental strengths and weaknesses in adolescents. It is administered in the form of a semistructured interview with questions about the adolescent's childhood play, socialization with the family, at school, and with peers, occupational choice, and future work goals and plans. Each question has specific scoring criteria to reduce subjectivity. The adolescent receives a score of plus (+) for appropriate responses, a minus (−) for inappropriate responses, and a zero (0) for answers that are vague or indicate marginal behavior. A majority of plus scores indicates appropriate behavior and developmental consistency, a majority of minus scores indicates inappropriate behavior and developmental inconsistency, and a large number of zero scores may indicate apathy or an unwillingness to participate in the assessment. A majority of plus and zero scores indicates no role impairment, whereas a majority of minus and zero scores signifies severe impairment in role behavior and indicates the need for treatment.[13]

The use of the adolescent role assessment in the identification of specific developmental inconsistencies provides the occupational therapy practitioner with a baseline for the establishment of goals. For example, if the adolescent receives scores of minus or zero on questions regarding family and school responsibilities, an appropriate treatment focus would be the development of responsible behaviors. Table 10-2 shows other structured assessments that may be useful in the evaluation process with children and adolescents.

TABLE 10-2

Assessments Appropriate for Use with Children and Adolescents with Psychosocial Dysfunctions

ASSESSMENT	APPROPRIATE AGES	PURPOSE
Vocational Interest Inventory Revised (VII-R)	High school students	Assesses vocational interests
Locus of Control for Children	School-age children	Assesses perception of control over personal actions
Self-Esteem Scale	Adolescents	Assesses attitudes about abilities and accomplishments
Stanford Preschool Internal-External Scale (SPIES)	Preschool-age children	Assesses perceptions of internal versus external control over behaviors and feelings
Tennessee Self-Concept Scale (TSCS)	12 yr and older	Assesses self-concept
AAMR Adaptive Behavior Scale—Residential and Community, Second Edition (ABS-RC:2); AAMR Adaptive Behavior Scale—School, second edition (ABS-S:2)	3 yr and older	Assesses the ability to cope with environmental demands in mentally retarded, emotionally impaired, and developmentally disabled individuals
Coping Inventory	3-16 yr	Assesses the ability to cope with environmental demands
Social Climate Scale: Family Environment Scale, third edition (FES)	5 yr and older	Assesses strengths and problems of families
Canadian Occupational Performance Measure, second edition (COPM)	7 yr and older	Assesses self-perception of changes in and satisfaction with occupational performance over time
Occupational Performance History Interview (OPHI)	Adolescents and adults	Gathers historical information and perceptions regarding occupational performance based on the Model of Human Occupation
Occupational Questionnaire	Adolescents and adults	Assesses use of time based on the Model of Human Occupation
Self-Assessment of Occupational Functioning (SAOF); Children's Self-Assessment of Occupational Functioning	10 yr and older	Self assessment that assesses level of functioning, strengths and priorities, based on the Model of Human Occupation
Kohlman Evaluation of Living Skills (KELS), third edition	Adolescents and adults	Assesses ability to perform living skills and independence of clients in short-term psychiatric settings
Interest Checklist	Adolescents and adults (including older adults)	Assesses leisure interests and participation in leisure activities
Allen Cognitive Level Test (ACL)	All ages (must be old enough to follow instructions)	Assesses cognitive function according to Allen's cognitive levels of function in any psychiatric population
Cognitive Adaptive Skills Evaluation	Adolescents and adults	Assesses cognitive function
Goodenough-Harris Drawing Test	3-15 yr	Assesses conceptual maturity (which, according to the author, can indicate intellectual ability)
Assessment of Communication and Interaction Skills (ACIS)	All ages	Assesses personal communication and group interaction skills in individuals with psychiatric disorders
Assessment of Motor Skills and Process Skills (AMPS)	5 yr and older	Assesses ADL and IADL skills

Modified from Asher IE, *Occupational therapy assessment tools: an annotated index*, ed 2, Bethesda, Md, 1996, American Occupational Therapy Association.

INTERVENTION PLANNING AND IMPLEMENTATION

The intervention plan is developed following completion of the evaluation. According to AOTA's "Standards of Practice for Occupational Therapy," the intervention planning process includes identifying strengths and weaknesses, estimating rehabilitation potential, developing long- and short-term goals, developing methods and activities to accomplish the goals, collaborating with the client and other appropriate individuals, determining frequency and duration of treatment, planning for reevaluation, and planning for discharge from treatment.[2] Although the OTR is ultimately responsible for the intervention plan, the COTA can contribute to all above steps of the intervention planning.

Strengths and weaknesses can be identified using the data gathered during evaluation. Health care professionals tend to focus on the child or adolescent's deficits rather than strengths; however, if treatment is to be effective it is critical to identify and capitalize on these strengths when developing goals and determining treatment activities. It is equally important to develop goals based on the child or adolescent's interests, cultural environment, and needs.

As discussed in Chapter 12, long-term goals identify the desired treatment outcome and short-term goals identify steps toward achievement of the long-term goal. Goals must always relate to function and be designed to improve one or more areas of occupational performance. For example, one desired treatment outcome for a child or adolescent with major depressive disorder displaying apathy and anhedonia may be to increase purposeful activities. This long-term goal directly relates to the ability to develop the competence needed to be effective in occupational performance roles, because children and adolescents explore and master their environment through purposeful activities.

Short-term goals are the building blocks to the achievement of the long-term goal and must be specific and measurable. Short-term goals for the child or adolescent with apathy and anhedonia symptoms may be increased participation in ADLs and leisure activities and increased ability to follow a daily schedule independently. Box 10-2 provides an example of a long-term goal and short-term goals. Reassessment must be an ongoing process with all clients; and goals must be continuously reviewed for appropriateness and modified as needed.

Treatment must be structured to provide an opportunity to experience and practice impaired skills. Treatment for children and adolescents may occur individually or in group settings, although most occupational therapy intervention with this population occurs in group settings. Well-designed occupational therapy treatment groups provide the optimal environment for achieving treatment goals, facilitating interaction, and developing competence. Regardless of whether treatment occurs individually or in groups, intervention must address specific concerns including structure and consistency, opportunities for interactions with others, and characteristics of treatment activities.

According to Cara and McRae, structure and consistency are of utmost importance in the treatment of children and adolescents with psychosocial disorders.[7] In this context, structure refers to the specific design of the environment, such as stating the rules, expectations, and consequences for inappropriate behavior at the beginning of each session. Consistency refers to the enforcement of the stated rules, expectations, and consequences in every instance. Behavioral expectations and consequences for occupational therapy sessions must be outlined at the beginning of treatment and consistently enforced.[9]

The treatment environment must be structured to provide opportunities for the child or adolescent to practice social skills. In an individual session the therapist should encourage and reinforce communication and appropriate social skills. Group sessions should be designed to facilitate interactions with both the therapist and peers. The sharing of tools and materials with other group members during activities or participation in a group activity such as baking cookies facilitates interactions among peers and provides opportunities for the development of teamwork and group cooperation skills. The occupational therapy practitioner should encourage socialization between group members working on individual activities.

BOX 10-2

Goals for a Child or Adolescent with Major Depressive Disorder Exhibiting Apathy and Anhedonia

LONG-TERM GOAL
By discharge, client will demonstrate increased participation in purposeful activities.

Short-Term Goal #1
By the end of Week 1, client will participate in 2 previously enjoyed leisure activities.

Short-Term Goal #2
By the end of Week 1, client will independently perform daily personal hygiene tasks (shower, comb hair, and brush teeth).

Short-Term Goal #3
By the end of Week 1, client will arrive daily at occupational therapy clinic at scheduled time without prompting.

Activities should be carefully analyzed to ensure they will promote developmentally appropriate skills and facilitate goal accomplishment. Activities may include toys, games, and crafts that are developmentally appropriate, interesting, fun, and provide a challenge. Creative arts and role playing also are useful activities. Cara and MacRae address four issues of consideration when planning activities for children and adolescents: (1) whether the activity is age-appropriate, (2) the ability of the activity to be broken down into understandable steps, (3) whether each step is age-appropriate and can be completed independently, and (4) whether the occupational therapy practitioner wants the child to do the activity independently or ask for assistance.[7]

As mentioned, group treatment sessions are extremely effective with this population. In addition to providing opportunities for clients to learn and practice skills and interact with their peers, groups allow occupational therapy practitioners to maintain productivity by simultaneously providing quality treatment for multiple clients.

Group sessions are usually designed to address specific problem areas or age groups. For example, in a school setting the occupational therapy practitioner may design a task group for children in first through third grades who have difficulty attending to a task or demonstrate poor work skills. Children can develop or improve the skills needed to complete tasks effectively by working on individual craft projects. During group sessions the occupational therapy practitioner can adapt the planned activities to provide opportunities for success and facilitate the development of social skills, coping skills, and self-esteem. Table 10-3 provides sample occupational therapy groups for this population.

TABLE 10-3

Sample Occupational Therapy Groups for Children or Adolescents with Psychosocial Dysfunction

GROUP TITLE	PURPOSE	GOALS	METHODS	APPROPRIATE POPULATION
KIDS CAN COOK GROUP	To encourage, promote, and teach basic independent living skills and age-appropriate interpersonal skills	Provide opportunities to accomplish the following: • Increase the ability to plan, organize, follow directions, and carry out a task • Learn and practice cooperation and teamwork • Learn and practice good manners and sharing skills • Learn and practice safety and health in ADLs	Small-group cooking and eating activities	Children 4-11 yr who meet the following criteria: • Function on a developmentally appropriate level, both cognitively and intellectually • Are able to comply with and follow directions without disrupting the group process
IMAGINATION GROUP	To teach and reinforce concepts and skills important to the achievement of the developmental tasks of childhood	Provide opportunities to accomplish the following: • Learn to distinguish between right and wrong and begin to develop a conscience, morality, and values • Improve peer interactions • Work toward age-appropriate independence	Group storytelling sessions; audiovisual aids, puppetry, and role play activities	Children 3-11 yr who meet the following criteria: • Function on a developmentally appropriate level, both cognitively and intellectually • Are able to comply with and follow directions without disrupting the group process

Data courtesy Mary Beth Brock, Institute of Psychiatry, Medical University of South Carolina, Charleston, SC.

Continued

TABLE 10-3

Sample Occupational Therapy Groups for Children or Adolescents with Psychosocial Dysfunction—cont'd

GROUP TITLE	PURPOSE	GOALS	METHODS	APPROPRIATE POPULATION
IMAGINATION GROUP— cont'd		• Develop wholesome, positive attitudes toward self and others • Develop healthy attitudes toward social groups, institutions, and authority figures		
TASK SKILLS GROUP	To teach the fundamentals of task performance and to improve the ability to successfully carry out task activities	Provide opportunities to improve the following task skills: • Neatness and attention to detail • Task organization, planning, and implementation • Ability to follow directions • Task completion • Recognition of errors and problem-solving skills • Preparation of materials and clean up of work area Provide opportunities to improve or learn coping skills in the following problem areas: • Short attention span • Poor impulse control • Excessive motor activity • Decreased memory skills • Distractibility • Low frustration tolerance • Difficulty delaying gratification Provide opportunities to increase self-esteem and self-confidence	Short-term therapeutic media (craft activities); short-term creative art activities	Children and adolescents 3-18 yr who meet the following criteria: • Function on a developmentally appropriate level, both cognitively and intellectually • Are able to comply with and follow directions without disrupting the group process • Are able to handle tools, materials, and supplies safely and appropriately

Data courtesy Mary Beth Brock, Institute of Psychiatry, Medical University of South Carolina, Charleston, SC.

TABLE 10-3

Sample Occupational Therapy Groups for Children or Adolescents with Psychosocial Dysfunction—cont'd

GROUP TITLE	PURPOSE	GOALS	METHODS	APPROPRIATE POPULATION
TASK SKILLS GROUP— cont'd		Provide opportunities to increase social skills and the ability to share space and materials in a group setting Provide opportunities to explore and develop healthy leisure interests		
COMMUNI-CATION SKILLS GROUP	To provide concrete activities that enhance and encourage the development of more effective interpersonal communication skills	Increase awareness of existing communication style and the impact of this style on others Enhance interpersonal and social skills Increase assertiveness Improve spontaneity and self-confidence when expressing self in the presence of others	Group activities, including verbal and nonverbal techniques, such as pencil and paper tasks, creative art activities, games, role playing, leader presentations, and audiovisuals	Adolescents 13-18 yr who meet the following criteria: • Function on a developmentally appropriate level, both cognitively and intellectually • Are able to comply with and follow directions without disrupting the group process
SELF-AWARENESS	To provide concrete activities that increase insight and self-awareness	Teach feelings identification and increase feelings vocabulary	Group activities, including verbal and nonverbal techniques such as pencil and paper tasks, creative art activities, games, roles play, leader presentations, and audiovisual activities	Adolescents 13-18 yr who meet the following criteria: • Function on a developmentally appropriate level, both cognitively and intellectually • Are able to comply with and follow directions without disrupting the group process • Are able to emotionally cope with personal exploration and self-discovery

SUMMARY

Children and adolescents can have a variety of mental disorders that affect every area of occupational performance and interfere with normal development. Occupational therapy practitioners may encounter children and adolescents with psychosocial dysfunction in several settings. In many children and adolescents, physical dysfunction often accompanies mental disorders. The occupational therapy practitioner should have the skills to treat psychosocial and physical needs for every child and adolescent.

References

1. Adults should heed teens' warning signs, *USA Today Magazine* 126:4 1997.
2. American Occupational Therapy Association: Standards of practice for occupational therapy. In American Occupational Therapy Association: *Reference manual of the official documents of the American Occupational Therapy Association*, ed 6, Bethesda, Md, 1996, The Association.
3. American Occupational Therapy Association: Uniform terminology for occupational therapy, ed 3, *Am J Occup Ther* 48:1047, 1994.
4. American Psychiatric Association: *Diagnostic and statistical manual of mental disorders*, ed 4, Washington, DC, 1994, The Association.
5. Asher IE: *Occupational therapy assessment tools: an annotated index*, ed 2, Bethesda, Md, 1996, American Occupational Therapy Association.
6. Bonder BR: *Psychopathology and function*, ed 2, Thorofare, NJ, 1995, Slack.
7. Cara E, MacRae A: Psychosocial occupational therapy: a clinical practice, Albany, NY, 1998, Delmar.
8. Early MB: *Mental health concepts and techniques for the occupational therapy assistant*, ed 2, New York, 1993, Raven.
9. Florey L: Psychosocial dysfunction in childhood and adolescence. In Neistadt ME, Crepeau EB: *Willard and Spackman's occupational therapy*, ed 9, Philadelphia, 1998, Lippincott.
10. Gutkind L: *Stuck in time: the tragedy of childhood mental illness*, New York, 1993, Henry Holt.
11. Hafen BQ, Frandsen KJ: *Youth suicide: depression and loneliness*, Evergreen, Col, 1984, Cordillera.
12. Harrison PA, Fulkerson JA, Beebe TJ: DSM-IV substance use disorder criteria for adolescents: a critical examination based on a statewide school survey, *Am J Psychiatry* 155:486, 1998.
13. Hemphill BJ, editor: *The evaluative process in psychosocial occupational therapy*, Thorofare, NJ, 1982, Slack.
14. Hermes, P: *A time to listen: preventing youth suicide*, San Diego, 1987, Harcourt Brace Jovanovich.
15. Piers EV: *Piers-Harris children's self-concept scale*, rev ed, Los Angeles, 1984, Western Psychological Services.
16. Sherry CJ: *Inhalants*, New York, 1994, Rosen.
17. Winter PA, editor: *Teen addiction*, San Diego, 1997, Greenhaven.

REVIEW *Questions*

1. What is a mental disorder and in what way does it affect a child or an adolescent's participation in purposeful activity?
2. Briefly describe the primary symptoms of each of the following disorders: conduct disorder, oppositional defiant disorder, separation anxiety disorder, Tourette's syndrome, anorexia nervosa and bulimia nervosa, major depressive disorder, and substance dependence.
3. Briefly describe the way each disorder in Question 4 affects occupational performance.
4. List appropriate methods for gathering data when evaluating children and adolescents with mental disorders.
5. Describe important considerations when designing intervention for this population.

SUGGESTED *Activities*

1. Visit day-care centers and observe children engaged in educational or play activities. Note normal psychosocial behavior and behaviors that may indicate dysfunction, such as aggression, isolation, and poor attention span.
2. Visit a place where adolescents gather such as a mall. Note interactions among adolescents.
3. Many videos that depict mental disorders in children and adolescents are available through campus learning resource centers. Watch videos on the disorders discussed in this chapter and imagine the way you would feel if the child or adolescent were a member of your family. List the questions and concerns that come to mind.
4. Contact the National Alliance for the Mentally Ill (1-800-950-6264) for information on family support.

Other Common Pediatric Disorders

GRETCHEN EVANS PARKER

CHAPTER *Objectives*

After studying this chapter, the reader will be able to accomplish the following:

- Understand the reason having a broad knowledge base of pediatric conditions is important
- Understand the reason knowing the child's diagnosis aids in treatment planning
- Recognize which organ systems specific conditions affect
- Describe the ways different conditions affect children
- Understand that each condition has common specific treatments needs, which aids in treatment planning
- Describe basic treatment precautions for specific pediatric conditions
- Describe the roles of the COTA and OTR in treatment in the discussed conditions

KEY TERMS

Orthopedic conditions
Amputation
Arthrogryposis
Juvenile rheumatoid arthritis
Genetic conditions
Duchenne muscular dystrophy
Down syndrome
Neurological conditions
Spina bifida
Shaken baby syndrome
Seizures
Sensory system conditions
Vision impairments
Hearing impairments
General sensory disorganization
Fussy baby
Environmentally induced and
acquired conditions
Fetal alcohol syndrome
Acquired immunodeficiency
syndrome

CHAPTER OUTLINE

ORTHOPEDIC CONDITIONS
Amputation
Arthrogryposis
Juvenile Rheumatoid Arthritis
Osteoporosis

GENETIC CONDITIONS
Muscular Dystrophy
Down Syndrome
Chronic Fatigue Immune Dysfunction Syndrome and Fibromyalgia

NEUROLOGICAL CONDITIONS
Spina Bifida
Shaken Baby Syndrome
Erb's Palsy
Seizures

SENSORY SYSTEM CONDITIONS
Vision Impairments
Hearing Impairments

GENERAL SENSORY DISORGANIZATION
Fussy Baby
Language Delay and Language Impairments

ENVIRONMENTALLY INDUCED AND ACQUIRED CONDITIONS
Failure to Thrive
Fetal Alcohol Syndrome
Effects of Cocaine Use
Human Immunodeficiency Virus
Latex Allergies
Lead Poisoning
Allergies to Foods or Chemicals

ROLE OF COTA AND OTR IN ASSESSMENT AND INTERVENTION

SUMMARY

This chapter explores pediatric conditions; it is organized by organ systems and the way the child acquires the condition being discussed. Its design gives the reader a better understanding of the many types of pediatric conditions encountered by occupational therapy practitioners and an understanding of the major symptoms and signs of the more common diagnoses. Knowing the basic characteristics of a specific condition serves as a framework for assessment and treatment of the child. Understanding the characteristics of different pediatric conditions enables the practitioner to be a better equipped member of the child's intervention team.

This chapter focuses on a hypothetical certified occupational therapy assistant (COTA) named Jill as she and her direct supervisor, Margaret, a registered occupational therapist (OTR), evaluate and treat children at the clinic where they work. One day a week, Jill and Margaret visit the school around the corner. There they consult with the teachers who have students with disabilities in their classes. They also help with the vocational readiness program in the class for students with developmental delays. Margaret meets with Jill weekly to review charts and discuss any needed updates to the children's therapy goals. Additionally, Margaret and Jill cotreat the children on Jill's caseload every seventh visit.

Once a month, Margaret indulges her love of horses by consulting at the therapeutic horseback riding program in the neighboring town. There she provides supervision for a COTA, Greg, who is involved in a therapeutic riding class that is focused on children with a variety of health-related problems, including orthopedic conditions and sensory processing problems.

ORTHOPEDIC CONDITIONS

Orthopedic conditions involve bones, joints, and muscles. Frequently, functional deficits are also present in the performance areas of activities of daily living (ADLs), play and leisure, and work and productive skills because of the orthopedic problems.

Amputation

Beth was born with an above elbow **amputation** *(Table 11-1). At the age of 3 months, she had her first occupational therapy appointment. Margaret, her OTR, did a developmental evaluation at that time and determined that Beth was achieving all her developmental milestones. Margaret and Beth's mother, Melanie, discussed the pros and cons of fitting Beth with a prosthesis. Margaret told Melanie that most children with congenital upper extremity amputations choose to use a prosthesis as a tool some of the time, but they learn adaptive techniques for performing many activities without it. Small children often use the*

sensations in their stump for learning about the environment. Margaret gave Melanie some books as well as phone numbers of other parents with children who had congenital upper extremity amputations. She suggested that Melanie and her husband spend some time talking to other people who had experienced raising a child with an upper extremity amputation. After a lot of research, Beth's parents decided to wait to have her fitted with a prosthesis until 2 years of age because she could then begin to understand its use as a tool. They also thought that at 2 years her language skill level would make it easier to learn to use the prosthesis. They felt that Beth would gradually learn whether to do things with or without it. Her first prosthesis had a friction elbow that did not lock and a rubber mitt. Later an adept hand was added. Made of plastic, it had one C-shaped "finger" with an indentation in the end for the opposing "thumb" to fit into. The adept hand opened until she chose to close it by pulling on a cable attached to a shoulder harness.

Beth is now 7 years old. She has had two surgeries for the end of the bone in her stump. Every year she has a prosthesis revision, and small details are added or changed. Now that she is older, Beth's parents include her in the decisions for changes. The family has learned that Beth usually knows what works for her better than anyone else on her treatment team. Whenever a change is made, Jill, the COTA, spends a few occupational therapy sessions with

TABLE 11-1

Types of Congenital Upper Extremity Amputations

TYPE OF DEFICIENCY	MISSING SKELETAL PARTS
TRANSVERSE AMELIA Forequarter amputation	All or most of the arm is missing from the shoulder and below.
TRANSVERSE HEMIMELIA Below elbow	All of the arm is missing from amputation the elbow and below.
LONGITUDINAL HEMIMELIA Partial amputation	One of the long bones of the forearm is missing. Fingers or thumb may or may not be missing.
PHOCOMELIA	Bones of the upper or lower arm are missing. All or part of the hand remains.

Modified from Rothstein JM, Roy HR, Wolf SL: *The rehabilitation specialist's handbook,* ed 2, Philadelphia, 1998, FA Davis.

Beth exploring the new uses and operation of the updated prosthesis. During these sessions, Jill and Margaret work closely together; training requires a specific understanding of the way the prosthesis components work and function. Margaret always directs Beth and Jill's interactions during these sessions because she has more experience. Jill's role is to implement the therapy goals Margaret has planned. Jill reports Beth's progress to Margaret, as well as any needs for change in treatment.

An infant born missing all or part of a limb has a congenital amputation. A traumatic amputation is the result of an accident, an infection, or cancer. About 2 to 8 children in 10,000 are born missing all or part of a limb each year. Types of amputations vary greatly (see Table 11-1). Thumb and below elbow amputations are the most common types of upper extremity congenital amputations.[31]

CLINICAL *Pearl*

Therapy for an older child who has lost a limb as a result of trauma or surgery is different than therapy for a child with a congenital amputation. A child who loses a limb later in childhood benefits from having a prosthesis fitted as soon as possible for psychological and rehabilitation reasons.

Fitting a prosthesis on a child with a congenital amputation at a very young age allows the child to reach developmental milestones on time. It is less likely to be rejected when the child is older if it becomes a part of the child's body concept early in life. With a less severe congenital amputation a child often does well without a prosthesis until older. Sometimes the child does not use a prosthesis at all. Use of any prosthesis depends on the severity of the amputation and whether one or both arms are involved.

Arthrogryposis

Courtney is a 4-year-old girl with a beautiful face and a vocabulary that is large for a child of her age. Her arms and legs have a tubular shape; the skin between her fingers and in the fold of her knees and elbows is webbed. During her first 2 years of life, Courtney could not sit on the floor to play because her hips and knees did not bend, and her feet turned in so much that the soles faced each other (that is, she had clubbed feet). To get from place to place, she rolled along the floor using the normal movement of her trunk. Her shoulders and forearms turned inward so that the back of her hands always touched her sides. She currently cannot bend her elbows, and her wrists are permanently bent toward her forearms. Her finger movement is very limited and weak, leaving her with no functional pinching ability. The palms of her hands are narrow and almost fold together.

Because her hips and knees would not bend, Courtney had surgery at the age of 2 years. Her clubbed feet were also surgically repaired so that she could place the sole of her foot on the floor. Before the surgery, she stood on the sides of her feet; now she can stand for short periods but cannot get to a standing position without help. To keep her legs stable while standing, she wears braces on her knees and ankles. Seated at a table of the right height, Courtney can move toys that are moderately sized and not too heavy. She grasps small things by pressing them between the backs of her wrists.

During Courtney's infancy the COTA saw her daily for many months to stretch her muscles and maintain the joint motion she had at birth. The stretching was very painful. Courtney's cries during therapy would often drive her mother from the clinic. To gain maximum increases in joint mobility, the stretching was begun immediately after Courtney was born and continued for several months.[4] Stretching requires great care to avoid damaging joint, muscle, and bone tissue. Jill worked closely with Margaret to determine the amount of stretching to be done. Jill made resting pan splints for Courtney to wear to encourage functional wrist and hand positioning. Because her triceps constantly pulled her elbows straight, Jill also made soft fabric bands to hold Courtney's elbows bent for 10 to 15 minutes at a time throughout the day, which also helped reduce her elbow extension contractures.

CLINICAL *Pearl*

Parents of a newborn with **arthrogryposis** have a lot to learn in a short period. Functional gains are made only in the early months of life. To maintain the gains in joint movement made during therapy, a clearly written home program should be created so that the parents have easy-to-follow guidelines. The program should include specific exercises, precautions, and a clearly written splint-wearing schedule.

CLINICAL *Pearl*

A dynamic elbow flexion splint for an infant with arthrogryposis can be made with elastic and orthoplast. The elbow straightens against the pull of elastic; the elastic then pulls the elbow into flexion, allowing hand-to-mouth movement. The dynamic elbow flexion splint allows infants to do activities such as eat finger foods or blow bubbles.

Ongoing therapy is important for helping children with arthrogryposis meet educational, self-care, and play needs. Because of the multiple physical limitations, activities in all areas of their life require adaptations. Technology can provide many play, education, and environmental adaptations (see Chapter 16). Close consultation with family members and school personnel enhances the team approach to treatment and case management.

Arthrogryposis is not genetic; the cause is usually never known. In its classic form, all the joints of the extremities are stiff (but the spine is not affected). The shoulders are turned in, elbows are straight, and wrists are flexed with ulnar deviation. The hips may be dislocated and the knees straight with the feet turned in. Arm and leg muscles are small and difficult to see, with webbed skin covering some or all of the joints. The condition is the worst at birth, so any increases in range of motion (ROM) or joint motion are improvements.[4] In typical cases all the joints of the arms and legs are fixed in one position, which is partly caused by muscle imbalance or lack of muscle development during gestation.

Juvenile Rheumatoid Arthritis

Five-year-old Amber is a cheerful kindergartner who loves riding her bike. Occasionally she becomes irritable, and her mom knows it is time for Amber to take a break from riding the bike. Amber has pauciarticular arthritis, a type of **juvenile rheumatoid arthritis** *(JRA) (Table 11-2), and her joints can become painful, hot, and swollen. Once a month, Amber visits Jill, the COTA, at the clinic to review her home program of passive and active stretching and strengthening activities. During each visit the OTR, Margaret, measures all of Amber's joints with a goniometer to be sure Amber's ROM is not deteriorating.*

By the time they are adults, 75% of individuals with JRA have permanent remission.[31] There are three types of JRA: Still's disease (20% of JRA cases), pauciarticular arthritis (40% of JRA cases), and polyarticular arthritis (40% of JRA cases)[4] (see Table 11-2). Children with JRA experience exacerbations and remissions of symptoms. During exacerbations, or "flare ups," symptoms worsen and the joints become hot and painful; joint damage can

TABLE II-2

Three Types of Juvenile Rheumatoid Arthritis

TYPE	LIMB INVOLVEMENT	FUNCTIONAL IMPLICATIONS
PAUCIARTICULAR (FEW JOINTS) Affects four or fewer joints Comprises approximately 40% of JRA cases	Only a few unmatched joints are affected. Leg joints are usually affected, but elbows can also be affected. Children often recover in 1-2 yr. Children can develop an eye inflammation called *iritis* that can lead to blindness unless it is treated early.	Pain and joint stiffness may limit activities. Contractures can develop. Splints may be needed. Work simplification may be needed. Adaptive equipment may be needed. Climbing stairs may be difficult.
POLYARTICULAR (MANY JOINTS) Comprises approximately 30% of JRA cases Five or more joints affected Girls more commonly affected than boys	Onset is fast. The symmetrical joints of legs, wrists, hands, and sometimes the neck are affected.	Functional implications are the same as those for pauciarticular arthritis but also include the following: Activities can be limited by fatigue Difficulty with fine motor activities
STILL'S DISEASE Affects joints as well as internal organs Comprises approximately 20% of JRA cases	The onset speed and affected limbs are the same as those for polyarticular arthritis. Other organs such as the spleen and lymph system may also be affected. Bone damage may affect growth.	Functional implications are the same as those for polyarticular arthritis but also include the following: Rash and fever may develop, last for weeks, and require bed confinement.

Modified from Case-Smith J, Allen AS, Pratt PN: *Occupational therapy for children,* St Louis, 1996, Mosby; Arthritis Foundation: *www.arthritis.org.*

occur. During flare ups, children need joint protection (Boxes 11-1 and 11-2). During remission, or pain-free periods, more normal activities can be resumed. Joint protection efforts should be encouraged even during periods of remission so that their use becomes a habit.

Osteoporosis

Austin has multiple handicaps, is blind, and does not speak. He is 6 years old and can walk if someone holds his hand; he refuses to walk on his own, partly because of his blindness. He cries and falls when he is left standing with no support. Austin prefers to sit and scoot on his bottom, but his hips and knees are becoming stiff from sitting so much. Beginning contractures of the hips and knees are limiting his ability to stand up straight. Because of his blindness, he constantly alternates between pushing on his eyeballs or mouthing his hands. (See Visual Impairments section in this chapter.) These "blindisms," or self-stimulating behaviors, could cause elbow flexion contractures that would limit his ability to straighten his elbows. His pediatrician thinks standing independently and walking with a walker for stability would benefit Austin physically as well as make him easier to care for. His doctor has prescribed occupational therapy to his increase arm ROM and make elbow splints to maintain the ROM gained during therapy. The splints will also limit the self-stimulation activities. During his first stretching session, Austin's arm bone snapped and broke as Margaret began gentle stretching.

CLINICAL *Pearl*

To avoid causing fractures, use care when handling and doing ROM exercises with severely affected, inactive children. Maintaining good joint mobility with daily careful passive stretching and proper positioning that are initiated during infancy helps control osteoporosis.

In children with disabilities, osteoporosis is caused by a lack of weightbearing activities such as crawling or standing. The bones are weakened as a result of mineral loss; weightbearing activities and muscles pulling on bones during movement makes bone strong. Children who develop osteoporosis are usually severely affected as a result of some other condition such as cerebral palsy. They are usually very inactive and unable to stand; their bones can become so brittle that simple dressing activities could cause a fracture.

CLINICAL *Pearl*

With proper joint management, children can be placed in prone or supine standers for weightbearing activities. Standing is good not only for bone growth and strengthening but also for body functions such as circulation and digestion.

GENETIC CONDITIONS

Humans have 23 pairs of chromosomes, which are tiny, thread-shaped structures found in each cell of the body. Each chromosome is made up of tiny sections called *genes*. Half of the genes come from the mother through her egg, and others come from the father through the sperm. The genes are mixed together and determine every aspect of a

---

BOX 11-1

Rules of Joint Protection for Children with Juvenile Rheumatoid Arthritis

- If joints are warm and swollen, encourage children to use them carefully during all activities and to continue to do ROM exercises as much as they are able.
- Because tired muscles cannot protect joints, teach children that they should not remain in the same position, such as holding a pencil to write, for long periods without stretching or taking a break.
- Larger muscles are found around big joints, so teach children the way to use big joints for heavy work. For example, they can balance a lunch tray on their forearms, wear a backpack on both shoulders, or carry a purse over a shoulder rather than in a hand.
- If children become tired or are in pain, stop the activity.
- Proper positioning prevents contractures and deformities. Teach children that they should always use good posture.

BOX 11-2

Treatment for Juvenile Rheumatoid Arthritis

Splinting to prevent development of contractures
AROM and PROM exercises to maintain ROM
Careful monitoring of each joint to maintain functional level and prevent deformity
Exercises to maintain or increase strength
Teaching the importance of joint protection during all activities to prevent deformities or contractures

person's characteristics. Sometimes a gene carrying a specific problem can be passed from one or both parents to the child. Problems can develop when the mother and father's normal genes mix and match improperly or when an infant receives a gene with a mutation (that is, a gene that has been damaged or is abnormal in some way). **Genetic conditions** cause characteristic patterns of physical involvement and progression. Knowing whether a child has a genetic condition aids in determining the types of treatment interventions from which the child may benefit. About 30% of developmental disabilities result from inheriting a gene that causes the disability or one that has a particular mutation. Fifty percent of major hearing and vision problems are caused by genetic syndromes.[31] The more common conditions seen by the occupational therapy practitioner are discussed in this section. Children

with other genetic disorders may occasionally be seen as well. Descriptions for some of the additional genetic disorders are found in Table 11-3.

Muscular Dystrophy

Kevin has started second grade in a regular classroom, and his teacher is worried. When seated at his desk, he looks like the rest of students in the class, although his arms and legs look chubby. Though he is bright, he is having trouble keeping up with his classmates. He struggles to write, and his handwriting is hard to read. Recently he started to walk his fingers across the desk to get his pencil. It is hard for him to raise his hand to ask a question or get his books out of his desk. When the class goes to other parts of the school for gym or music, Kevin can easily be spotted by his waddling

TABLE 11-3

Additional Genetic Conditions

CONDITION AND GENETIC CAUSE	INCIDENCE	COMMON SYMPTOMS AND SIGNS	FUNCTIONAL IMPLICATIONS
TUBEROUS SCLEROSIS Autosomal dominant gene or mutation	1 in 20,000 births[22]	Very mild to severe symptoms Tumors in the brain; can cause seizures, mental retardation, delayed language skills, and motor problems (which is rare) Tumors in the heart, kidneys, eyes, or other organs; can (but may not) cause problems	Possible learning disabilities Possible aggressive or hyperactive behavior Possible inability to speak and need for alternative communication Possible severe delays in gross and fine motor skills Mild to severe delays in self help skills
ANGELMAN'S SYNDROME Deletion of mother's chromosome 15[14]	1 in 25,000[13]	Microcephaly (see Table 11-4) Tremors and jerky gait Developmental delays Severe language impairment; nonverbal or severe speech delay Very happy mood (happy puppet syndrome) Possible seizure disorder	Gross and fine motor delays, delayed walking skills Severely delayed self-care skills Inability to speak but possible use of alternative communication Sleep disorders (can be very disruptive to family life) Severe sensory processing problems Behavior problems such as biting, hair pulling, stubbornness, screaming

Continued

TABLE 11-3

Additional Genetic Conditions—cont'd

CONDITION AND GENETIC CAUSE	INCIDENCE	COMMON SYMPTOMS AND SIGNS	FUNCTIONAL IMPLICATIONS
PRADER-WILLI SYNDROME Deletion of father's chromosome 15[24]	1 in 15,000[24]	Growth failure related to poor suck-swallow reflex in infancy Obsession with food, possibly causing obesity (must lock all kitchen cabinets; PRECAUTION: may eat *anything*) Developmental delays, low intelligence Hypotonia and poor reflexes Speech problems related to hypotonia Laid back attitude but possible stubbornness and violent tantrums Severe stress on families resulting from behavior problems	Obsession with eating (can be dangerous during treatment) Gross and fine motor delays Delayed development of self-help skills Difficulty walking resulting from obesity or low muscle tone Possible need for alternative communication Possible benefits from prevocational and vocational training
RHETT SYNDROME Undetermined genetic cause[20]	Seen only in girls	Normal or near normal development first 6-18 mo of life Loss of skills and functional use of hands beginning at approximately 18 mo Loss or severely impaired ability to speak Development of repetitive, almost constant hand movements such as hand washing and wringing, clapping, and mouthing Shakiness in trunk and limbs Unsteady, wide-based, stiff-legged walking	Gross and fine motor problems Lacking or delayed development of self-help skills Difficulty walking or inability to walk Delayed response to requests, possibly taking up to 2 min to respond Possible need for alternative communication
FRAGILE X SYNDROME Mutation on X chromosome (most common genetic disease in humans)[15]	1 in 2000 males and 1 in 4000 females[15]	Boys more severely affected than girls Possible hyperactivity Low muscle tone Sensory processing problems involving touch and sound Possible autistic behavior Language delays (more common in boys); possible dysfunctional speech Intelligence problems ranging from learning disabilities to severe mental retardation	Mobility problems; delayed walking skills Gross and fine motor delays Delayed development of self-help skills Possible learning problems ranging from learning disabilities and ADD to mental retardation Possible need for alternative communication in boys (unusual for girls) Possible benefits from prevocational and vocational training

gait. He has lordosis (Figure 11-1) and to keep from falling forward, he carries his shoulders and head back. His gait looks like a slow march because he has to pick his feet up high so that his toes do not drag. He falls a lot. To get up from sitting, he "walks" his hands up his legs (Gower's sign). Kevin has **Duchenne muscular dystrophy** (MD).

The COTA, Jill, visits Kevin's school weekly. During a recent visit, Kevin's teacher met with Jill to tell her what was happening. Fortunately Jill already knew Kevin from the clinic and was able to give the teacher suggestions to help him meet his classroom needs. Jill suggested that Kevin start using a computer for his written work. She also suggested that rather than sitting at a regular school desk, he sit at a larger table and have all his books within easy reach.

Kevin's family brings him to the clinic several times a year so that Jill and Margaret can check on his adaptive equipment needs. Because his ability to move has decreased, Jill has taught the family ROM exercises to keep his joints loose, making it easier to dress and bathe him. She teaches them about proper body positioning to prevent contractures or scoliosis from developing (Figure 11-2). She has also given Kevin a list of strengthening exercises that will help him function independently for as long as possible. Jill knows that usually by the age of 9 years, children with Duchenne MD use a wheelchair at least part time.

MD comprises a group of muscle disorders. One of the more common types is Duchenne, or pseudohypertrophic (which literally means "false overgrowth"). In children with Duchenne-type MD, muscle breaks down and is replaced with fat and scar tissue, making the muscles, espe-

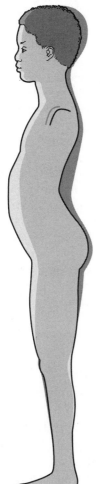

FIGURE 11-1 Lordosis—an increased forward curve of the lower back. Abdomen falls forward and the knees lock backward. Posture shifts weight forward; to balance weight, child tends to carry head and shoulders back farther than normal. This posture is common in children with hypotonia.

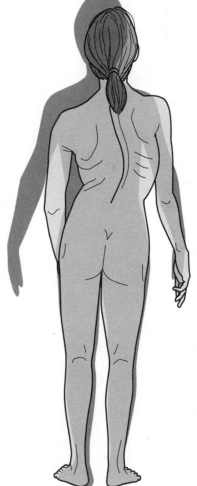

FIGURE 11-2 Scoliosis—a sideways bending of the vertebral column. In severe cases, ribs are rotated, compressing lungs and reducing their function.

BOX 11-3

Progression of Functional Losses in Children with Duchenne Muscular Dystrophy

LEVEL 1
Initially independent but has progressive functional losses over a period of several years: for example, walks independently but then loses stair-climbing ability, then needs leg braces to walk, then needs assistance to get up from a chair

LEVEL 2
In wheelchair: sits erect and is able to roll chair and perform ADLs such as upper extremity dressing, eating, and brushing the teeth in bed or chair

LEVEL 3
In wheelchair: sits erect but is unable to perform ADLs in bed or chair such as placing equipment conveniently or rolling over without assistance

LEVEL 4
In wheelchair: sits erect with support and can do minimal ADLs (such as brushing teeth or eating using adapted equipment)

LEVEL 5
In bed: can do no ADLs without assistance

Modified from Rothstein JM, Roy HR, Wolf SL: *The rehabilitation specialist's handbook*, ed 2, Philadelphia, 1998, FA Davis.

cially the calf muscles, look unusually large. Several other forms of MD also affect boys and girls but usually at a later age. Duchenne-type MD is only seen in boys. About 3 individuals per 100,000 develop the condition.[31] Most children with Duchenne MD survive until they are in their 20s, and a few live until they are in their 30s. The cause of death is usually cardiopulmonary system (heart and lung) complications that lead to pneumonia.

Parents with a child who has Duchenne MD usually begin to suspect something is wrong when the infant begins to walk on his toes at about 1 year of age (Box 11-3). The diagnosis is usually made by the age of 4 after a muscle biopsy is performed. By then, the child's calves look large, and progressive weakness has begun, especially in the joints closest to the body.

Scoliosis (see Figure 11-2) can develop because of muscle weakness, especially during growth spurts. Proper wheelchair positioning and support are important for preventing scoliosis. Older children with MD may have to use a ventilator, so good body alignment is important for maintaining the vital chest capacity needed for breathing.

Down Syndrome

*Dennis has **Down syndrome**. When he was 12 years old, Jill, the COTA, gave him a prevocational assessment at the OTR's request (see Chapter 11 Appendix A). Based on the results, Jill and Margaret developed a plan of care in which Dennis's prevocational skills could be improved in his vocational readiness classes at school. Dennis is now 15 years old and works as a bagger at the local grocery store 2 half days a week. The work is part of the vocational training program run by the local high school. When he carefully sorts and places items in grocery sacks, his short, stubby fingers and hands move slowly. His tongue sometimes protrudes as he works; it seems large for his mouth. His face is full and round. Behind his glasses is a fold of skin on either side of his nose that gives his eyes an Asian appearance. Dennis is about 5 feet 6 inches tall. His chest is round, and his body is chunky (Box 11-4). When he pushes grocery carts to cars, he walks with a wider base of support than normal, and his feet roll in. He politely chats with the customers he helps. Dennis is a confident young man and seems to like his work.*

One of 2000 live infants born to women who are less than 40 years of age have Down syndrome; one of 40 infants born to women who are more than 40 have the syndrome. Although inherited abnormal genes or accidental genetic mutations can cause Down syndrome, about 95% of individuals with Down syndrome have an extra twenty-first chromosome. The extra chromosome comes from the father 25% to 30% of the time.[4] Genetic counseling is very important to help parents determine the origin of the syndrome and with future family planning.

Through early intervention and ongoing treatment, occupational therapy is an important part of helping children who have Down syndrome reach their maximum potential. Recent research indicates that early intervention, including teaching families ways to enrich their children's environment, helps reduce developmental delays.[26] Constant monitoring and changes in treatment also help keep children progressing developmentally.

Chronic Fatigue Immune Dysfunction Syndrome and Fibromyalgia

In the past, 14-year-old Rachel had some growing pains and felt under the weather. Lately she has begun waking up tired every morning. Her symptoms started with a flulike illness and sore throat that would not go away. Now she has tremendous difficulty just getting through each day; she falls asleep every time she sits down. In spite of her fatigue, she cannot sleep more than an hour or two at night before muscle jerks awaken her and she is covered with sweat. Every morning she gets out of bed feeling shaky. Some days she experiences sudden weak spells and sweats. Sometimes

BOX 11-4

Physical Characteristics of Down Syndrome

- Shortened limbs and fingers
- Slanted eye skin fold over nasal corners of eyes
- Small mouth, protruding tongue
- Straight line across palm of hand (simian line)
- Heart defects (congenital, high incidence)
- Mental retardation (usually mild or moderate)
- Atloaxoid instability (important factor for children who engage in sports); can cause quadriplegia after minor neck injuries
- Floppy muscle tone
- Hyperextensibility of hips, limbs, and fingers
- Sensory processing problems
    Diffuse tactile discrimination difficulties
    Tactile sensitivity
    Gravitational insecurity
    Hyperactive postrotary nystagmus
    Poor bilateral motor coordination
- Changes in developmental reflexes in infants (caused by altered sensory processing)
    Reduced suck reflex
    Increased gag reflex (eventually resulting in food selectivity or intolerance and chewing problems)
    Diminished palmar grasp reflex
    Prolonged and exaggerated startle reflex
    Prolonged flexor withdrawal and avoidance reactions in hands and feet
    Delayed placing response in hands and feet
    Lack of primary standing or air response*
    Poor optical righting
    Poor body-on-body righting delayed equilibrium responses, particularly in quadruped and standing

Modified from Crepeau EB, Neistadt ME, editors: *Willard and Spackman's occupational therapy,* ed 6, 1998, Philadelphia, JB Lippincott-Raven.
*Normally, when infants' feet touch a supporting surface, they support their body weight against the surface with their feet. Infants with Down syndrome pull their feet away from the supporting surface.

she feels like she will pass out. Other times her heart races, and she feels like she is having a panic attack. She has begun having problems with irritable bowel and alternates between having constipation and loose stools. She also started having trouble with bladder infections and reduced bladder control. Many days her muscles feel stiff and sore. Nothing the family doctor tried has helped her.

One day her brother found a website describing Rachel's condition perfectly; it was called fibromyalgia syndrome (FMS). The family doctor agreed with the diagnosis and said that Rachel was also one of the 40% of people with chronic fatigue immune dysfunction syndrome (CFIDS) and FMS

(CFIDS/FMS) who also had reactive hypoglycemia. Hypoglycemia is a low blood glucose level; this caused Rachel's panic attacks, sweats, shakiness, and feelings of weakness.

Realizing Rachel fatigued easily and that repetitive motions such as those used for writing could be painful, the doctor recommended an occupational therapy consultation. Margaret met with Rachel's teacher and recommended that Rachel write less by photocopying a classmate's notes. Rachel was given a second set of books for home use and an elevator pass so that she would not have to climb the stairs. Margaret also ordered Rachel a built-up pen to help reduce her muscle fatigue while writing.

More children are beginning to be recognized as having CFIDS, FMS, or CFIDS/FMS. Emerging research indicates that these conditions are similar enough to have the same cause, with the only difference being some of the symptoms.[3] The exact diagnosis (that is, CFIDS, FMS, or CFIDS/FMS) given to a child may depend more on the specialist who is making the diagnosis than on the child's symptoms because the symptoms of the diseases are very similar. The symptoms (Box 11-5) can develop gradually or linger after a case of the flu. Suspect CFIDS/FMS in a child if a parent has been identified as having one of the syndromes. At least half of the children born to parents with one of the syndromes are suspected to also be affected.

Forty percent of people with CFIDS/FMS also have reactive hypoglycemia.[30] Hypoglycemia can cause individuals to feel like they are having panic attacks or like they are simply anxious. It can also cause their heart to race, shakiness, and fatigue.[31] A promising medical treatment is being developed that puts this combination of conditions into remission in both children and adults.

Children with CFIDS/FMS may be referred to occupational therapy for treatment of attention deficit disorder (ADD) or attention deficit hyperactivity disorder (ADHD) (Box 11-6). The ADD or ADHD associated with FMS/CFIDS is probably caused more by the pain and fatigue characteristic of CFIDS/FMS than the sensory processing deficits and difficulties typical of children with true ADD or ADHD. Children who have had pain for a long period may not consider it abnormal. The pain or fatigue may cause them move around more than others to alleviate the pain or to wake up. The constant pain and need to move may distract them from their schoolwork and activities.

Often children with CFIDS/FMS need help with work simplification, self-care skills, or adaptive equipment because of fatigue, cognitive problems, or pain. Once the condition is identified, children may benefit from using built-up pencils to ease finger pain and fatigue. Fatigue and pain interfere with performance of repetitive activities and may cause writing to become difficult.

BOX 11-5

Symptoms of Chronic Fatigue Immune Dysfunction Syndrome and Fibromyalgia

Children may have several or all of the following symptoms or conditions:
- Growing pains
- Frequent periods of not feeling well
- ADD
- Sleep disturbances or insomnia
- Irritable bowel syndrome
  - Gas or bloating
  - Periods of alternating constipation and diarrhea or loose stools
- Urinary tract problems
  - Reduced bladder control
  - Bladder infections
  - Painful urination
- Deep aches in calves and other muscles
- Frequent, severe headaches
- Lack of stamina
- Short-term memory loss
- Neurological problems
  - Shooting leg pains
  - Restless leg syndrome (feeling a constant need to move the legs)
  - Muscle tics or twitches
  - Numbness
- Reactive hypoglycemia
  - Racing heart beat
  - Shakiness
  - Blacking out
  - Sweats
  - Anxiety or panic attacks

Data from St Amand RP: March, 1998, Personal communication; Williamson ME: *Fibromyalgia: a comprehensive approach,* New York, 1996, Walker.

BOX 11-6

Characteristics of Children with Attention Deficit Disorder or Attention Deficit Hyperactivity Disorder

Very active or fidgety
Impulsive; act without thinking of consequences
Have racing thoughts
Inattentive during activities they consider boring or unexciting (which often include doing schoolwork)
Slow to wake up in morning; are disorganized or grumpy unless anticipating an exciting activity
Slow to fall asleep
Spatially dyslexic (write mirror-image reversals of letters; have difficulty with left-right discrimination; have difficulty properly sequencing letter, words, or numbers)
Have episodic temper tantrums that include hitting, biting, and kicking
Bedwetters
Unexplainably emotionally negative

Modified from Attention Deficit Disorder Medical Treatment Center of Santa Clara Valley: www.addmtc.com/clinical.html.

BOX 11-7

Signs of a Blocked Shunt

Headache
Nausea or vomiting
Irritability
Changes in behavior or school performance
Temperature elevation
Pallor
Visual perception difficulties

NEUROLOGICAL CONDITIONS

Children born with problems in the brain or spine (the central nervous system) have congenital **neurological conditions.** Neurological conditions may also be acquired from trauma or infection at the time of birth or in the early months of life. Neurological conditions may affect the central nervous system or the peripheral nerves (the nerves outside of the brain). The more common neurological conditions seen by the occupational therapy practitioner are discussed in depth. Table 11-4 describes other central nervous system conditions.

Spina Bifida

Yesterday, 10-year-old Niki was on the school playground playing catch when she began to feel ill. Today she is in the hospital recovering from surgery to repair a shunt that was previously placed to control her hydrocephalus. Her father had rushed her to the emergency room when she got off the bus with a fever and headache (Box 11-7). Niki was born with **spina bifida** *and has had many surgeries, most of which were to repair her shunt. Others were to repair the hole in her back and her congenital clubbed feet. Her legs are paralyzed, and she has no bowel or bladder control. She has learned to use a catheter to empty her bladder and uses a special bowel program to eliminate. When she was younger, Niki walked with crutches and braces but was always frightened of being on her feet. As she got older, she gained weight, which made it hard to walk. Now Niki uses a manual wheelchair to move around.*

TABLE 11-4

Other Common Central Nervous System Conditions

CONDITION	SYMPTOMS OR SIGNS
AGENESIS OF THE CORPUS CALLOSUM Absence or poor development of the central part of the brain that connects the two hemispheres	Deficits ranging from mild learning problems to severe physical and mental problems Possible vision or hearing problems Possible sensory processing problems Possible eye-hand coordination problems Mental retardation and epilepsy (common)
MICROCEPHALY Literally, "small head"	Head that appears small for body Moderate to severe mental retardation Moderate to severe motor problems Possible seizure disorder

There are three types of spina bifida classifications: (1) occulta, (2) meningocele, and (3) myelomeningocele (Figure 11-3). Spina bifida, a condition in which one or more of the vertebrae are not formed properly, is the most common type of congenital spinal abnormality.[6] The meninges (the covering of the spinal cord) or the meninges *and* the spinal cord push out through an abnormal opening in the vertebra in the meningocele and myelomeningocele types, respectively. The amount of resulting disability can range from minimal, as it is in individuals with spina bifida occulta, to severe, as it is in individuals who have a myelomeningocele. Typically the occupational therapy practitioner sees children with the myelomeningocele type because their limitations and disabilities are the most severe of the three types. (NOTE: The terms *spina bifida* and *myelomeningocele* are used synonymously in the remainder of this section.)

Spina bifida occurs in about 1 of 1000 births. Its cause may be genetic or result from high maternal temperatures or insufficient folic acid in the mother's diet. The amount of resulting physical disability is related to the size and location of the defect.[31] The higher the level of the spinal opening, the greater the disability (see Figure 11-3). Eighty percent of children born with spina bifida have hydrocephalus caused by excess cerebrospinal fluid. To drain the fluid, a shunt is placed in the ventricles of the brain. The tube (which is similar to small aquarium tubing) runs down the neck to the abdomen where the extra fluid drains. Scoliosis or kyphosis may be present at birth or develop later (see Figures 11-2 and 11-4), and both conditions are complex to treat. In the early months, proper positioning of the paralyzed legs is important to prevent the development of contractures. Because of the lack of mobility, children are not able to engage in the normal developmental sensorimotor experiences.

This is an important area of treatment in occupational therapy for older infants. The lack of sensorimotor experience may contribute to poor development of body concept, fear of movement, tactile sensitivity, poor eye-hand control, and poor motor planning (see Chapter 15). Infants and toddlers with spina bifida benefit from a good sensory enrichment home program that is related to the therapy provided in the clinic.

Shaken Baby Syndrome

The young parents of 7-month-old Tony sat nervously in the hospital waiting room wondering how a day that started so normally could be ending like this. That morning Tony's mother had been called in to work unexpectedly and did not have time to get him to his regular sitter, so she called her neighbor to watch him.

When Tony's mother got home that afternoon, she found Tony in a deep sleep. When she finally woke him, he forcefully vomited his lunch. She became very frightened when she noticed that his left arm and leg seemed floppy. When his whole body suddenly began to jerk uncontrollably, Tony's mother frantically called 911, and the paramedics carried him by ambulance to the nearest hospital.

When the doctor finally spoke with the Tony's parents, he told them that Tony had received an emergency tracheotomy, a surgical procedure in which a hole is made in the throat to allow an individual to breathe. After a computerized axial tomography (CAT) scan of the head showed bleeding on one side of the brain, the doctor had given Tony phenobarbital to stop his seizures. The bleeding is what had caused his arm and leg to seem hemiplegic (floppy). Tony had a head trauma caused by an extremely rapid, forceful movement. Tony's brain had started to swell, and the pressure inside his head was dangerously high

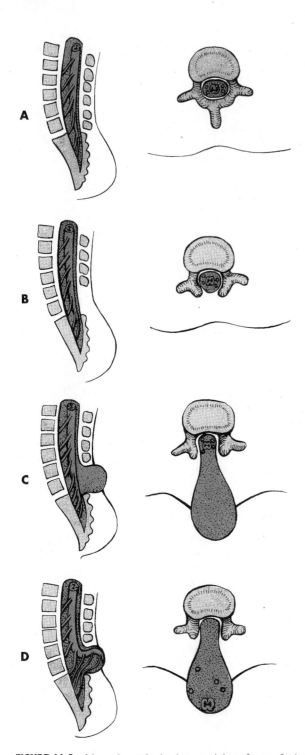

FIGURE 11-3   Normal vertebral column and three forms of spina bifida. **A,** Normal: intact vertebral column, meninges, and spinal cord. **B,** Spina bifida occulta: bony defect in vertebral column. This type of spina bifida can only be diagnosed by x-ray and often goes undetected. **C,** Meningocele: bony defect in which meninges fill with spinal fluid and protrude through opening in vertebral column. **D,** Myelomeningocele: bony defect in which meninges fill with spinal fluid and portion of spinal cord with its nerves protrude through opening in vertebral column. This type of spina bifida is the most severe and can be detected at birth. (From Wong D et al: *Whaley and Wong's nursing care of infants and children,* ed 6, 1999, St Louis, Mosby.)

FIGURE 11-4   Congenital kyphosis—a backward rounding of spine in chest area that can be caused by malformed vertebrae. Changes in spine cause head and shoulders to be carried forward. Front of body bends forward, compressing the internal organs.[33]

(Box 11-8). *A neurosurgeon put a drain in his head to control the pressure. An ophthalmologist confirmed that Tony had bleeding behind both eyes. The doctor told Tony's parents that usually the eyes heal with time, but sometimes shaken infants can become completely blind.*

Tony's mother was stunned to hear that her child had been shaken. The police soon arrived to question her. She told them that her neighbor had cared for Tony that day. A background check at the police station revealed that she had been previously charged with shaking her own grandchild.

Infants who are violently shaken by adults sustain serious brain damage. **Shaken baby syndrome** causes the brain to hit the inside of the skull so hard that it bruises the brain or causes bleeding. The damage caused by shak-

BOX 11-8

Possible Injuries from Shaken Baby Syndrome

Injuries inside the brain
Brain swelling
Diffuse nerve cell damage
Shear injury
Bleeding
Injuries outside the brain
Retinal bleeding (75% to 90%)
Rib fractures
Bruises
Abdominal injuries

Modified from Alexander RC, Smith WL: Shaken baby syndrome, *Inf Young Children* 10(3):3, 1998.

CLINICAL *Pearl*

It is not unusual for children with cortical blindness to need corrective lenses or glasses because they are nearsighted or farsighted. A developmental optometrist can determine whether glasses would be beneficial.

ing is proportional to the size of the child; larger children are harder to shake. To give a proportional size comparison, an adult shaking a child is similar to a 2000-lb gorilla shaking a grown man.[1] The exact numbers of shaken baby cases is not known because of a lack of information in general about child abuse cases. Subtle cases may go undetected. Many cases show that the children have suffered previous abuse. Men are responsible for 60% of shaken baby syndrome cases; 15% involve baby sitters of either sex. However, mothers may also be at high risk for shaking a baby too hard. Members of lower socioeconomic groups and younger adults are more likely to shake infants too hard, and the person shaking the infant has usually been previously abused. Most of the cases of shaken baby syndrome involve children less than 2 years of age; about 25% of these children die. Only a small percentage of infants who survive a severe shaking are almost normal after the abuse.[1] Children with disabilities are at greater risk for being abused and neglected; they are at least twice as likely to be mistreated than children without disabilities. Another major risk factor involves the number of caregivers an infant has. A normal child averages three caregivers besides the parents, but an infant with disabilities could have as many as 27.[11]

Children with shaken baby syndrome can have developmental delays, visual impairments, and neurological damage, which can result in mild learning problems or profound mental impairments. Brain injuries usually involve bleeding or lack of oxygen. Loss of muscle control or cerebral palsy is a common result (see Chapter 8). The eyes often heal within weeks or months if the retinas remain attached. If the brain is damaged in the area involving vision, visual impairments or cortical blindness can result. Because the eyes are not actually damaged in children with cortical blindness, the children see images as if they were looking through several layers of plastic wrap.

Treatment of children with shaken baby syndrome involves monitoring for developmental delays to ensure their development continues and is progressing at an age-appropriate level. Assessment of vision begins with clinical observations to determine whether children require large objects or specific color contrasts to interact with their surroundings. As the children develops, they may need to learn the many skills used by individuals who are legally blind to improve independence (see Vision Impairments section in this chapter). When children have motor impairments or cerebral palsy, a careful assessment of movement patterns must be made to determine which normal and abnormal movement patterns are present. Usually, if parents and caregivers handle the children properly, many abnormal movement patterns can be prevented, allowing more normal movements to develop. Parents, teachers, and caregivers must be taught correct handling and positioning techniques because they have the most contact with the child (see Chapter 17).

Erb's Palsy

As her anxious father watched, Kira's mother, Debbie, laid the sleeping 7-day-old infant on the mat in the clinic. When Debbie unwrapped the receiving blanket, Kira began to waken, gave a lusty yawn, and stretched. Her right arm reached out as her back arched and she awakened. The other arm lay lifelessly at her side, and her left shoulder fell back against the mat. As she finished stretching, her right arm flexed against her chest, bringing her fist under her chin; the left one still did not move.

Kira's birth had been difficult. Weighing more than 9 lb, she became lodged in the birth canal because her shoulders were too wide for Debbie's narrow pelvis. The left shoulder was stuck, which stretched the nerve roots of the brachial plexus (the nerves from the neck area of the spinal cord that supply the arm). As the OTR, Margaret, examined Kira's arm, it felt as limp in her hands and had no muscle tone. Her left fingers did not reflexively curl around Margaret's finger as Margaret laid her finger across Kira's palm. Gentle pinches on Kira's left arm showed she that she felt nothing. The infant quietly watched Margaret as she moved Kira's arm through its ROM. No joint tightness or limitations were present. Margaret would have referred Kira for x-rays had she begun crying; Margaret knew that Kira would experience pain if she had an undetected fracture of the humerus or clavicle or any tissue tearing in the shoulder joint.

Erb's palsy occurs in about 2% of births.[25] During birth, stretching or tearing of peripheral nerves that supply the arm and shoulder can cause Erb's palsy. Infants who are born feet first or are too large for the birth canal are at risk for this type of injury. Erb's palsy can generally be diagnosed in the first 24 hours after birth. The paralysis usually goes away untreated in a few days or weeks. During the first 2 weeks of life, 40% of infants recover; 35% worsen by the time they are 18 months old. By 18 months, gross and fine motor skill development are also delayed.[25] The infants who have not been treated in the early months of life develop elbow flexion contractures, and the affected arm is noticeably shorter than the other one.

Older children who have not had good early care or have not completely recovered may benefit from instruction in ADL skills. A residual strength assessment may indicate that a home strengthening program would be beneficial. Designing strengthening programs for children requires creativity and diversity to engage children and keep them interested long enough to yield benefits. Any home program must include attention to active ROM (AROM) and passive range of motion (PROM). Until full balanced muscle strength or full growth is attained, contracture development is possible.

After assessing Kira's function, the parents were taught ways to physically handle her at home to prevent further damage. The therapist showed them how to support her arm so that it would not flop away from her body as they picked her up.

They were taught how to use ROM exercises with all of the left arm joints, including the shoulder, to prevent stiffness and increase mobility. While Margaret was finishing Kira's assessment, Jill made a small sling to make holding Kira easier; soft cotton tubing was placed over her arm and pinned to her shirt, a design that worked well (Figure 11-5).

In addition to helping the parents hold Kira, the sling actually served another function. Because Kira felt almost no sensation in her affected arm, Jill positioned the sling so that Kira's left hand rested under her chin next to her right hand. This allowed Kira to explore her hands and become accustomed to having a left hand. As children with brachial plexus injuries grow, they often ignore the affected hand and arm because it feels little or no physical sensations. The therapist instructed the parents to talk to Kira about her two hands and to hold them together to help her touch and feel them. Infants begin to explore their physical bodies by mouthing their hands. By placing an affected hand in the mouth, infants begin to explore the shapes of their fingers with their tongue. This also helps the mouth to become accustomed to feeling new sensations. Margaret encouraged the parents to put Kira's hands in Kira's mouth.

As Kira grew older and stronger, Margaret checked for return of muscle activity every week. The shoulder was the first to show tiny movements. By then, Kira could hold up her head to play while on her tummy with a rolled towel under her shoulders. During her therapy sessions, Kira was placed in supported, upper-extremity weightbearing positions to encourage use of her returning strength and encourage bone growth and improved bone density, reducing the chance of developing osteoporosis in the arm. By putting Kira in upper-extremity weightbearing positions, the practitioner hoped to avoid noticeable growth differences between the two arms as Kira got older. When her biceps

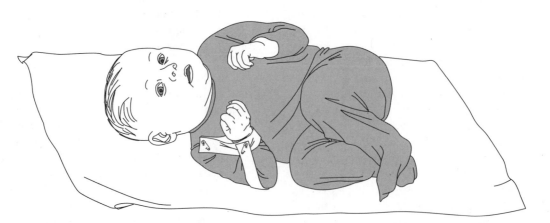

FIGURE 11-5   Sling for infant with Erb's palsy. Sling is made of cotton stockinette and safety pins. It is pinned to infant's shirt at shoulder in position that keeps affected hand near infant's face.

became active, Kira was encouraged to bend her elbow to suck on her left fingers and hold them in her mouth independently. The parents were instructed to put bits of food Kira liked on her left hand while gently restraining her right arm to encourage her to bring her left hand to her mouth. As each muscle group began to show activity, new and appropriate weightbearing and play activities were introduced to Kira's home program to encourage her to strengthen her left arm (see Chapter 17).

At 1 year of age, Kira had movement of muscles throughout her entire arm. The shoulder and elbow muscles were strongest, but all of the muscle groups remained unbalanced and weaker than those in the right arm. At the age of 2, the parents enrolled Kira in a parent-toddler gymnastics class to encourage her to use her affected arm in bilateral activities. The parents were very knowledgeable by then and found an instructor who was willing to meet Kira's needs. To make the classes even more productive, Margaret met with the teacher to discuss Kira's needs and limitations. Gymnastics was very motivating to Kira, and in her attempt to keep up with the class her strength continued to improve. The gymnastic routines stretched her tight joints as well. Kira is now 6, and although her left arm is a little smaller than her right and she has mild weakness in her elbow and the muscles below it, her left arm weakness is not noticeable to those unaware of her problem. Because bone grows faster than muscle, Margaret continues to monitor Kira's progress every few months to be sure no further contractures are developing and to adjust her home program.

Seizures

Ryan is a 6 year old who had right hemiplegic cerebral palsy and a seizure disorder. During a busy day in the clinic, Ryan and Jill were working on putting on a shirt. Ryan had just gotten tangled up in the shirt when he gave a high-pitched cry, his head went back, and he fell off his stool. Jill knew Ryan had a history of uncontrolled seizures and knew right away what had happened (Box 11-9). She immediately removed

the stool from the area so that he would not bump it with his flailing arms and legs. She turned his head to the side and tucked a cushion under it. She carefully watched his breathing and skin color as she waited for the seizure to subside. In a few minutes, Ryan began to regain consciousness but was groggy. Jill knew the occupational therapy session for that day was over and that Ryan needed a nap.

About 2% of the general population experience **seizures** of some type.[4] One fourth of those have ongoing repeated seizures or epilepsy. Epilepsy occurs more often in children than adults, and many children outgrow their seizures.[31] Most people with seizures have only one type, which is usually grand mal (Table 11-5). About a third have both grand mal and petit mal.[4] Children with congenital brain damage, including those with cerebral palsy (particularly hemiplegia), spina bifida, or microcephaly, can have seizures.

SENSORY SYSTEM CONDITONS

Sensory system conditions include those involving **vision impairments** (seeing impairments) and auditory system impairments **(hearing impairments).** Children may also have processing problems or deficits in other sensory systems including the tactile (touch) system, the vestibular (balance and movement) system, and the proprioceptive (position sense) system (see Chapter 6).

Vision Impairments

Evan was born 3 weeks late and weighed 8½ lb. During his first 12 months, he was a happy, busy baby and met all his developmental milestones on schedule. By his first birthday, he had shown no interest in walking. If placed on his feet with nothing to hold on to, Evan would scream from fear and drop down to his bottom immediately. His grandmother assumed his ankles were weak and bought

---

BOX 11-9

Caring for a Child Who is Having a Seizure

If the child is flailing, make sure nothing is close by that could cause an injury if hit with the child's body.
Place something soft under the head.
Do not place anything in the mouth; it may damage the teeth.
Do not put a finger in the mouth. It will be bitten—hard.
Roll the child on the side to avoid inhaling vomit.
Call for emergency medical help if the child's skin begins to turn blue.

TABLE 11-5

Seizures

TYPE OF SEIZURE	CHARACTERISTICS
Grand mal seizures	Possible crying out or mood change before the seizure Loss of consciousness for 2-5 min Fall; shaking arms, legs, and body Possible loss of control of bowels and bladder Afterward, possible deep sleep headache, or muscle soreness
Absence (petit mal) seizures	Mostly in children Most likely to occur many times a day Brief loss of consciousness for 10-30 s Possible eye or muscle fluttering No loss of muscle tone Sudden cessation of activity; restarts a few seconds later
Febrile seizures	Mostly in children 3 mo-5 yr Most common in children with existing neurological problems In individuals with fever but no brain infection Varying duration; brief or up to 15 min
Infantile spasms (salaam seizures)	Seen in children under 3 yr with obvious brain damage A few seconds in duration but occur several times each day Sudden flexion of arms, extension of legs, and forward flexion of the trunk
Akinetic (drop) seizures	Brief and sudden Complete loss of consciousness and muscle tone Danger of head injury because child will suddenly fall to the ground

Data from Berkow R, editor: *The Merck manual,* ed 17, Rahway, NJ, 1999, Merck.

him ankle-high leather tennis shoes. Evan still had no interest in walking. At 18 months he finally began walking, and at the same time, the "terrible twos" began. His cheerful personality disappeared, and he was frustrated most of the time. He only seemed happy when left sitting quietly in his room playing with his construction toys. He hated playing on playground equipment; merry-go-rounds terrified him. Evan remained fearful and stubborn long past the terrible twos stage. At 4 years old, he still could only climb stairs one at a time. Temper tantrums were a daily event. He refused to join the neighborhood boys in gross motor play. He could not catch a ball but loved his big-wheel tricycle. He could not hop or even stand on one foot, and his running was clumsy. Interactions with other children his age always turned into confrontations. He still sat for hours playing with building toys. His mother never noticed that one eye turned in slightly or that he always sat very close to the television to watch videos.

One day when he was almost 5, Evan's vision was tested at his cooperative nursery. His mother was shocked that he could not pass even a simple distance vision test. She immediately made an appointment with a developmental optometrist (a children's eye doctor) and was even more shocked to find out that Evan was legally blind. The doctor explained that Evan had used his normal intelligence to compensate for his poor vision. Because he was born with poor eyesight, Evan did not know what normal vision was. He had started walking later than normal because when he stood up, he could no longer see the floor. He could not catch a ball because he could not see it coming. He was frustrated all the time because he knew that he was not as capable as his friends at playing neighborhood games.

The day that Evan put on his first pair of glasses, he stood at the kitchen window and was amazed he could see the garden. Almost 5 of the most precious years of gross motor and social development had been severely affected by his lack of clear vision. Those lost visual experiences continued to affect his development in later years. He always had trouble interpreting the emotional expressions on people's faces and understanding nonverbal language. Sports were never a favorite of his, and it took time for his gross motor skills to catch up to his chronological age, but he loved his first computer and excelled in school.

TABLE 11-6

Suggestions for Working with Blind Children and Children with Vision Impairments

METHOD TO USE	PURPOSE OF APPROACH
Use children's names.	Helps reduce the feeling of isolation; alerts children that they are included in what is going on around them
Explain what is going to occur.	Helps to create a relationship as well as helps them understand what is going on
Describe the room.	Helps children associate sounds, smells, and shapes
Walk children to locations when possible.	Helps children develop space perception
Reduce extra noise.	Helps children identify sound clues
Use touch to introduce new things; brush objects on the back of their hand first.	Helps identify location and function of objects; helps develop independence and teach children that their actions have a cause and effect
Explain new activities and surroundings.	Helps calm children who do not understand a new activity; helps them understand what is going to happen
Talk *to* children, not about them.	Helps prevent you from underestimating children's ability to understand what is said to them
Never assume children with vision impairments sees something.	Helps prevent you from assuming children can see and understand you

Data from Harrell L: Touch the baby. Blind and visually impaired children as patients: helping them respond to care, New York, 1984, American Foundation for the Blind.

CLINICAL *Pearl*

All children should have their eyes examined by age 3. A visual evoked response test that detects brain activity during visual stimulation can be administered for infants who are suspected of having vision problems.

BOX 11-10

Signs of Undetected Visual Problems

Parents notice the child does not focus on their face or toys.
The child holds objects close to his face.
Gross or fine motor skills are poor.
The child has crossed eyes or jerky eye movements.
The child closes one eye to focus on an object.
The child tilts his head while looking at specific objects.
The older child performs poorly in school.

Data from Case-Smith J, Allen AS, Pratt PN: *Occupational therapy for children*, St Louis, 1996, Mosby.

About 1 in 4000 children is legally blind. One in 20 has significant but less severe vision problems. Thirty percent of children with multiple handicaps have some sort of vision problem.[31] Because a large portion of children who have handicaps also have vision problems, the vision of all children with special needs should be monitored closely (Box 11-10). Discovering vision problems early can alert practitioners and family members to the need for appropriate intervention. Glasses may ease developmental and motor delays if the problem is detected early. Children who are identified early as having a vision problem may be referred to special organizations for help (see Chapter 11 Appendix B).

Children who are legally blind may be able to see objects if they are close enough. People who are totally blind have no perception of light. Children with cortical blindness have physically functional eyes, but the visual processing part of their brain has been damaged in some way, resulting in images that look as if they are being seen through several layers of plastic wrap. Less severe vision problems must be considered during therapy as well. Visual perception is the understanding of what is being seen. It can affect eye-hand coordination. Crossed eyes cause double vision because the image seen by each eye does not fuse into one image. A lazy eye can affect depth perception because only one eye at a time is working. Many of the more minor problems can be improved using eye exercises prescribed by a developmental optometrist. These minor problems are identified in 80% of children with reading problems.[8]

The treatment plan for children who have vision impairments depends on the severity of the impairment (Table 11-6). Legally blind children may be able to see quite well with corrective lenses; often, many of the interventions used for totally blind children also benefit legally blind children. If the impairment has been discovered after late infancy (that is, after about 18 months), legally blind children will probably have problems with sensory integration, particularly with tactile defensiveness (being extremely sensitive to certain textures) and vestibular processing. It can be assumed that totally blind children will have these problems as well. Playing with various textured materials helps to normalize the feeling of different textures in the hands and reduce the aversion to touch.

Opportunities to experience movement are important. To help children who are blind tolerate movement, start with gross motor activities that involve little movement and increase movement amount slowly. Many playground toys can be adapted for this purpose by the practitioner. Blind infants and younger children do not know to reach out for objects in the environment. By tying toys to strollers, chairs, or cribs and teaching the infants to feel for objects with their hands, they learn to "look" for objects around them. Teaching children to look for objects in larger and larger areas can increase this skill.

Vision is a learned skill. Any residual vision a child has should be used. The more a child uses the visual pathways, the better the vision becomes. Treating a child in a darkened room with a spotlight on the activity helps the child see better by reducing other visual distractions. Emphasizing the visual contrasts in the surfaces of objects also increases the child's ability to see. For example, outlining a container's opening with a dark marker, sewing a bright ribbon around the neck and arm openings of a shirt, or reducing clutter on a desk surface are ways to improve contrast.

CLINICAL *Pearl*

A fun and useful game children with vision impairments is "flashlight hide-and-seek." Darken a room and "hide" toys around the room. Shine a flashlight on one of the toys, and ask a child to go get it. The team who finds the most toys wins. This is a great competitive game and a good way to stimulate children's visual pathways.

Children with total blindness often fill the void left by lack of visual stimulation with other forms of sensory self-stimulation called *blindisms*. Blindisms are consistent, repetitive movements and are proportional to the degree of blindness. Blindisms can take the form of body rocking or head shaking, which stimulates the vestibular system, or eye poking, which stimulates the optic nerve. These activities can become socially unacceptable, so more accepted forms of stimulation should be taught to these children.

Hearing Impairments

Eighteen-month-old Sam was born with a genetic syndrome and was developmentally delayed. For that reason, he was attending weekly occupational therapy sessions. The COTA, Jill, was always exhausted after his treatment sessions because he never followed directions and was hyperactive and distractible. His genetic syndrome made speech difficult, so the therapist was beginning to use age-appropriate sign language to help him identify objects and express his needs. His parents found that using sign language at home reduced his frustration.

Everyone working with Sam feared he could have mental retardation, yet when shown a complex age-appropriate game, he could play it well. Sam's mother was frustrated because he was frequently stubborn. Sometimes he would withdraw to his room for hours and play alone; other times he would scream in frustration as he tried to communicate his desires.

One day Sam was playing in the yard near the driveway when his teenage brother started his car. The car backfired loudly, and Sam's mother was so startled that she jumped and dropped what she was holding. She rushed to Sam assuming that he was also frightened. She was shocked to find him playing in the sandbox, unaware that anything had happened. That night the family reflected on Sam's response and began to suspect that he had a hearing loss.

Sam was soon fitted with hearing aids for both ears. He began learning to understand spoken language extremely rapidly. His development quickly began to catch up to that of the peers in his age group. Because his genetic condition had limited his speech, Sam continued to learn sign language, but his family his family was amazed at how quickly he learned to understand what was said to him.

CLINICAL *Pearl*

It may be helpful to attach a child's hearing aids to the back of the child's shirt with clear fishing line and a safety pin to keep the child from losing them.

Sam had a considerable developmental delays because of his undetected lack of hearing. His progress needed to be continually followed to monitor and update his occupational therapy program. Although he seemed to have mental retardation when he was first brought into the clinic, once his hearing improved Sam began to perform more age-appropriate tasks with less frustration.

About 28 million Americans have a hearing loss, and about 2 million are profoundly deaf.[30] Few occupational therapists work with people who are deaf unless those in-

BOX 11-11

Possible Indications of Hearing Loss in Infants and Children

Newborn has no startle reflex when hearing a loud noise.
Three month old does not turn head toward toys that make noise.
Infant stops babbling around 6 months of age.
Infants between 8 and 12 month old does not turn toward sounds coming from behind.
Two year old does not use words.
Two year old does not respond to requests such as "show me the ball."
Three year old's speech is mostly unintelligible.
Three year old skips beginning consonants of words.
Three year old does not use two- to three- word sentences.
Three year old uses mostly vowels.
Child of any age speaks too loudly or too softly; voice has poor quality.
Child always sounds like a person who has a cold.

Modified from Case-Smith J, Allen AS, Pratt PN: *Occupational therapy for children*, ed 3, St Louis, 1996, Mosby.

BOX 11-12

Suggestions for Total Communication

Face the child at eye level.
Be directly in front of the child so that your face and hands can be easily seen.
Get the child's attention.
Use good overhead lighting.
Use a normal tone of voice.
Speak a word and sign it at the same time.
Use appropriate pauses.
Sit close to the child.
Keep instructions simple.
Be consistent.
Talk to the child. Deaf children need to "hear" the same amount of language as an average child.

Modified from Case-Smith J, Allen AS, Pratt PN: *Occupational therapy for children*, ed 3, St Louis, 1996, Mosby

dividuals have other disabling conditions. Hearing loss accompanies many other developmental problems and can be caused by maternal infection during pregnancy. An undetected hearing loss causes developmental delays. Because a crucial time exists for the acquisition of language skills, early detection of a hearing loss is very important.

Most occupational therapy services for individuals with hearing impairments address the related developmental delays. The first 4 years of life are the most important for language development. Impaired language skills affect all other areas of development, including social and environmental interactions and identification of objects. Early detection and treatment of hearing loss are essential for normal development in these areas.[23] A vigilant therapist is aware of and able to identify the signs of hearing loss in children (Box 11-11). Parents often begin to suspect their infant has a hearing loss when the infant is not wakened by loud noises or does not turn toward a noisy toy. Older infants who do not hear well will not pay attention to simple commands or give feedback to questions. Any infant or child who is suspected of having a hearing loss should be referred for hearing testing. Younger infants can be given an evoked response audiometry test, which is a record of brain waves that occur in response to test sounds.

Several methods of communication can be used with the deaf. "Total communication" includes lip reading, using oral speech, signing, and using gestures (Box 11-12).

In the book *Signing Exact English*, Tom Spradley states that "Language is something that is caught, not taught."[17] American sign language (ASL) is a rich and unique language but is often difficult for parents who are not deaf to learn. Tom Spradley recommends that deaf children "catch" ASL from deaf friends at school and "catch" English from parents by signing exact English (SEE), which is completely different from ASL.[17] Learning the seemingly foreign language of ASL is a huge task for new parents of deaf children. While they learn it, the vocabulary available from SEE enables communication between parent and child. Parents who know their infants have hearing impairments can begin using SEE in the early months of life. This allows the infant to "catch" English from the parents, making the infant bilingual as ASL is learned. (See Figure 11-6 for examples of SEE.) Occupational therapy aids this process by using the signs taught in the home and introducing new signs for identifying new objects or activities during therapy. The signs chosen should relate to items or ideas the child understands, such as objects the child can see or touch or actions such eating and dressing. Constant communication between the practitioner and parents is vital for preventing confusion and fostering language growth for the child and everyone who is working with the child.

Helping a child to accept using a new hearing aid may be difficult because of tactile defensiveness (a physical and tactile overreaction to the objects). The head is often the most sensitive part of a child's body. The younger a child is fitted with hearing aids, the easier it is for the child to accept them. The aids must be thought of as clothing—necessary items that are put on each morning. An older child may need to start using new hearing aids during quiet times in speech-related activities. Hearing aids have recently undergone significant changes. Audiologists can now make more precise fittings to accommodate certain types of hearing loss. The aids are programmable and can be adjusted for factors such as background noise or voice levels. Because hearing aids are sensitive pieces of equipment, practitioners must be able to recognize their common malfunctions. Batteries often die in approximately a week depending on how much they are used. Batteries can also stop working because of corrosion or incorrect installation. An audible squeal coming from the hearing aid can be caused by a loose ear mold or incorrectly set switches. Ear molds often become plugged with wax, which block sound transmission.

GENERAL SENSORY DISORGANIZATION

In some conditions, children's entire sensory systems transmit information poorly, causing their perception of the world to be frightening. Changes in any one of the sensory systems affect development, making it difficult for children to make sense of gross or fine motor activities or even their surroundings. For example, one way that infants learn about their mothers is through the sense of touch; if the perception of touch is not normal, the infants may perceive touch as painful or frightening. If the vestibular system (which detects movement) is not responsive, infants may only be happy when they are moving or someone is holding them while walking. If several sensory systems are not functioning properly, behavior and development can be adversely affected, as can the relationship between infants and their parents or caregivers.

Fussy Baby

Leigh was born 3 weeks early. By the time she was 3 months of age, she would scream for hours at a time. Leigh was only happy when her mother, Gayle, held her and walked around. No one but Gayle could calm her; she was tired and frustrated. After Gayle took Leigh to the pediatrician several times, the doctor concluded that nothing was seriously wrong, and Leigh just had colic. All Leigh's tests were normal, and changing her formula and prescribing medication did nothing. The only assurance the doctor could give Gayle was that Leigh would grow out of the screaming episodes.

At 8 months Leigh still cried most of the time. She could only be comforted by being tucked into a fabric baby carrier on Gayle's shoulders. During a well-baby checkup, the doctor told Gayle that she and Leigh may not have bonded. Gayle adored Leigh and knew that bonding was not the problem.

Long after Leigh should have been accustomed to eating solid foods, they still made her gag. Leigh hated fuzzy toys and shivered when she touched one. The noise from squeaky toys made her jump and scream in fear. Leigh would become startled and scream when she was picked up from behind.

Leigh did not walk until she was 14 months old and then she fell more than normal. When she learned to run, her gait was clumsy, and she did not like climbing on playground toys. Temper tantrums were Leigh's way of showing that she did not want to do something.

The tantrums continued well into her elementary-school years. Although Leigh did well in school, at home she was stubborn and refused to cooperate with anyone. When she became a teenager her grades fell sharply; she began to use drugs and alcohol and skip classes in school. Leigh was almost killed several times in car wrecks. In desperation, her parents took her to a psychologist who finally diagnosed attention deficit disorder (ADD) (see Box 11-6).

Infants can be fussy for many reasons including maternal drug or alcohol abuse during pregnancy. (See sections on Cocaine Abuse and Fetal Alcohol Syndrome in this chapter.) Infants with genetic problems such as Down or Angelman's syndrome may have **general sensory disorganization.** Children with a history of ADD, ADHD, or learning disabilities were often fussy infants. Infants with autism are often also fussy infants (Box 11-13). Families who already have members with have learning disabilities, ADD, or ADHD (see Box 11-6) are more likely to have fussy infants.[4,12,13]

The formal assessment for a **fussy baby** who is between the ages of 4 and 18 months is the test of sensory functions in infants (TSFI). TSFI measures infants' reactions to touch or movement and their use of vision to locate the source of touch or respond to objects in their visual field. The test also evaluates infants' ability to move their body while playing. The results indicate how well infants use sensation to understand their environments and bodies. The level functioning in the tested areas can affect all areas of learning throughout life.

Infants who cry constantly, particularly past the age of 3 months, may have problems with sensory regulation (see Chapter 15) and not colic. Some characteristics of fussy babies are listed in Box 11-14. If the characteristics are recognized early, treatment can help the infant become calmer. The results from the TSFI will give a good indication of the level at which treatment should begin, but observing infants who are less than 4 months old and questioning their parents is also helpful. In some cases, trial and error coupled with educated guessing is the only method to determine the way to calm an infant (Table 11-7).

Language Delay and Language Impairments

As the COTA, Jill, was taking a case history during Tommy's first visit to the clinic, a look that he gave her caused her to question his diagnosis. Nancy, his mother, had

BOX 11-13

Signs of Autism or Pervasive Developmental Delay

INFANTS

Stiffen when picked up or do not mold to the adult's body when held

Do not calm when held; may prefer to lay in the crib

Startle easily when touched or bed is bumped

Hate baths, dressing, or diaper changing

Have poor sucking ability or are hard to feed

Have poor muscle tone; bodies feels floppy

Do not have age-appropriate head control or age-appropriate ability to sit, crawl, or walk

CHILDREN

Seem unaware of surroundings

Do not make eye contact

Have general learning problems

Do not relate to others

Only eat certain food textures

CHILDREN—cont'd

Refuse to touch certain textures (for example, mud, sand)

Have sleep problems such as difficulty getting to sleep or difficulty staying asleep

Are hyperactive

Are withdrawn, miserable, anxious, or afraid

Display repetitive behavior or speech patterns

Fixate on one object or body part

Compulsively touch smooth objects

Show fascination with lights

Flap arms when excited

Frequently jump, rock, or spin self or objects

Walk on tiptoes

Giggle or scream for no apparent reason

Eat strange substances (for example, soil, paper, toothpaste, soap, rubber.)

BOX 11-14

Characteristics of a Fussy Baby

Sleep problems

Infant takes more than 20 minutes to fall asleep and wakes up several times a night.

Difficult to calm

Infant cannot calm self by putting hand in mouth or by looking at or listening to toys such as mobiles or music boxes.

Infant is difficult to calm, and mother spends many hours doing so during the day.

Feeding problems

Infant has no eating schedule.

Infant vomits, refuses food, or has other problems unrelated to allergies.

Overarousal

New types of stimulation or situations cause the infant to become overwhelmed and appear intense, wide-eyed, or jittery.

Data from DeGangi GA, Greenspan SI: *Test of sensory functions in infants,* Los Angeles, 1989, Western Psychological Services.

TABLE 11-7

Common Problems and Ideas for Treating Fussy Babies

REACTION (PROBLEM)	POSSIBLE CAUSE	TREATMENT
Pulls away from the nipple	Very sensitive to touch in mouth	Use infant's fingers to rub infant's lips, working into mouth and to gums and tongue. Eventually begin using own finger or a cloth to do same procedure.
Flails arms and legs and screams	Frightened by movement	Swaddle infant with baby blanket.
Hates windup swing, stroller or other moving things; has a strong startle reaction to movement during activities such as dressing; scares self when moves independently	Frightened by movement	Swing infant in "blanket hammock." Start with tiny swings and build up slowly to larger ones. Sit on therapy ball, hold infant snugly against chest facing you, and bounce or roll ball slowly under hips. Start with tiny movements and increase slowly to larger ones.
Wants bottle but is not hungry	Reduced feeling of sensation in mouth	Offer pacifier or heavily textured toys for chewing. Touch gums and tongue with pressure using cloth-wrapped finger.
Seems frightened or gags when touching some things with hands or feet	Feels the sensation too strongly or not strongly enough	Play in large pans of various materials like rice or beans. First allow infant to watch play. Slowly encourage infant to touch items in pan. Goal is to get infant's entire body in pan.

just been told he had pervasive developmental delay (PDD) (Box 11-15), a condition that is very much like autism. Nancy stated that Tommy, who was almost 3 years old, did not speak at all (even in single words). He was frustrated all the time. He would throw a tantrum when a person interrupted anything he was doing. His only play activity was lining cars end to end. He would lie on his mother's bed for hours and trace the stripes on the sheets with his finger. He always had a toy car in each hand wherever he went. He preferred to wear only a diaper but would wear one particular sweat suit when his mother insisted. When a person other than a family member came near him, he would begin screaming. Nancy said her house was in a shambles because Tommy never stopped running, climbing, jumping, and throwing. The only thing that calmed him was country music videos; he insisted that the television volume be extremely loud all day. He refused to eat most foods and was very small for his age. Nancy could force him to eat yogurt or animal crackers in small portions.

When Tommy looked at Jill as she was taking the history, he seemed to be trying to communicate. His occupational therapy evaluation indicated that he had a severe sensory processing disorder and showed tactile defensiveness all over his body. His mouth was so sensitive to touch that he could not eat because he could not stand the feel of food in his mouth. He carried cars so that he did not have to touch other things. He like the country music to be loud because it blocked out other sounds that confused him. He lined up cars and traced stripes to give himself some sort of visual organization and control. Tommy progressed using a combination of sensory integration therapy, speech

therapy, horseback riding therapy, intervention from a preschool teacher who was knowledgeable about sensory processing problems, and a good home program. At the age of 6, his speech was labored and not always clear but was improving. He had also begun to relate to people other than family members as his social skills improved.

CLINICAL *Pearl*

Adding spices to foods often reduces oral defensiveness. Decreasing the texture of food by blending it or adding texture by including crisp cereal could make it easier for children to tolerate the food.

Children develop language problems for many reasons. Some children do eventually learn to talk, other children may only learn a few sentences, and some children may never learn any words at all. Children are often nonverbal because of other developmental problems caused by genetic disorders or because of neurological conditions such as cerebral palsy. Major language delays seem to occur more in boys, who often have several areas of sensory processing problems. Children with language delays can develop learning problems later.

Always be patient with children who do not talk or have trouble understanding speech. All children use "prelanguage" before they start using speech as a form of communication; they point to an object to indicate that they want it or pull a parent to the cookie jar to indicate they want a cookie. Children who are physically unable to move their limbs may indicate their needs with a smile or an eye gaze. An understanding of language develops before the ability to speak.

Other forms of communication can be used to reduce frustration while oral speech is developing. Children with fair or good hand control can learn words in ASL to aid in communication. Using signs during therapy sessions and at home may be the most convenient way for children to communicate (see Figure 11-6). Choose signs that have meaning in the child's everyday life. Another alternative for communication is a simple poster board with taped-on pictures of people and objects commonly encountered in a particular child's everyday life (see Chapter 5). For young children, colored shapes of green and red could be substituted for the words "yes" and "no," which are important for indicating choices. A more portable communication system can be created using a small photo album with single pictures on each page.

BOX 11-15

Pervasive Developmental Delay

A child is given the diagnosis of PDD when the child's precise diagnosis is not clear. A child given this diagnosis may receive valuable treatments that are appropriate for the actual undiagnosed condition. Subgroups and related conditions that may not be diagnosed in a child who is identified as having PDD include the following:
- Angelman syndrome
- Apraxia
- Asperger syndrome
- Attention deficit disorder
- Fragile X syndrome
- Landau-Kleffner syndrome
- Language delay
- Prader-Willi syndrome
- Rett syndrome

Modified from Autism Research Institute: 1998, *www.autism.com/.*

Facilitated communication

The administrators at Aaron's school recommended that he be placed in a class for children with multiple handicaps because he seemed to understand little of what was said to him and was nonverbal. Aaron's parents knew he could understand everything that was said to him. They insisted he be placed with students his own age in a regular classroom. To avoid a potential lawsuit by the parents, the school administrators placed Aaron in a regular classroom and moved him up a grade each year. Aaron sat in class every day doing no written work but seeming to listen. When he was 13 years old, he learned to use facilitated communication with a tiny keyboard communicator to express his thoughts. He began relating amazing perceptions about his past, classmates, and family as well as current events. His teachers were finally able to administer tests and discovered that Aaron was reading and doing math at his appropriate grade level.

Facilitated communication is a controversial approach to helping children who have many different types of developmental communication delays. With the help of a another person (a facilitator), children can point to letters, words, or pictures on a computer or some other communication device.[5] Children using facilitated communication have the facilitator help them point their finger, control tremors, and slow down movements. The approach is controversial because the facilitators have the ability to influence the children, which could cause them to communicate the facilitators' thoughts instead of the children's. Under the right circumstances and with a trustworthy facilitator, this means of communication is the only way some nonverbal intelligent children can express themselves. This method of communication is used for some children with developmental dyspraxia (Box 11-16) or autism (see Box 11-13).

BOX 11-16

Developmental Dyspraxia

Developmental dyspraxia is the inability or difficulty to initiate voluntary movement. Children with this problem may have trouble starting or stopping a movement. They may be able to do routine activities but have trouble with new ones. Sometimes the force of their movements are too strong or weak to be effective.

Modified from Miller N: *Dyspraxia and its management,* Rockville, Md, 1985, Aspen.

ENVIRONMENTALLY INDUCED AND ACQUIRED CONDITIONS

Environmentally induced and acquired conditions can develop before or after birth and are directly related to factors found in the environment. Contributing factors include drugs, toxic chemicals, allergens, and viruses.

Failure to Thrive

Nathan was born 5 weeks early and weighed only 3 lb. He was resuscitated twice in the delivery room because his breathing had stopped. He left the delivery room in an incubator and on his arrival in the neonatal intensive care unit (NICU), he was put on a respirator. Because he was too weak to suckle, he was fed through his nose by a tube that went from his nose to his stomach (a nasogastric, or NG, tube). Wires were taped to his chest to monitor his heartbeat and to his head to measure brain activity. When Nathan was born, he was too ill to be held by anyone, including his parents. Four weeks after he was born, Nathan had not grown in length and had gained only a few ounces. After consulting with the medical team, the parents agreed to remove Nathan from the respirator because they were told he had no chance of survival. After all his equipment was removed, Nathan was handed to his mother for the first time. She rocked and sang to him in the NICU. Two months later, after his parents had spent every day touching, rocking, and talking to him, Nathan weighed 4½ lb and was able to go home with his parents.

Failure to thrive can be a symptom of another acute or chronic condition or can be a condition in its own right. When failure to thrive is a symptom of another condition, it is usually obvious by the age of 6 months. Weight gain is the most accurate indicator of an infant's nutritional status. Delayed height growth usually indicates more severe and prolonged poor nutrition. A reduced head growth rate suggests severe malnutrition because the body provides energy to the brain before any other organ[4] (Box 11-17).

BOX 11-17

Signs of Possible Failure to Thrive

Weight persistently less than 3% on growth charts
Weight less than 80% of ideal for height and age
Progressive loss of weight to below third percentile
Decrease in expected growth rate compared to previous pattern

Data from Berkow R, editor: *The Merck manual,* ed 17, Rahway, NJ, 1999, Merck.

When infants fail to thrive but have no other physical conditions (that is, they are physically normal at birth and have contracted no illnesses after birth), the problem is caused by neglect or lack of appropriate stimulation. This type of failure to thrive can occur at any age. Hospitalized infants or children may fail to thrive because of a lack of social stimulation; an infant of a parent who is depressed or has poor parenting skills may fail to thrive as may a fussy baby whose mother is under significant stress or is mentally ill.

Another group of infants who may experience failure to thrive includes premature infants and infants with feeding problems caused by neurological or orthopedic factors (such as cleft palate) or a poor sucking ability caused by cerebral palsy or sensory problems.

Fetal Alcohol Syndrome

The use of alcohol during pregnancy is the most common cause of birth defects. **Fetal alcohol syndrome** (FAS) occurs in 2 to 6 births out of 1000.[31] Infants of chronic drinkers are most severely affected. Alcohol consumption during pregnancy causes mental retardation, microencephaly, small facial features, poor development of the corpus callosum (see Table 11-4), and heart defects. Characteristic facial features include a turned-up nose and small jaw; a cleft lip or palate may also develop. Children with FAS may also experience a failure to thrive and be fussy. One or more of these problems can result in a developmental delay. Hyperactivity can develop and adversely affect attention span and learning. Children with FAS are frequently hypotonic, have poor coordination, and may have sensory processing difficulties.[31] Infants or children with milder cases of FAS may be referred for occupational therapy treatment of hyperactivity caused by a sensory processing disorder. The infants may also have related learning problems as they grow older. Fine motor and visual perception skills must be assessed before the treatment intervention plan can be determined (see Chapter 12).

Effects of Cocaine Use

Cocaine use during pregnancy may produce malformations of the fetus' arms, legs, bowel, bladder, or genitals. It can cause poor blood flow to the placenta, causing a miscarriage or neurological damage to developing infants. Some infants may experience bleeding in the brain at birth. Infants of mothers who used cocaine near the time of birth will go through withdrawal after birth. Symptoms of withdrawal include vomiting and diarrhea, irritability, sweating, convulsions, and hyperventilation. Wrapping these infants tightly and feeding them frequently to calm them can help alleviate the symptoms of mild withdrawal.[4]

Infants who have been exposed to cocaine before birth can be unpredictable. A careful assessment of all developmental areas must be done to determine areas needing intervention. Because of the possible neurological involvement, sensory integration evaluation and monitoring should be included. Treatment is highly individualized so that it meets each child's unique needs. Long-term follow-up clarifies whether the child will develop learning disabilities or emotional or behavioral difficulties.

Human Immunodeficiency Virus

The human immunodeficiency virus (HIV) causes the immune system to break down, resulting in many different problems as early as the first 1 or 2 years of life. Early symptoms may be failure to thrive, fever, and diarrhea. Half of all HIV-infected infants develop full-blown **acquired immunodeficiency syndrome** (AIDS) by the age of 3.[4] A woman infected with HIV can pass the virus on to her infant during pregnancy, birth, or breastfeeding. Infants born to women who are infected before or during pregnancy and receive no medical treatment have about one chance in four of being born with the HIV infection. Medical treatment with zidovudine (AZT) during pregnancy and labor may reduce the risk of infant infection to about 1 in 12. HIV-infected mothers *must not* breastfeed. Treating infants with AZT for the first several weeks of life can reduce but not prevent their risk of infection.[7]

Children with AIDS may have delayed motor or cognitive development. They may not meet developmental milestones or attain certain intellectual skills and may develop microencephaly. Loss of social skills and language occurs in about 20% of children with AIDS. Paralysis, tremors, spasticity, and balance problems can also develop; major organ systems are damaged. Half of the infants born with AIDS develop pneumonia by 15 months, a common cause of death.[4] Children with AIDS-related complex (ARC) are infected with HIV and have some symptoms but have not had serious infections.[31] In the United States, 2% of all individuals with AIDS are children or adolescents. In 90% of pediatric AIDS cases, children have gotten the virus at birth from their mother. From 1993 to 1996, 4325 children had AIDS or an HIV infection that was acquired at birth. By 1996 the Centers for Disease Control (CDC) reported 7476 cases of AIDS in children (Boxes 11-18 and 11-19).[31]

CLINICAL *Pearl*

Monitoring for developmental delays is one of the main goals of occupational therapy for children with AIDS. Because their mothers are frequently ill as well, the occupational therapist coordinates care for the mothers and their children.

BOX 11-18

Precautions for Working with Children Who Have Infectious Diseases

Wear gloves when coming into contact with blood or secretions.

Mix 1 oz of bleach with 10 oz of water and disinfect surfaces.

Bandage all cuts and sores.

Wash hands and or body parts immediately after contact with blood.

Use sharp instruments only when necessary.

Modified from Centers for Disease Control National AIDS Clearing-house: *www.cdcnac.org.*

BOX 11-19

Transmission of Human Immunodeficiency Virus

HIV does not survive well in the environment. Simply drying a surface contaminated with HIV kills 90% to 99% of the virus. HIV exists in different concentrations in blood, semen, vaginal fluid, breast milk, saliva, and tears. Infection occurs when blood or body secretions that could contain visible blood (such as urine, vomit, or feces) come into contact with an open wound or mucous membranes (which are found inside the mouth, nose, eyes, vagina, and rectum). The concentration of the virus in saliva, sweat, and tears is low, and no case of HIV infection through these fluids has been documented.

Modified from Centers for Disease Control National AIDS Clearing-house: *www.cdcnac.org.*

Latex Allergies

Children with spina bifida, children who need frequent surgery, and children who must use catheters for congenital urinary tract problems are the most likely children to become allergic to latex. Between 18% and 40% of the mentioned children will develop sensitivity to latex.[27] However, anyone who has frequent exposure to latex through work or surgery can develop an allergy. A reaction can occur after breathing latex dust from an open package or contact between latex and skin, mucous membranes, open lesions, or blood. Coming into contact with a person or object that has just been in contact with latex can cause a reaction. Symptoms include watery eyes, wheezing, hives, rash, and swelling. Severe reactions can result in anaphylaxis, a system-wide body reaction that affects the heart rate and ability to breathe; anaphylaxis can be fatal.[27]

CLINICAL *Pearl*

Children who are allergic to latex may also be allergic to bananas, avocados, and kiwi fruit because they are all in the same plant family as latex. Being around latex and consuming any of these fruits may heighten the reaction.

The number of children seen who have or develop an allergy to latex is increasing for several reasons. Universal precautions require the use of latex gloves to prevent spread of infection, and latex is used in many health care products such as tape, bottle nipples, and catheters.

To avoid developing a latex allergy, try to use it as little as possible. During play activities, substitute Mylar balloons for latex balloons. Vinyl gloves can be used instead of latex gloves. Check labels of tapes or any other substances that may contain rubber products. During assessments, always ask parents or caregivers about possible allergies, which not only makes the rehabilitation team aware of possible problems but also teaches the parents symptoms to be aware of should an allergy develop.

Lead Poisoning

It is estimated that about 4 million children in the United States have high enough lead levels to slow their development.[18] Although many environmental toxins exist, lead is the one that most commonly affects children. Children living in older homes have a greater risk for exposure to peeling paint containing lead (which children sometimes eat) and lead used in plumbing. Lead is no longer used in these materials; however, children can eat or breathe lead from contaminated air, food, water, or soil as well. Some industries, such as battery manufacturing, produce higher air and dust levels of lead than other industries. Parents working in these industries can carry lead home from work on their clothing. Mothers with high lead levels can pass it on to their infants during gestation. Mild toxicity produces muscle aches and fatigue, and moderate levels cause fatigue, headaches, cramping, vomiting, and weight loss. High toxicity levels cause mental retardation, behavior problems, seizures, and sometimes death. Even low toxicity levels can affect intelligence and behavior.[31]

Allergies to Foods or Chemicals

The use of art supplies, construction materials, and food during pediatric therapy should be carefully assessed so that children's developing bodies are not unnecessarily exposed to toxic chemicals, toxic materials, or allergy-producing foods. Always check with parents or guardians about their children's food allergies before using food for

BOX 11-20

Most Common Foods Associated with Food Allergies

Wheat	Soy
Corn	Eggs
Cane sugar	Milk
Citrus foods	Peanuts

BOX 11-21

Signs of a Hidden Food Allergy

Pale skin color
Dark shadows or wrinkles under eyes
Nose congestion
Crease across nose (caused by the child pushing up
    the tip of the nose as it drips)
Breathing by mouth
Face and body rashes
Chapped lips
Spots on tongue that resemble a map
Hyperactivity
Fatigue
Clumsiness

Modified from Crook WG: *Solving the puzzle of your hard-to-raise child,* 1987, New York, Random House.

BOX 11-22

Reasons Children are More Susceptible to Allergic Reactions

In relationship to their weight, children have a large
    body surface, which allows them to absorb more
    elements through the skin.
Children have higher metabolic rates.
Children breathe twice as much air per pound of
    body weight as adults.
Children have not yet developed detoxification
    enzymes.
Children put numerous items in their mouths.

Modified from Gorman C, Dickson MH: *Less-toxic alternatives,* Dekalb, Tex, 1997, Optimum Publishing.

an art project or feeding therapy (Box 11-20). Sometimes children have "hidden" food or chemical allergies because they eat the foods or are exposed to the chemicals daily (Box 11-21). Toxic chemical fumes or materials may cause asthma, skin irritation, anaphylaxis, or other unseen damage that can accumulate over time. Risk factors are listed in Box 11-22. Always ensure that materials used

in therapy are nontoxic. Avoid using latex products when another substitute is available.

CLINICAL *Pearl*

Styrofoam packing peanuts are fun to play with but can emit formaldehyde fumes or be accidentally eaten. Never allow children to play in a pile so large that they could immerse their body or head. Styrofoam peanuts are very light weight and can be easily inhaled and block breathing.

ROLE OF COTA AND OTR IN ASSESSMENT AND INTERVENTION

Greg has been a COTA for 10 years. He is also a North American Riding for the Handicapped Association* (NARHA) certified riding instructor for the therapeutic riding program in his town. He has ridden all his life and shows horses as often as he can. In his therapeutic riding sessions, he uses horses to treat children with sensory processing problems and motor delays. By analyzing all of the activities involved in caring for and riding horses, Greg has developed a comprehensive treatment program for each child he treats. Margaret, the OTR, is not certified by NARHA. She has her own horse and loves to ride. Margaret contracts through the riding program to supervise Greg on a monthly basis.

Six-year-old Emily was referred to the riding program by her pediatrician. The doctor's referral said he suspected Emily had ADD (see Box 11-6), sensory processing problems, and a possible learning disability. Based on the pediatrician's referral, Margaret told Greg to administer the Miller Preschool Assessment (see Chapter 11 Appendix A). Margaret and Greg will discuss the results of the test during their next monthly meeting. Together they will write a plan of care for Greg to follow. Greg will use the plan to choose the activities Emily will use in her horseback riding therapy sessions.

An OTR must supervise a COTA in any work setting where a COTA provides occupational therapy services to infants and children. The level of supervision varies and depends on many variables. The OTR is responsible for the provision of occupational therapy services (which includes the assessment and intervention processes) while working with children and adolescents with physical dysfunctions. The COTA assists the OTR in data collection and evaluation during the assessment process using standardized or simply structured tests and interviews.

---

*NARHA provides information on and sets standards for therapeutic riding and certifies therapists as horseback riding instructors (see Chapter 11 Appendix B).

The COTA directly provides services for children with physical dysfunctions. The occupational therapy practitioners work together to develop a plan of care. While providing services to a child or adolescent, the COTA follows a documented care plan under the supervision of the OTR. The level of supervision depends on the COTA's level of experience and service competency.

SUMMARY

Working with children can be a rewarding experience for occupational therapy practitioners. Meeting the needs of children is a complex task. Not only must practitioners meet the needs of their clients, but they must also educate the family and caregivers. Occupational therapy practitioners' role takes on added dimension when they join a school's educational team to treat school-age children. Knowing the common characteristics of children's conditions helps focus the initial assessment and treatment plan. The assessment and treatment reveal that although conditions have common characteristics, the needs of children and their families are unique and must be addressed.

References

1. Alexander RC, Smith WL: Shaken baby syndrome, *Inf Young Children* 10(3):1, 1998.
2. Arthritis Foundation: *www.arthritis.org.*
3. Bell DS, Bell KM, Cheney PR: Primary juvenile fibromyalgia syndrome and chronic fatigue syndrome in adolescents, *Clin Infect Dis* 18(1):21, 1994.
4. Berkow R, editor: *The Merck manual,* ed 17, Rahway, NJ, 1999, Merck.
5. Biklen D: Questions and answers about facilitated communication, *Facil Comm Dig* 2(1):10, 1993.
6. Case-Smith J, Allen AS, Pratt PN: *Occupational therapy for children,* St Louis, 1996, Mosby.
7. Centers for Disease Control National AIDS Clearinghouse: *www.cdcnac.org.*
8. Cohen A: The efficacy of optometric vision therapy, *J Am Optom Assoc* 59(2):39, 1988.
9. Corn KN: *Idiopathic scoliosis: potential interaction of neurological variables as causation,* Master's thesis, Modesto, Calif, 1998, University of the Pacific.
10. Crook WG: *Solving the puzzle of your hard-to-raise child,* 1987, New York, Random House.
11. Crosse, SB, Kaye E, Ratnofsky AC: *Report on the maltreatment of children with disabilities,* National Center on Child Abuse and Neglect, Washington, DC, 1993, US Department on Health and Human Services.
12. DeGangi GA, Greenspan SI: *Test of sensory functions in infants,* Los Angeles, 1989, Western Psychological Services.
13. Edelson SM: *Angelman syndrome,* 1995, *www.autism.org. angel.html.*
14. Facts About Angelman Syndrome: *www.asclepius.com/ angel/asfinfo.html#Chromosome 15.*
15. Fragile-X Research Foundation: *www.fraxa.org.*
16. Gorman C, Dickson MH: *Less-toxic alternatives,* 1997, Dekalb, Tex, Optimum Publishing.
17. Gustason G et al: *Signing exact English,* Los Alamitos, Calif, 1980, Modern Signs Press.
18. Haan MN, Gerson M, Zishka BA: Identification of children at risk for lead poisoning: an evaluation of routine pediatric blood lead screening in an HMO-insured population, *Am Acad Pediatrics* 97(1):84, 1996.
19. Harrell L: *Touch the baby. Blind and visually impaired children as patients: helping them respond to care,* New York, 1984, American Foundation for the Blind.
20. International Rhett's Syndrome Association: *www.paltech. com/irsa/irsa.htm.*
21. Miller N: *Dyspraxia and its management,* 1985, Rockville, Md, Aspen.
22. National Institute of Neurological Disorders and Stroke: *www.ninds.nih.gov.*
23. Neistadt ME, Crepeau EB, editors: *Willard and Spackman's occupational therapy,* ed 9, 1998, Philadelphia, JB Lippincott-Raven.
24. Prader-Willie Syndrome Association: *www.pwsausa.org.*
25. Pronsati MP: *Erb's palsy, Adv Occup Ther* 7(21):19, 1991.
26. Pueschel SM: *Down syndrome,* 1992, *www.thearc.org/faqs/ down.html.*
27. Romanczuk A: Latex use with infants and children: it can cause problems, *Maternal Child Nurs* 18(4):208, 1993.
28. Rothstein JM, Roy HR, Wolf SL: *The rehabilitation specialist's handbook,* ed 2, Philadelphia, 1998, FA Davis.
29. St Amand RP: April, 1998, Personal communication.
30. Stancliff B: Silent services: treating deaf clients, *OT Practice* 3(2):27, 1998.
31. Wallace HM et al: *Mosby's resource guide to children with disabilities and chronic illness,* St Louis, 1997, Mosby.
32. Williamson ME: *Fibromyalgia: a comprehensive approach,* New York, 1996, Walker.
33. Winter RB, Hall JE: Kyphosis in childhood and adolescence, *Spine* 3:285, 1978.

Recommended Reading

American Occupational Therapy Association: *Rheumatoid arthritis: caring for your hands,* 1995, Bethesda, Md, The Association.

Dunn MK: *Pre-sign language skills,* San Antonio, 1982, Therapy Skill Builders.

Erhardt RP: *Developmental visual dysfunction,* San Antonio, 1993, Therapy Skill Builders.

Frick SM et al: *"Out of the mouths of babes." Discovering the developmental significance of the mouth,* San Antonio, 1996, Therapy Skill Builders.

Gross MA: *The ADD brain: diagnosis, treatment and science of attention deficit disorder (ADD/ADHD) in adults, teenagers and children,* 1997, Nova Science Publishers.

Gustason G, Pfetzizng D, Zawolkow E: *Signing exact English,* Los Alamitos, Calif, 1980, Modern Signs Press.

Puttkammer CH: *Working with substance exposed children,* San Antonio, 1994, Therapy Skill Builders.

Williams MS, Shellengerger S: *How does your engine run?* Albuquerque, NM, 1994, Therapy Works.

REVIEW *Questions*

1. Explain the difference between a central and a peripheral nervous system condition.
2. What are the three types of juvenile rheumatoid arthritis? Describe them. Which functional limitations do each cause?
3. Name the four spine conditions discussed in this chapter. In what way does each affect the functional performance of the child?
4. Describe the reason a COTA must have a good understanding of the symptoms and signs of a child's condition before doing the initial assessment. In what way does this aid in treatment?
5. Describe two genetic syndromes. Explain the way they affect the child's ADL skills.
6. Using information you have learned about the sensory systems, explain why it is so important to treat sensory system problems early.
7. What are the differences among legal blindness, total blindness, and cortical blindness? In what ways are they the same? In what ways can you make learning easier for a child who has vision impairments?
8. In what ways does an undetected hearing loss affect a child's early development?
9. Name three avoidable environmental factors that affect infants either before or after birth. Explain the way these factors can cause developmental delays.
10. Describe arthrogryposis. In what ways it can affect the child's daily functioning?
11. Why is it important to watch for signs of abuse in children who are disabled?
12. What is total communication? In what ways could it be used during a therapy session?

SUGGESTED *Activities*

1. Visit a classroom for children who have special needs and observe the children at work. During your visit observe and keep a list of the way each child's condition affects the ability to do schoolwork. Later, make a list of suggestions you think might improve each child's ability to do schoolwork.
2. Spend some time at an outpatient clinic observing the children receiving occupational therapy services. Make a list of characteristics observed in individual children. Later, try to identify each child's possible condition or which of the systems is involved.
3. Spend some time observing a child playing who has a disability. Write down ways that the child's specific condition affects the ability to play.
4. Interview a COTA who works in a school system. Ask in what ways knowing a student's condition helps the COTA decide what information to obtain during the evaluation and intervention process. Make notes during your visit; later, come up with ideas of your own to add to the list.
5. Talk with a family who has a child with a disability. Before the interview, use the knowledge you have gained from this chapter to make a list of the way you would expect the child's disability to affect the family. During the interview, make notes on the family's comments. Later, compare your initial list to the family's comments. How accurate were your expectations?

CHAPTER 11 APPENDIX A

Commonly Used Pediatric Assessments

TEST NAME	AREAS TESTED	AGE
Alberta Infant Motor Scale (AIMS)	*Motor:* Assesses postural control in supine prone, sitting, and standing positions	0-18 mo
Ayres Clinical Observations	*Sensory and motor:* Assesses postural and motor control and planning and sensory reactions	3-18 yr
Bayley Scales of Infant Development II	*Developmental:* Assesses mental, motor, and behavioral development	0-42 mo
Bruininks-Oseretsky Test of Motor Proficiency	*Developmental:* Assesses gross and fine motor proficiency upper limb coordination	4½-14½ yr
The Carolina Curriculum for Infants and Toddlers with Special Needs	*Behavioral:* Assesses mental, communication, self-help, and gross and fine motor skills	0-3 yr
DeGangi-Berk Test of Sensory Integration (TSI)	*Sensory:* Assesses underlying sensory motor mechanisms; postural control bilateral motor integration and reflex integration	3-5 yr
Denver II	*Developmental:* Detects possible gross and fine motor developmental problems; assesses language and personal social skills	2 wk-6 yr
Developmental Test of Visual-Motor Integration (VMI)	*Developmental:* Assesses visual motor skills	2-15 yr
Erhardt Developmental Prehension Assessment	*Developmental:* Describes details of grip patterns, involuntary hand and arm patterns, early voluntary hand and arm movements, and prewriting skills	0-15 mo
Erhardt Developmental Vision Assessment	*Developmental:* Assesses involuntary and voluntary eye control	0-teenage years
Functional Independence Measure for Children (Wee-FIM)	*Functional:* Measures severity of disability; assesses self-care, mobility, gross and fine motor, language, and social skills	6 mo-7 yr
Gesell Preschool Assessment	*Developmental:* Assesses motor, adaptive, language, and personal social skills	2½-6 yr
Hawaii Early Learning Profile (HELP)	*Behavioral:* Determines developmental level; assesses cognitive, language, gross and fine motor, social, and self-help skills	0-3 yr
Miller Assessment of Preschoolers (MAP)	*Developmental:* Identifies children with mild to moderate delays; assesses sensorimotor and cognitive skills	33-68 mo
National Children's Medical Center Prevocational Capabilities Assessment	*Developmental and sensory motor:* Assesses cognition, gross and fine motor function, and sensory processing	12-19 yr
Peabody Developmental Motor Scales	*Developmental:* Assesses reflexes and gross and fine motor skills	0-83 mo
Sensory Integration and Praxis Test (SIPT)	*Sensory motor:* Assesses general sensory organization, coordination of right and left, motor planning, visual-motor coordination, and perception	4-8 yr
Test of Sensory Functions in Infants (TSFI)	*Sensory:* Assesses tactile and deep pressure functions, visual-tactile integration, adaptive motor function, ocular-motor function, and reactivity to vestibular stimulation	4-18 mo
Test of Visual-Perceptual Skills (TVPS) (Nonmotor)	*Developmental:* Assesses visual form discrimination, memory, spatial relationships, form constancy, sequencing, and figure-ground discrimination.	4-13 yr
Transdisciplinary Play Based Assessment	*Developmental:* Determines developmental skill level, learning style, and interaction through structured play; assesses cognitive, communication, sensory motor, and social skills	6 mo-6 yr

Modified from Rothstein JM, Roy SH, Wolf SL: *The rehabilitation specialist's handbook,* Philadelphia, 1998, FA Davis.

Organizations and Websites for Information on Pediatric Conditions and Disorders

The Agenesis of the Corpus Callosum (ACC) Network
5749 Merrill Hall, Room 18
University of Maine
Orono, ME 04469-5749
(207) 581-3119
Fax: (207) 581-3120
Website: *http://www.FAMILYVILLAGE.WISC.EDU/lib_agcc.htm*

American Foundation for the Blind
15 West 16th Street
New York, NY 10011
(212) 502-7600
Website: *http://www.afb.org/afb/index.html*

Angelman's Syndrome Foundation
PO Box 12437
Gainesville, FL 32604
(904) 332-3303
(800) 432-6435
Website: *http://medhlp.netusa.net/agsg/agsg47.htm*

The Arc
PO Box 1047
Arlington, TX 76004
(800) 433-5255
Website: *http://thearc.org/welcome.html*

Arthritis Foundation
1330 West Peachtree Street
Atlanta, GA 30309
(404) 872-7100
Arthritis Answers:
(800) 283-7800
Website: *http://www.arthritis.org/*

Autism Research Institute
4182 Adams Avenue
San Diego, CA 92116
Website: *http://www.autism.com/ari*

Autism Society of America
7910 Woodmont Avenue, Suite 650
Bethesda, MD 20814
(800) 328-8476
Website: *http://www.autism-society.org/*

Centers for Disease Control: CDC National AIDS Clearinghouse
PO Box 6003
Rockville, MD 20849-6003
Website: *http://www.cdcnac.org/*
CDC National AIDS Hotline
(800) 342-AIDS (2437)
Spanish: (800) 344-SIDA (7432)
Deaf: (800) 243-7889

Epilepsy Foundation
4351 Garden City Drive
Landover, MD 20785
(800) EFA-1000
Website: *http://www.efa.org/*

Erb's Palsy Information and Research Group
1313 Ridview St
Mesquite, TX 75149
(972) 329-6860
Website: *http://www.erbspalsy.org/index.html*

Facilitated Communication Institute
370 Huntington Hall
Syracuse University
Syracuse, NY 13244-2340
(315) 443-9657
Fax: (315) 443-2274
Website: *http://soeweb.syr.edu/thefci/*

International Rett Syndrome Association
9121 Piscataway Road, Suite 2-B
Clinton, MD 20735
(301) 856-3334
(800) 818-RETT
Fax: (301) 856-3336
Website: *http://www2.paltech.com/irsa/irsa.htm*

Muscular Dystrophy Association
3300 East Sunrise Drive
Tucson, AZ 85718
(602) 529-2000
Website: *http://www.mdausa.org/*

Organizations and Websites for Information on Pediatric Conditions and Disorders—cont'd

National Council on Disability
800 Independence Avenue, SW, Suite 814
Washington, DC 20591
(202) 267-3846

National Down Syndrome Congress
1605 Chantilly Drive, Suite 250
Atlanta, GA 30324
(800) 232-6372
Website: *http://members.CAROI.NET/NDSC*

National Down Syndrome Society
666 Broadway
New York, NY 10012
(800) 221-4602
Website: *http://www.babycenter.com/refcap/1446.html*

National Fragile X Foundation
PO Box 30023
Denver, CO 80203
(800) 688-8765
(303) 333-6155
Website: *http://www.nfxf.org/*

National Information Center for Children and Youth with Disabilities
PO Box 1492
Washington, DC 20013-1492
(800) 695-0285 (Voice/TT)
(202) 884-8200 (Voice/TT)
(800) 999-5599
Website: *http://www.kidsource.com/NICHCY/index.html*

National Information Center on Deafness
Gallaudet University
800 Florida Avenue, NE
Washington, DC 20002
(202) 651-5051
(202) 651-5052 (TDD)
Fax: (202) 651-5054
Website: *http://www.gallaudet.edu/-nicd/*

National Organization for Rare Disorders, Inc
PO Box 8923
New Fairfield, CT
(203) 746-6518
Website: *http://www.pcnet.com/~orphan/*

National Pediatric HIV Resource Center
HIV Resource Center
15 South Ninth Street
Newark, NJ 07107
(800) 362-0071
Website: *http://www.pedhivaids.org*

National Tuberous Sclerosis Association
8181 Professional Place, Suite 110
Landover, MD 20785
(301) 459-9888
(800) 225-NTSA
Fax: (301) 459-0394
Website: *http://www.ntsa.org/*

North American Riding for the Handicapped Association (NARHA)
PO Box 33150
Denver, CO 80233
(800) 369-RIDE (7433)
(303) 452-1212
Fax: (303) 252-4610
Website: *http://www.NARHA.org/*

The Prader-Willi Syndrome Association (USA)
5700 Midnight Pass Road
Sarasota, FL
(800) 926-4797
(941) 312-0400
Fax: (941) 312-0142
Website: *http://www.pwsausa.org*

Spina Bifida Association of America
4590 MacArthur Boulevard, NW, Suite 250
Washington, DC 20007
(800) 621-3141
Website: *http://www.sbaa.org/toc.htm*

United Cerebral Palsy Association
1522 K Street, NW, Suite 1112
Washington, DC 20005
(800) USA-5UCP
Website: *http://www.irsc.org/cerebral.htm*

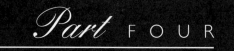
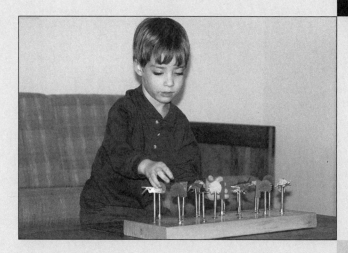

Part FOUR

Occupational Therapy Process

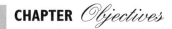

General Treatment Considerations

ANGELA M. PERALTA

PAULA KRAMER

CHAPTER *Objectives*

After studying this chapter the reader will be able to accomplish the following:

- Explain the way assessment relates to program planning and treatment implementation
- Differentiate among long-term goals, short-term objectives, and mini objectives
- Apply activity analysis to treatment sessions
- Apply the knowledge of activity adaptation for a given case
- Describe the discrete trial method of measuring performance

This chapter discusses specific treatment considerations that arise during the occupational therapy process. This process begins with the referral, screening and evaluation; continues with the intervention plan, goal setting, and treatment implementation; and moves to reevaluation and discharge planning.

The occupational therapy process is somewhat different for the registered occupational therapist (OTR) than it is for the certified occupational therapy assistant (COTA). The OTR is responsible for selection of the assessments used during the evaluation, interpretation of results, and development of the intervention plan. The COTA may gather evaluative data under the supervision of an OTR using an approved structured format. The COTA is not responsible for the interpretation of the assessment results but should contribute any knowledge of the client gained during the assessment process.

REFERRAL, SCREENING, AND EVALUATION

The referral, screening, and evaluation aspect of the occupational therapy process is referred to as the *evaluation period*. During the evaluation period the occupational therapy practitioner meets the child to collect information that will assist in setting goals and developing an activity configuration for the child.

Referral

A **referral** is the usual method through which a client is introduced to occupational therapy. The specific need for a referral depends on the individual state licensure law or regulations within the area of practice. It is incumbent on the OTR and the COTA to know the laws and regulations that govern their area of practice. A physician or a nurse practitioner generally gives the referral, again depending on the state's laws; it is called a *physician's referral* or *doctor's orders*. Some states require a referral before an occupational therapy practitioner sees a client. Other states require a referral only for the intervention process.

According to the *Standards of Practice for Occupational Therapy* published by the American Occupational Therapy Association (AOTA) in 1998,[1] only the OTR may accept a referral for assessment.[1] COTAs, if given a referral, are responsible for forwarding the referral to a supervising OTR and for educating "current and potential referral sources about the scope of occupational therapy services and the process of initiating occupational therapy referrals."[1] A COTA may acknowledge requests for services from any source. However, COTAs do not accept and begin working on cases at their own professional discretion without the supervision and collaboration of the OTR.

Screening

Another way that clients may come to occupational therapy is through a mass **screening.** Both OTRs and COTAs can conduct such screenings. For example, a COTA or a teacher may be hired to screen children in a well-baby clinic or an incoming kindergarten class to determine the need for additional evaluation before entering school. Once the COTA has identified the need for a more complete evaluation, the OTR determines the specific evaluation or format to be used. Data gathered by the COTA is interpreted by the OTR. A COTA "may contribute to this process under the supervision of a registered occupational therapist."[1]

Evaluation

The **evaluation** is a critical component of the occupational therapy process. It is usually initiated in response to a referral. The OTR is responsible for determining the type and scope of the evaluation. An evaluation includes assessments of an individual's performance areas, performance components, and performance context. According to the AOTA's *Occupational Therapy Roles*, an entry level COTA "assists with data collection and evaluation under the supervision of the occupational therapist" (see Chapter 1, "Scope of Practice").[2] An intermediate or advanced level COTA "administers standardized tests under the supervision of an occupational therapist after service competency has been established."[2] Although the COTA may participate in the evaluation process, it is the responsibility of the OTR to interpret the results of the assessments and develop an intervention plan for the client. The evaluation determines the child's strengths and limitations and should give the occupational therapy practitioner an understanding of the child's level of performance.

Levels of performance
Functional independence
A child is considered to be functionally independent when the child is able to complete an age-appropriate activity with or without the use of assistive devices and without human assistance (for example, eat independently with an offset spoon).

Assisted performance
Assisted performance refers to a child's participation in a specific task with some assistance from the caregiver (for example, putting on a shirt and receiving assistance with buttoning).

Dependent performance
Dependent performance occurs when a child's is unable to perform a specific age-appropriate task. A caregiver is

required to perform the task for the child (for example, hold a cup for a child with cerebral palsy who is unable to drink from a cup).

INTERVENTION PLAN, GOAL SETTING, AND TREATMENT IMPLEMENTATION

Intervention Plan

The OTR develops the **intervention plan** after the evaluation is complete. The intervention plan includes a list of the client's limitations and strengths. It identifies the client's rehabilitation potential, long-term goals and short-term objectives. It identifies the type of media (that is, specific types of materials) and modalities (that is, intervention tools) that will be used and the frequency and duration of treatment. The intervention plan also includes plans for reevaluation and discharge. The intervention plan should also classify the level of personnel that will be providing the intervention.[1]

The strength of the COTA lies in the intervention process. Though following an intervention plan developed by the OTR, the COTA understands the process of **activity analysis;** selection, gradation, and adaptation of activities. The COTA is knowledgeable about treatment implementation and can identify the need for reevaluation during the intervention process. The intervention is executed in collaboration with a supervising OTR, but the COTA is a proficient contributor to the intervention process.

Legitimate tools

Legitimate tools are the instruments or tools that a profession uses to bring about change. Legitimate tools change over time based on the growing knowledge of the profession, technological advances in society, and the needs and values of both the profession and society.[11] Occupational therapy practitioners use various tools to bring about change. Some of the critical tools used when working with children are purposeful activities, activity analysis, and activity synthesis.

Purposeful activities

An important principle of occupational therapy is that occupation must have a purposeful goal to be effective in the treatment of physical and mental disabilities. Purposeful activity is defined by the AOTA as goal-directed behaviors or tasks that comprise occupations.[7] An activity is considered purposeful if the individual is a voluntary, active participant and the activity is directed toward a goal that the individual considers meaningful. Occupational therapy practitioners use purposeful activity to evaluate, facilitate, restore, or maintain individuals' abilities to function in their daily occupations.

Purposeful activity provides opportunities for persons to achieve mastery of their environment, and successful performance promotes feelings of personal competence. A person involved in purposeful activities directs attention toward the goal rather than the processes required for achievement of the goal. Engagement in purposeful activity within the context of interpersonal, cultural, physical, and other environmental conditions requires and elicits coordination among the individual's sensorimotor, cognitive, and psychosocial systems. Purposeful activities cannot be prescribed on the basis of analysis of their inherent characteristics alone. By definition prescription of purposeful activity is specific to the individual. An occupational therapy practitioner grades or adapts a chosen activity for an individual to promote successful performance or to elicit a particular response.[7]

Activity analysis

Activity analysis refers to the process of analyzing an activity to determine how and when it should be used with a particular client. Activity analysis is the identification of the components of an activity.[9] Several methods are used to analyze activity, two of which are discussed in this chapter.

The first method is the task-focused activity analysis. This method of analyzing activity is geared toward the identification of components of a specific task. It identifies the materials needed for the activity and the required sequential steps of the activity. Task-focused activity analysis identifies the most important and the least important performance components needed to complete the activity. It also identifies the physical, social, and cultural influences the activity may have. In this type of analysis the occupational therapy practitioner identifies how the activity may be graded, adapted, and synthesized and also considers potential safety hazards of the activity.

Task-focused activity analysis is used to understand the activity, the skills required to complete the activity, and the cultural meaning of the activity. It helps the occupational therapy practitioner understand how the activity can be use therapeutically. Task-focused activity analysis enables the occupational therapy practitioner to quickly identify the demand of an activity (Figure 12-1).[5]

The second method is the child- and family-focused activity analysis (Figure 12-2). The occupational therapy practitioner is focused on the actual treatment implementation with this method. The practitioner identifies the child and family's strengths and weaknesses. The practitioner then identifies the objectives and plans activities that are specifically designed to meet those objectives. The practitioner describes the types of materials, supplies, and equipment that will be needed; identifies the position of the child and the occupational therapy practitioner during intervention; and cites expected results or any rec-

TASK-FOCUSED ACTIVITY ANALYSIS

CHILD'S NAME: _Kellie Peralta_   DATE: _12/30/98_

ACTIVITY DESCRIPTION: _Closing Velcro tabs on shoes_

SUPPLIES/EQUIPMENT: _Socks, shoes, chair_

STEPS OF ACTIVITY:

1) _Prepare work area with chair, socks, and shoes._
2) _Position child on chair._
3) _Put socks and shoes on._
4) _Demonstrate how to close tabs._
5) _Allow the child to practice closing tabs with hand-over-hand assistance._
6) _Allow child to begin practicing closing tabs._

LIST THE MOST IMPORTANT PERFORMANCE COMPONENTS REQUIRED FOR THIS ACTIVITY:

Sensorimotor	Cognitive	Psychosocial/Psychological
1) Sensory awareness	1) Level of arousal	1) Values
2) Tactile	2) Attention span	2) Interests
3) Proprioception	3) Sequencing	3) Role performance
4) Kinesthesia	4) Learning	4) Self-expression
5) Fine coordination/dexterity	5) Concept formation	5) Coping skills

LIST THE LEAST IMPORTANT PERFORMANCE COMPONENTS REQUIRED FOR THIS ACTIVITY:

Sensorimotor	Cognitive	Psychosocial/Psychological
1) Oral-motor control	1) Orientation	1) Self-concept
2) Reflexes	2) Recognition	2) Social conduct
3) Pain response	3) Categorization	3) Interpersonal skills
4) Olfactory	4) Spatial operations	4) Time management skills
5) Gustatory	5) Problem-solving skills	5) Self-control

ENVIRONMENTAL CONTEXTS:

1. Physical	2. Social	3. Cultural
Activity can be done in the child's room or another room in the home. Area should be well lighted. Child can sit on chair or floor.	Practitioner and child will work together until task is learned. Mother will practice with child.	In our culture, people are expected to wear shoes.

Gradation	Adaptation	Safety Hazards
Method of instruction can vary to accommodate child's learning needs. Task can be taught using hand-over-hand method	D rings can be placed on tip of tabs to facilitate grasping the tabs.	None

FIGURE 12-1 Task-focused activity analysis form for Kellie Peralta.

CHILD- AND FAMILY-FOCUSED ACTIVITY ANALYSIS

DATE: *12/30/98*

CHILD'S NAME: *Kellie Peralta*   AGE: *2 years, 7 months*

DIAGNOSIS: *Pervasive Developmental Disorder—Autism*

SETTING: *Home based*   FREQUENCY OF OT: *5 times per week*

DURATION: *1 hour per session*

Strengths	Limitations
Strong family support system	*Decreased eye contact*
Enjoys proprioceptive activities	*Delays in fine motor skills*
Enjoys vestibular activities	*Delays in gross motor skills*
	Delays with self-care skills

OBJECTIVE: *Kellie will be able to engage in at least three activities without tantrums within 6 months.*

Planned Activities	Materials	Supplies and Equipment
1) Hair brushing *2) Vestibular activities* *3) Dressing activities*		*1) Hair brush* *2) Therapy ball* *3) Clothing, shoes*
Position of Child and Practitioner	**Performance Results**	**Recommendations**
1) Child sits on floor in front of therapist.	*1) Child had difficulty tolerating hairbrushing.*	*1) Continue with deep pressure hairbrushing with corn brush. Allow child to initiate hairbrushing activity.*
2) Child initially sits on a 9-inch ball. Practitioner is positioned behind child and supports child at hips.	*2) Child was able to tolerate sitting on ball. She was able to carry out a task while sitting on a ball.*	*2) Introduce a 12-inch ball during next session.*
3) Child sits on floor in front of practitioner. Practitioner also sits on floor.	*3) Child was receptive and able to follow directions. Hand-over-hand assistance was required.*	*3) Mother should practice activity with child every day. Discrete trial teaching will be used during therapy sessions.*

FIGURE 12-2   Child- and family-focused activity analysis form for Kellie Peralta.

ommendations indicated. It is assumed that an occupational therapy practitioner will know of several activities and will have analyzed these activities using the task-focused activity analysis.

It should be noted that some degree of overlap exists between the two types of activity analysis. They are not mutually exclusive, though each emphasizes distinct as-

pects of activity. Both methods require the practitioner to understand the needs of the child, a variety of theoretical approaches, and the context of intervention.

Activity synthesis

Activity synthesis is another legitimate tool used by occupational therapy practitioners. Activity synthesis includes adapting, grading, and reconfiguring activities into a whole.

Activity adaptation is the process of changing specific steps during an activity so that the client is able to engage in it. Activities are adapted by modifying or changing the sequence of the activity, the way the materials are presented, the way the child is positioned, or by presenting the activity so that the child is expected to perform only certain aspects of it. Activities can also be adapted by changing the characteristics of the materials that are used (such as the size, shape, texture or weight of the materials).[11] For example, for a child who is fearful of movement and needs to improve or develop righting reactions, the practitioner could place the child on a therapy ball to elicit righting reactions. However, because of the child's fear of movement, the practitioner could begin the intervention with a smaller ball that allows the child's feet to stay on the ground and provides slow, controlled movements. The practitioner can make the activity easier or more difficult to find the right challenge for the child.

Grading an activity is another legitimate tool used by occupational therapy practitioners and is a form of adaptation. Grading refers to the process of arranging the steps of an activity in a sequential series to change or progress, allowing for gradual improvement by increasing demands for a higher level of performance as the child's abilities increase. The type and extent of grading is determined by professional judgment. Graded activities provide clients with the opportunity to perform an activity in tolerable increments and thereby change their level of performance. Once the practitioner has adapted and graded an activity, the activity is presented in its "real" form, thus synthesizing the analysis, adaptation, and grading into the activity itself.[10] For example, as a child is learning to self-feed, finger feeding is acceptable. The activity is then adapted by the introduction of a utensil. Initially, it would be acceptable for the child to hold the utensil and attempt to use it to scoop or spear food. Ultimately, the practitioner expects the child to grasp the utensil, spear the food, and bring the food to the mouth, thus synthesizing the activity of self-feeding into the child's repertoire of abilities.

Activity configuration

Activity configuration is the process of selecting specific activities to use during the intervention process based on the child's age, interests, and abilities. For example, a long-term goal may be that a child will be able to feed independently. One short-term goal may be that the child will be able to scoop with a spoon. A session objective may be that the child will learn how to control grasp and release of a spoon.

Therapeutic use of self

Therapeutic use of self refers to the ability of occupational therapy practitioners to be aware of their own personal feelings and to clearly communicate with the child and the child's family or caregivers.

Pediatric occupational therapy can be considered a subspecialty in occupational therapy, and practitioners planning to work in this area need to be knowledgeable about family dynamics, the impact of cultural and ethnic concepts on service provision, and family systems (see Chapter 2). Practitioners also need to be familiar with federal laws and have the ability to work with an interdisciplinary team (see Chapters 4 and 16).[8]

In a therapeutic relationship the practitioner is expected to help the child and the family without any expectation of the help being reciprocated. The practitioner is responsible for developing and maintaining a good relationship with the child and the family.[4] As Suzanne Peloquin said, ". . . concern for the patient as a person remains essential to effective practice."[12] Occupational therapy practitioners recognize that a child is seldom treated without consideration for environmental factors. All intervention needs to be geared toward both the child and the family or caregivers. The practitioner's role is to create an atmosphere of freedom and appropriate challenge within the structure of the intervention. The intervention should not be so simple that the child becomes bored or so difficult that the child feels inadequate. The practitioner should prepare a setting in which the child's needs are being met and the practitioner can guide the child toward mastery of the skill that is being taught.[12]

When working with children, especially those who have recently entered to the health care setting, practitioners must also work with the family and guide them as they care for the child. The families are often experiencing emotional turmoil caused by the child's diagnosis or undergoing a change in their traditional or expected roles. As a result, the parents may not be able to participate in the therapeutic process. They may feel that their "beautiful baby" is damaged, or they may simply view a diagnosis as catastrophic. They may not be ready to help the child on the road to recovery.

In pediatric practice, practitioners commonly encounter parents or caregivers who are in denial of their child's condition or appear uncaring. It can be frustrating for a practitioner who spends time discussing, instructing, and offering suggestions for the home to discover that the parents are doing nothing or are doing too much. Practitioners need to accept parents as they are and be willing to work with them rather than impose expectations. Occupational therapy practitioners need to work on goals with the parents and be sensitive to parents who are having difficulty accepting their child's disability and therefore not following the practitioner's recommendations.

Research about the way parents respond to being taught indicates that parents often find it overwhelming to absorb all of the information the occupational therapy practitioner expects them to remember.[7] Parents have reported that they sometimes learn more easily by observing the practitioner work with the child. Being able to ask questions helps them to use new routines or handling techniques that often require a change in the family life. Parents have also reported that just having general conversations about the child is helpful to the family. Practitioners should be aware of family dynamics and not place demands on the family that are impossible to meet.[5,7] The practitioner needs to provide intervention that assists the parents or caregiver with providing the best care possible for the child. Practitioners can assist caregivers by creating a realistic plan for them to assume new roles, which will help them meet the needs of the disabled child.[5]

A child with a disability influences the roles, values and relationships of the family in the same way that the family influences the child.[4] Occupational therapy practitioners play a major role in helping the child and the family adjust to a disability by providing strategies for meeting the needs of both the child and family.

Occupational therapy practitioners should be aware of the way their own feelings can affect treatment. Some practitioners find it difficult to treat a child who has a terminal illness, noticeable deformities, or severe behavioral problems. The practitioner should discuss these feelings with a supervisor to facilitate the implementation of an objective and effective intervention.

Family-centered intervention for children is emphasized in the Individual with Disabilities Education Act (IDEA). One of the primary mechanisms for ensuring the needs of infants and toddlers less than 3 years of age and their families are met is the individual family's service plan (IFSP). The individual education plan (IEP) is used for children older than age 3 (see Chapters 2 and 4). These plans address the child's current health status, family concerns, therapy goals, and outcomes that are important for the child and their families.

Multicultural implications

The increasingly diverse population of the United States demands that occupational therapy practitioners consider cultural differences between themselves and the children they serve. The consequences of dismissing cultural values when planning intervention can lead to a breakdown in communication between the practitioner and the family. Rapport may be difficult to establish and as a result the practitioner may find that the child or the caregiver may not trust the intervention and does not follow through with recommendations. When this happens, the lack of compliance and satisfaction generally makes the therapy process ineffective. The practitioner should plan the intervention within the context of the child and family's culture.

Goal Setting

The COTA should collaborate with the OTR on the development of long-term goals and short-term objectives for any child that they are treating. Through this collaborative process, the OTR and COTA can agree on the needs of the child as well as the appropriate sequence for intervention. This makes the intervention process more efficient and effective and leads to a better understanding of the child. Based on the evaluation, the occupational therapy practitioners can collaborate to develop realistic goals for the child.

Long-term goals

Long-term goals are statements that describe the terminal functional skills the client should achieve after intervention. Long-term goals should be measurable, observable, and clear. They should be written in behavioral terms. Goals need to be very specific and address the problems that have been identified. A practitioner can use the mnemonic **RUMBA criteria** method to evaluate the goal statements they write (Box 12-1).[6]

Short-term objectives

Short-term objectives are all the tasks that the client needs to be able to do to meet the long-term goal. They

---

BOX 12-1

RUMBA *Criteria*

R (RELEVANT)
A relevant goal reflects the client's life situation and future goals. Everyone involved with the client's care (client, therapist, family, and members of other disciplines) should agree on the goal.

U (UNDERSTANDABLE)
An understandable goal is stated in clear language. Jargon and very specialized or difficult words should be avoided.

M (MEASURABLE)
A measurable goal contains a criteria for success.

B (BEHAVIORAL)
A behavioral goal focuses on the behavior or skill the client must eventually demonstrate.

A (ACHIEVABLE)
An achievable goal describes a behavior or skill that the client should be able to accomplish in a reasonable period of time.

Modified from Early MB: *Mental health concepts and techniques for the occupational therapy assistant,* ed 2, New York, 1993, Raven Press.

are like sign posts that tell practitioners they are on the right track and moving closer to achieving the long-term goal. They are excellent indicators that progress toward the long-term goal is being made.

Short-term objectives are the interim steps that are used to reach the long-term goal. They are statements that describe skills that should be mastered in a relatively short period. For example, consider a client whose long-term goal is independent dressing. The short-term objectives may include the development of a pincer grasp for buttoning, learning to button, and the development of sequencing skills for dressing.

Treatment Implementation

Treatment implementation is the heart of the intervention process. It involves working within the system through which the child is receiving therapy, working with the family, and working directly with the child. Working with the child involves planning each session, developing and analyzing activities, and then grading and adapting activities as necessary. This process is geared toward reaching the short-term objectives first and then the long-term goals.

Treatment implementation is practice of the actual therapy. It includes the methods used to work toward meeting the goals and the media or activities that are used during the course of intervention. Treatment implementation also includes the periodic documentation of the child's progress or lack of progress and any revision to the plan.

Session, or mini, objectives

Mini objectives are the goals the practitioner has set for a specific treatment session. They are planned before the treatment session in collaboration with the child and parents. Sometimes mini objectives will last for several sessions because it may take more than one intervention to meet the objective.

Once the mini objectives are identified, the occupational therapy practitioner analyzes the activities that will facilitate meeting the objective. The practitioner may choose different types of analysis depending on the goals.

Working with the child

The OTR and COTA should collaborate during the development of the intervention plan. When the plan is developed, the OTR should be using a frame of reference for organizing the plan. The COTA must have a working understanding of the frame of reference to be able to carry out the plan.

Frames of reference are critical tools of occupational therapy. A frame of reference provides the conceptual framework for organizing practical material, outlining the theoretical concepts of a particular approach, providing guidelines for assessing functional capacities of the client, and providing a method for conceptualizing and initiating intervention. The occupational therapy practitioner is responsible for selecting the specific frame of reference used during intervention.

Various frames of reference are used in occupational therapy. Frames of reference are described in this and other occupational therapy texts. Occupational therapy practitioners should become familiar with several different frames of reference used in their practice arenas.

REEVALUATION AND DISCHARGE PLANNING

Reevaluation

Although it is the responsibility of the OTR to determine whether a reevaluation is indicated, the COTA is responsible for reporting any change in the child's condition to the supervisor. Therefore if the COTA observes changes, they must be brought to the attention of the OTR, and the COTA should suggest a reevaluation. The COTA participates in the reevaluation in collaboration with and under the supervision of the OTR.

Measuring performance

When a child is inconsistently able to perform a task independently (that is, requires assistance for a task periodically), the practitioner should document that the child needs assistance with the task.

The process of measuring performance is an evaluative task and requires the collaboration of the OTR and the COTA. This collaboration is a partnership between the OTR and the COTA based on respect, mutual trust, and knowledge of expectations. It is a two-way process, with both practitioners sharing the responsibility for maintaining and improving the relationship. Occupational therapy practitioners measure performance so that they can transition the child from simple to increasingly complex tasks. Several methods are used to measure performance, some of which are discussed in Chapters 13, 14, and 16. The **discrete trial** method of instruction is discussed here to illustrate one way performance can be measured.

Discrete trial teaching is a method of teaching used by behaviorists that uses repetition, prompting, and reinforcement procedures to strengthen the response and its lasting effects to teach a specific skill. The practitioner selects the specific activity or task that needs to be taught and breaks it down into minute components. Each component is then taught in isolation until the child masters it (Figure 12-3). The practitioner then assists the child in generalizing the uses of the activity and so that it can be

Program: Opening Velcro tabs on shoes

Date started: 9/20/98

Criteria: 90% over two trials

	9/20/98	9/21/98	9/22/98	9/23/98
	Opening Velcro Tabs	Opening Velcro Tabs	Opening Velcro Tabs	Opening Velcro Tabs
1	0	0	0	1
2	0	0	1	1
3	0	0	1	1
4	0	1	1	1
5	0	1	1	1
6	1	1	1	1
7	1	1	1	1
8	1	1	1	1
9	1	1	1	1
10	1	1	1	1
	50%	70%	90%	100%

0 = Incorrect response
1 = Correct response

FIGURE 12-3   Discrete trial worksheet for one task.

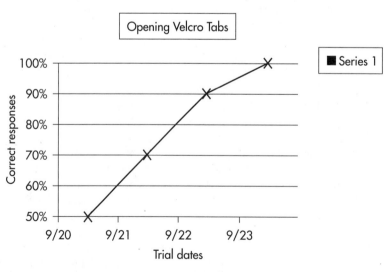

FIGURE 12-4   Discrete trials progress graph.

incorporated into the child's routine. This method is most effective with children who have processing deficits and is often used to teach skills to children with autism and mental retardation.

The information from the worksheet (see Figure 12-3) is then transferred to a graph so that the learning progress can be easily tracked by the occupational therapy practitioner, the child (if feasible), and the caregiver (Figure 12-4). It provides those involved in teaching the task with information about the rate of progress as well as when the child may be moved to the next task. Keep in mind that this is just one type of intervention and one way of measuring performance and change.

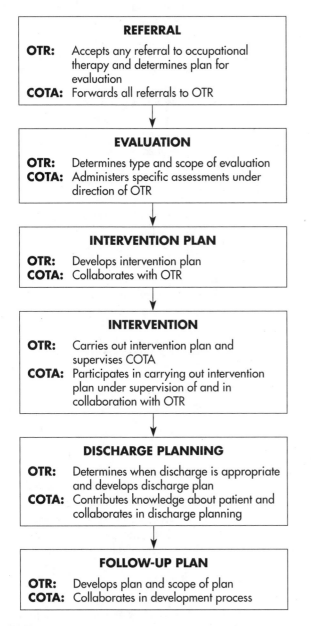

FIGURE 12-5 Responsibilities of OTR and COTA in occupational therapy intervention process.

Discharge Planning

In pediatric occupational therapy the discharge planning and date may be mandated by specific laws that govern the type of system in which the child receives occupational therapy services. Regardless of the system used with the child, the discontinuation process is the responsibility of the OTR. The COTA collaborates in the discontinuation process under the supervision of the OTR by reporting on the child's progress and making suggestions regarding future needs.

Discontinuation of services typically occurs once the child has met predetermined goals, has achieved maximum benefit from occupational therapy, or the parents or child determine that the child no longer wants to receive occupational therapy. The COTA may recommend discontinuation of services to the OTR when any of the mentioned conditions exist. Discontinuation plans should include a plan for follow up when indicated. Figure 12-5 provides a summary of the occupational therapy process from the referral to the follow-up plan.

GENERAL TREATMENT CONSIDERATIONS IN PEDIATRIC PRACTICE
Infection Control

Infection control is the responsibility of every practitioner. Occupational therapy practitioners must follow universal precautions when working with any client. Universal precautions are a set of rules set out by the Center for Disease Control in 1985 to address concerns regarding the transmission of the Human Immunodeficiency Virus (HIV) and the Hepatitis B Virus (HBV) to health care and public safety workers. Universal precautions are used when a person has the potential to be exposed to blood, certain other body fluids, or any other fluid visibly contaminated by blood. Health care workers must assume that all persons may be infected with HIV or HBV virus and follow universal precautions at all times.

Hand washing

Hand washing is the single most important component of infection control. Hands should be washed before and immediately after working with a client or whenever a person comes into contact with any type of body fluid. Hands should also be washed when gloves are removed.

Use of gloves

Gloves should be used by occupational therapy practitioners when the possibility exists of coming into contact with infected material, providing oral motor intervention that requires that the practitioners' fingers to enter the oral cavity, and changing diapers. Gloves should also be worn by occupational therapy practitioners who have scratches or other breaks in their skin.

Cleaning of equipment and toys

Occupational therapy practitioners need to maintain equipment and toys in clean, good working order. Although occupational therapy practitioners do not sterilize equipment and toys after children use them, all equipment and toys should be properly cleaned. The occupational therapy practitioner can also request that families provide the child's favorite toys for use during therapy. The practitioner can educate the families about the safest and most effective methods of cleaning their children's toys.

According to the U.S. Department of Labor, Occupational Safety and Health Administration (OSHA), facilities and agencies must provide their workers with policies and procedures for cleaning and disinfection.[13] These specific procedures are beyond the scope of this chapter. It is the responsibility of practitioners to become familiar with their facility's policies and procedures for disinfection.

Hepatitis B vaccination

The OSHA standard regarding bloodborne pathogens requires employers to offer a free three-injection hepatitis B vaccination series to all employees who are exposed to blood or any other potentially infectious materials as part of their job duties. This includes occupational therapy practitioners and other health care workers. Vaccinations must be offered within 10 days of initial assignment to a job in which exposure to blood or other potentially infectious materials can be "reasonably anticipated."[13]

CASE *Study*

Kellie is a 2-year 7-month-old girl with a diagnosis of pervasive developmental disorder. She was referred to an early intervention program for evaluation because of her parents concerns regarding her lack of speech development, difficulty tolerating self-care activities, and weak relationship with her siblings and peers.

The developmental specialist who initially evaluated Kellie recommended an occupational therapy evaluation.

Kellie was evaluated by an OTR on December 21, 1998. Findings are as follows:

Developmental History

Kellie was born at 9 months gestation after a normal pregnancy. There were no complications at birth, and Kellie was released from the hospital 4 days later. Her mother states that Kellie was a "very good baby." She was not fussy. She preferred her infant seat and often cried when she was picked up or was passed around from relative to relative. Her mother reports that Kellie met her developmental milestones as follows: (1) she was able to sit unsupported at 6 months; (2) she never crawled much and started walking at 9½ months (and currently rarely falls while walking); and (3) she started going up and down the stairs at about 11 months and was very careful doing so. Kellie is currently able to drink from a bottle but does not like to drink from a cup. She is very particular about the foods she eats and only likes very soft, almost liquid, types of food. Currently her food preferences include Cheerios with milk, pasta soup, and bland mashed potatoes. Kellie sometimes eats very ripe bananas. Her mother is concerned about the lack of variety in Kellie's diet. Kellie does not yet dress or undress independently and is fussy when bathed. She often hides when her mother announces that it is bath time. Her mother reports that Kellie only likes to wear long-sleeved shirts and leggings and refuses to walk around barefoot. Her mother is also concerned that Kellie often walks on her toes. Kellie sometimes enjoys going to the playground, especially when there are few or no other children around. She goes up and down the slide, sometimes as often as 30 times in an hour. She is terrified of the swing and refuses to go in the sand box. Kellie's mother is also concerned about Kellie's apparent lack of need for her mother, father, or siblings. Kellie's mother reports that Kellie prefers to sit in front of the television watching children's programs and does not play with toys. Kellie does not respond to her name when called despite having had a normal audiological examination. Kellie's eye contact is very limited. She does not verbalize her needs and instead takes her mother's hand to guide her to whatever she wants. She does not point or does look at her mom when requesting.

Occupational Therapy Evaluation Findings

Gross motor

Kellie is able to transition smoothly through all developmental postures up to and including standing. Kellie ambulates as her primary means of mobility. She occasionally walks on her toes when she is not wearing shoes. During testing some tightness was noted at both ankles, which may be caused by the toe walking, but passive range of motion (PROM) of both ankles remains within normal limits. Kellie has adequate equilibrium and protective responses for her age.

Kellie is able to walk up and down steps while holding a railing. She is able to climb onto an adult chair and sit. Kellie demonstrated poor posture while sitting and during some movement activities. She "W sits" and resumes this posture after it is corrected. She is able to run; however, her posturing during this activity is stiff, and she does not demonstrate appropriate arm swing or rotational movements. She maintains her scapula (shoulder blade) in a fixed position while running. She is unable to stand on one foot and or kick a ball. Kellie demonstrates low tone throughout her upper body and neck.

Kellie enjoys roughhousing with her father. She appears to enjoy being thrown up in the air and tickled.

Kellie demonstrates a 4- to 6-month delay in the development of her gross motor skills.

Fine motor

Kellie made good eye contact with the evaluator when she was first encountered, demonstrating her awareness of others. However, her eye contact during the evaluation was inconsistent, especially when given activities. She was able to visually track objects within the full range, but strabismus (a visual deficiency caused by an imbalance in the eye muscles) in the left eye was noted at times. Her mother states that this happens when she is tired and may be caused by weak eye muscles. It was unclear during the evaluation whether the strabismus interfered with her eye-hand coordination. Kellie demonstrated a short attention span during most activities except ones that she was familiar with and able to perform, such as playing with a pop-up toy. When she was unable to problem solve to complete an activity, she showed little frustration and just walked away from the activity.

Kellie possesses all the prerequisites for fine motor development but lacks the manipulation and problem-solving skills to integrate them functionally. She often likes to hold an object in each hand and visually examine them but does not usually manipulate them. She uses a pincer and tripod grasp to pick up objects. She has the finger isolation skills required for pointing and poking. Kellie was able to stack two blocks after a demonstration, with some incoordination noted; "normal" for her age is 8 to 10 blocks. She was able to pull three to four pegs out of the pegboard but unable to place one into the pegboard. She was unable to complete puzzles or sort shapes successfully and demonstrated deficits in spatial awareness, eye-hand coordination, and problem-solving skills. She did not attend to activities for very long. Kellie demonstrated delays in development of bilateral (two-handed) coordination skills. She was able to pull apart pop beads and attempted to put them together. She is unable to string large beads, even after demonstrations and verbal cues. Kellie did not follow one-step directions consistently, which may be related to her decreased attention span and eye contact. Presently, Kellie demonstrates an 11- to 12-month delay in development of her fine motor skills.

Oral motor

Kellie has increased tone in her facial muscles, resulting in a closed-mouth posture and decreased range of motion (ROM) in the jaw. Kellie has a retracted lower jaw, resulting in an overbite, which may be interfering with her oral mo-

bility. Her tongue is often retracted and elevated and has a cleft, which may indicate that she has a short frenum. (This was not evaluated because of her tactile defensiveness within the oral cavity.) Her mother reports it is hard to brush her teeth, and Kellie never really mouthed toys when she was younger. This limited her sensory exploration during the oral phase of development. Kellie rarely drooled when she was teething which is also an indication of extreme mouth closure caused by either high muscle tone or structural deficits. Kellie's mother was given the recommendation that Kellie be evaluated by a pediatric dentist or maxillofacial specialist to assess her facial structure.

Kellie is able to bite off a piece of a cookie and bring it to the chewing surface. She is able to lateralize her tongue but only toward the back of her mouth. She is unable to actively bring her tongue forward to meet her teeth. Her decreased tongue mobility is interfering with her feeding and speech skills. Kellie is able to drink from a spout cup and a straw.

Presently Kellie demonstrates oral motor skills in the 16- to 18-month level, about a 9- to 11-month delay.

Adaptive skills

Kellie is demonstrating delays in all areas of self-care. At 2 years of age, she was beginning to use a spoon but generally preferred using her fingers and was able to drink from a sippy cup independently. Although demonstrating the ability to use a spoon and spear with a fork, Kellie currently still prefers finger feeding.

Kellie is able to remove her socks. She is unable to remove slip-on shoes or unlace or unbuckle other shoes. She is unable to put on or take off pants, skirts, or shirts. Kellie is able to remove mittens, hats, and coats (after the coats are unzipped).

Kellie is presently demonstrating a 5- to 7-month delay in her development of adaptive skills.

CLINICAL *Pearl*

Children are expected to begin participating in self-care tasks in a progressive pattern. For example, when learning dressing skills, a child is generally expected to undress before they begin to dress. Shoes and socks are usually taken off before pants and shirts. Children usually learn to drink from a bottle before a sippy cup or an uncovered cup. Children usually finger feed before they are able to use spoon or a fork (see Chapter 13).

Sensory integration

Kellie demonstrates delays in her ability to integrate touch, vision, and vestibular input. She has a decreased tolerance for the feeling of different textures on her hands and feet and in her mouth. She does not tolerate handling or vestibular input. She demonstrates poor motor planning skills that are affected by her inability to integrate sensory stimuli.

Abbreviated Intervention Plan

PROBLEM LIST	INTERVENTION STRATEGIES
ADAPTIVE SKILLS	
Inability to put on and remove socks, shoes, pants, skirts, or shirts	Skill training and practice sessions to include all dressing and undressing tasks
Inability to manipulate closures	Fine motor skills practice sessions
Inability to use spoon or fork consistently	Discrete trial teaching method
GROSS MOTOR SKILLS	
Low muscle tone throughout upper body	Weightbearing activities for her upper body, such as wheelbarrow walking; pushing and pulling activities involving heavy objects, such as dragging the practitioner's bag across the floor from the door to the work area; use of equipment such as a ball, Theraband (for resistive pulling activities), therapy putty (for resistive kneading and pulling apart and making figures of animals); jumping activities such as jumping over obstacles and on trampoline while supported at her hands, progressive grading to independent jumping; running activities such as running toward the practitioner to be picked up and raised over the practitioner's head
Poor posturing during activities	Facilitation activities to increase trunk extension ans correction of "W sitting posture"
SENSORY INTEGRATION ACTIVITIES	
Tactile defensiveness and decreased proprioceptive awareness throughout body	Brushing program to decrease tactile defensiveness and to provide proprioceptive input
Generalized sensory disorganization	Sensory integration activities

Long-term goal
Kellie will be able to dress herself with verbal prompting within 6 months.

Short-term objectives
1. Will demonstrate bilateral coordination skills within two months
    - Will be able to put together 5 to 6 pop beads independently 3 out of 4 times
    - Will be able to string 1 to 2 beads with verbal cues 3 out of 4 times
    - Will be able to unbutton a shirt independently 3 out of 4 times
2. Will demonstrate manipulation and eye-hand coordination during activities
    - Will be able to stack 7 to 10 blocks consecutively 3 out of 4 times
    - Will be able to turn and manipulate a puzzle piece independently to fit into the correct space 3 out of 4 times
    - Will be able to maintain a tripod grasp on a crayon independently while she imitates drawing a vertical line independently 3 out of 4 times
    - Will be able to zip and unzip jacket independently 3 out of 4 times

Long-term goal
Will demonstrate increased muscle tone in facial musculature and increase ROM of the jaw and tongue required for independent feeding

Short-term objectives
1. Will tolerate oral motor stimulation from a Nuk toothbrush for 2 minutes 3 times per day by practitioner or parent
2. Will tolerate deep pressure to face by hands or washcloth, with the pressure applied evenly in a downward motion starting from the temporal mandibular joint to increase PROM of the jaw, 3 times per day for 2 to 3 minutes
3. Will be able to bring her tongue forward and elevate it to her upper lip to wipe off food three out of 4 times

Long-term goal
Will demonstrate the ability to adaptively respond and relate to people and stimuli in her environment via sensory based activities within 6 months.

Short-term objectives
1. Will tolerate touching various textures with her hands for approximately 10 to 20 seconds 3 out of 4 times per practitioner or parent observation
2. Will remove 4 to 5 objects from a rice or bean bath and attempt to identify them through sounds or gestures 3 out of 4 times per practitioner or parent observation

3. Will tolerate sitting on therapy ball without movement for approximately 2 to 3 minutes 3 out of 4 times per practitioner or parent observation
4. Will tolerate linear movement on a therapy ball for approximately 2 to 3 minutes and then engage in a fine motor task 3 out of 4 times per practitioner or parent observation

SUMMARY

Occupational therapy services may be provided to children from birth to 21 years of age. Before engaging in pediatric practice, the practitioner must be familiar with the profession's tools, the occupational therapy intervention process, and federal, state, and local laws to be able to effectively design and implement an occupational therapy program in various settings. Practitioners working in pediatrics should possess a general knowledge base and the special skills needed to work not only with the child but also with the family or caregiver. In addition, the practitioner must become familiar with various methods for measuring progress. Knowledge about infection control is also essential to the provision of occupational therapy

References

1. American Occupational Therapy Association: *Standards of practice for occupational therapy*, Bethesda, Md, 1998, The Association.
2. American Occupational Therapy Association: *Occupational therapy roles*, Bethesda, Md, 1994, The Association.
3. Blesedell-Crepeau E: Activity analysis: A way of thinking about occupational performance. In Neistadt ME, Crepeau EB, editors: *Willard & Spackman's Occupational Therapy*, ed 9, Philadelphia, 1998, Lippincott-Raven.
4. Case-Smith J: *Pediatric occupational therapy and early intervention*, ed 2, Boston, 1998, Butterworth-Heinemann.
5. Crowe T et al: Role perceptions of mothers with young children: the impact of a child's disability, *Am J Occup Ther* 51(8):651, 1997.
6. Early MB.: *Mental health concepts and techniques for the occupational therapy assistant*, ed 2, New York, 1993, Raven Press.
7. Hinojosa J, Sabari J, Pedretti LW: Purposeful activities, *Am J Occup Ther* 47(12):1081, 1993.
8. Humphry R, Link S: Preparation of occupational therapists to work in early intervention programs, *Am J Occup Ther* 44(8):28, 1990.
9. Hyde A, Jonkey B: Developing competency in the neonatal intensive care unit: a hospital training program, *Am J Occup Ther* 48(6):539, 1994.
10. Kramer P, Hinojosa J: Activity synthesis. In Hinojosa J, Blount M: *Purposeful activities*, Bethesda, Md, in press, American Occupational Therapy Association.
11. Luebben A, Hinojosa J, Kramer P: Legitimate tools of pediatric occupational therapy. In Kramer P, Hinojosa J: *Frames of reference in pediatric occupational therapy*, ed 2, Baltimore, 1999, Williams & Wilkins.
12. Peloquin S: The patient-therapist relationship in occupational therapy: understanding visions and images, *Am J Occup Ther* 44(1):13, 1990.
13. United States Department of Labor, Occupational Safety and Health Administration: *Bloodborne facts: hepatitis B vaccination for you*, Washington, DC, The Administration.

Recommended Reading

Carver C: Crossing thresholds, *OT Practice* 3(7):18, 1998.

Case-Smith J: Pediatric assessment, *OT Practice* 2(4):24, 1997.

Esdaile S: A play focused intervention involving mothers of preschoolers, *Am J Occup Ther* 50(2):113, 1996.

Fisher A, Murray E, Bundy A: *Sensory integration—theory and practice*, Philadelphia, 1991, FA Davis.

Haack L, Haldy M: *Making it easy—adapting home and school environments*, *OT Practice* 1(11):22, 1996.

Harris S, Weiss M: *Right from the start—behavioral intervention for young children with autism*, Bethesda, Md, 1998, Woodbine House.

Kranowitz C: *The out-of-sync child*, New York, 1998, Perigee.

Larson E: The story of Maricela and Miguel: a narrative analysis of dimensions of adaptation, *Am J Occup Ther* 50(4):286, 1996.

Maurice C: *Behavioral intervention for young children with autism*, Austin, 1996, Pro-ed.

Siegel B: *The world of the autistic child*, New York, 1996, Oxford University Press.

Stancliff B: Autism: defining the OT's role in treating this confusing disorder, *OT Practice* 1(7):18, 1996.

Stancliff B: Understanding the "whoops" children, *OT Practice* 3(11):18, 1998.

REVIEW *Questions*

1. In what way does assessment of a child guide the occupational therapy practitioner in the program planning and treatment implementation processes?
2. Define and differentiate among long-term goals, short-term objectives, and mini objectives.
3. What are the components of an activity analysis?
4. In what ways are activity analysis and adaptation used by the occupational therapy practitioner during program planning and treatment implementation?
5. What are the levels of performance?

SUGGESTED *Activities*

1. Using the task-focused activity analysis form as a guide, analyze the specific daily routines that you personally perform, such as brushing your teeth, getting dressed, or preparing lunch.
2. Visit a day-care center or observe a neighbor's child performing specific tasks. Analyze what you observe using the task-focused activity analysis.
3. Choose an activity that in which you typically engage, and experiment by changing your position and the materials used for the activity. For example, eat a bowl of ice cream while sitting at the table and then do the same thing on your stomach in front of the television. Try different sizes of bowls and spoons. Write down how the change in your position or in the bowl and spoon made a difference in your performance.
4. Identify at least one long-term personal goal. Write short-term objectives about the way you plan on reaching your goals. Consider what methods you will use in attaining the objectives and ultimately your goals. Long-term goals should be attainable within 12 months. Use the RUMBA criteria when writing your goals.

Occupational Performance Areas: Daily Living and Work and Productive Activities

LISE M.W. JONES

PEGGY ZAKS MACHOVER

CHAPTER *Objectives*

After studying this chapter, the reader will be able to accomplish the following:

- Describe therapeutic activities the certified occupational therapy assistant might use to address a variety of problems related to feeding, dressing, toileting, hygiene, grooming, communication, mobility, safety, and educational and prevocational skills

- Explain the ways sensory processing problems might interfere with independence in feeding, dressing, toileting, hygiene, and mobility and school skills

- Apply the occupational therapy tools of analyzing, grading, and adapting activities of daily living for specific children

- Give examples of the ways reading the child in context from moment to moment guides a treatment session

- Discuss the ways specific oculomotor problems can interfere with communication and educational skills and describe several intervention methods

- Identify ways the certified occupational therapy assistant works with children in a school setting to address postural control, sitting tolerance, attending to instructions, managing assignments, managing behavior, and handwriting

- Identify ways in which the certified occupational therapy assistant might work with children to address indoor and outdoor mobility, health maintenance, and prevocational skills

- Identify ways the certified occupational therapy assistant works with parents, caregivers, registered occupational therapist supervisors, agency administrators, and team members to address activities of daily living and work and productive activities for the child

KEY TERMS	CHAPTER OUTLINE

OCCUPATIONAL PERFORMANCE MODEL

The occupational therapy practitioner's primary goal is to help children maximize function and achieve independence in living. To accomplish this goal, occupational therapy practitioners determine priorities and plan and implement treatment. The **occupational performance model** provides a framework for this process. It views children as having the role, or occupation, of learning and developing competence in a variety of skills. Some of these skills include taking care of their own personal needs (such as feeding, dressing, grooming, and hygiene tasks), learning to socialize and communicate with others, learning to negotiate the physical environment at home and in the community, going to school and doing homework, and developing prevocational skills. The occupational performance model consists of the following three domains:

1. Performance areas
2. Performance components
3. Performance contexts

Performance areas include (1) activities of daily living (ADLs), (2) work and productive activities, and (3) play and leisure activities. Performance components are the underlying human skills needed to carry out the performance areas. Performance contexts include temporal (time-related) and environmental aspects affecting both performance areas and components.

When planning treatment within a specific performance area, the occupational therapy practitioner considers both performance components and performance contexts.[1] Funding agencies, parents, professionals, and administrators often view improvements in the performance areas as measures of occupational therapy success. For example, attaining toothbrushing or dressing independence or starting to use a pencil efficiently help show that therapy has worked for a child.

The registered occupational therapist (OTR) gathers information from the occupational therapy evaluation, reviews of available reports, and when possible, consultations with the child, parents, caregivers, team members, other occupational therapy practitioners or outside professionals. The OTR may then apply the occupational performance model to this information to help determine goals for a child.

Acknowledgments:
We would like to thank the following talented COTAs and OTRs who have worked with us in pediatric occupational therapy and have brought their enthusiasm, intelligence, ideas, and caring to the field and creation of this chapter: Alexandra Aristizabal, Dottie Bade (OTR), Andrea Brown, Andrea D'Aquino, Laura Falco, Darlie Faustin, Petal Fletcher, Louise Lear Greene, Doreen Torres Grey (OTR), Marge Lesser, Gloria Monroy, Felicity Reimold, Barbara Vaccaro (OTR). We would also like to thank Ike and Alexandra Machover for all their help.

While the OTR performs a complete evaluation, the certified occupational therapy assistant (COTA) may carry out an assessment of the performance area of ADLs. Certain subskills of ADLs, such as suck-swallow-breathe synchrony (see Feeding and Eating section in this chapter), warrant a more in-depth evaluation by the OTR. After instruction by the OTR, the COTA may also assess specific performance components (depending on the COTA's role at work). The COTA alerts the OTR to any complex issues and requests guidance for addressing them. To pinpoint areas of focus for intervention, the occupational performance model again provides a perspective for the COTA.

This chapter focuses on the first two performance areas: ADLs and work and productive activities. ADLs are tasks involved with taking care of the body and its needs (self-care) and interacting with the environment on a daily basis. Work and productive activities include home management, care of others, and educational and vocational activities. (See Chapter 7 for lists of the ages at which ADL skills develop.)

PLANNING AND IMPLEMENTING TREATMENT
Knowledge, Skills, and Attitudes

Early[11] suggests we think of learning in terms of three categories: **knowledge, skills,** and **attitudes.** "*Knowledge* is the acquisition of information or facts about reality."[11] For example, if a child does not have information about or understand the need for hand washing, a COTA may need to repeat explanations about why hand washing is necessary and how often it should be done. Instructions can be followed by questions; eventually the child can be asked to explain everything about hand washing.

"*Skills* are actions or behaviors that are learned."[11] Much of this chapter deals with techniques COTAs use to help clients learn ADL or work skills. For example, the COTA may use weightbearing on hands and thumb opposition games as techniques to help the child learn efficient pencil grasp patterns. A mature pencil grasp leads to better handwriting.

"*Attitudes* are learned feelings, values, and beliefs."[11] An adolescent may know exactly how to accomplish hygiene tasks, but negative feelings prevent the daily completion of these steps. Low self-esteem, hopelessness, boredom, expectations of failure, anger, frustration, anxiety, or a need to be nurtured and dependent are just some of the feelings that can interfere with performance.

Although learning needed skills is often the focus of treatment, clients may also need their attitudes gently shaped. Eliciting children's positive feelings and their desire to learn or carry out a skill can be much more difficult than teaching the skill sequence itself. The COTA can use the following techniques to shape positive attitudes and increase self-esteem:

1. Praise the child's attempts to learn a particular skill.[17,49]

2. Use a "matter-of-fact" approach when needed; this method may be especially helpful when treating adolescents.

3. A positive, concrete description of children's behavior tells them exactly what they have done right, even if their performance is not perfect.[17,49] For example, even if a child's handwriting is sloppy, the practitioner can still say, "You're working so hard," "I really like how you concentrated on that job," or "Wow, you finished the whole page without stopping!" Many children who have high cognitive skills but also have learning disabilities or motor impairments are painfully aware of their inability to perform like other children. Therefore be honest in your descriptions and comments; the children will know if you are not.

4. Avoid using the words "bad" or "good." Even the experienced practitioner works at choosing the right words to use. Although it is easy to understand why the word "bad" should not be used, it may seem strange that the word "good" is also avoided. Using the word "good" can imply that if performance is not "good" the child or performance is "bad."[49]

5. Never tell children to "be good" or ask them, "Were you good today?" All children want to be good, and adults can always consider them inherently good; only their behaviors may need to change. Children need to know what is expected of them. Make comments or give concrete instructions about exactly what positive behaviors are needed.[49] For example, say, "We're walking slowly to stay safe" or "Remember to follow directions and use nice words on the bus."

6. Avoid using words like "no" and "don't"; save them for dangerous situations when you must yell, "No!" or "Don't do that!" to prevent a child from getting injured. If used sparingly, children will heed these negative warnings more readily than if they are heard all the time. Instead, ensure that the last words the child hears explain the desired behavior, and the child may be more likely to listen. For example, "Yelling is finished. It's time to talk in a quiet indoor voice." The last words in the statement describe the desired behavior—to talk in a quiet indoor voice.[17] If you say, "Stop yelling!" the last word the child hears is "yelling"; the child has no description of a positive replacement behavior for the yelling and is therefore more likely to continue.

7. Being genuinely caring and having a sense of humor can really help at times. A positive social environment that includes opportunities to develop friend-ships and experience even small successes may motivate a child to perform independently. When you hear the child say, "Don't help me. I want to do it myself," you know you are on the right track.

CLINICAL *Pearl*

Promoting positive feelings is important for learning. Although obtaining certain skills is often the focus of treatment, children need gentle shaping of their attitudes to have positive feelings about performing the skills. Developing the desire to carry out a skill independently is much more difficult than simply learning the sequence and actions needed to attain a skill.

One of the biggest challenges for occupational therapy practitioners is to help children transfer new skills into everyday contexts. Independent performance of skills at school, at home, and in the community shows that children are using their knowledge, skills, and attitudes to truly maximize their ability to function in their environments. Occupational therapy practitioners are committed to this goal.

Analyzing, Grading, and Adapting Activities

To prioritize, plan, and implement effective treatments, occupational therapy practitioners (1) analyze, grade, and adapt activities and (2) carefully read the child in context. (See Chapter 12 for more information on occupational therapy tools.)

Activity analysis

Activity analysis is a process that breaks down an activity by examining every aspect involved. The characteristics of specific activities are determined by considering each performance component and each performance context involved in relation to the child's unique capabilities and situation.

Activity analysis requires the occupational therapy practitioner to (1) explore each aspect of a desired functional activity to determine what is required for it to be independently performed, (2) examine the way the child currently performs the desired activity to determine which of the child's capabilities help or interfere with performance, (3) explore activities to determine which therapeutic activities fit the strengths, limitations, and interests of the child, (4) examine the therapeutic activities during treatment to determine whether they provide the right level of challenge for the child, need to be modified, and help the child increase function.

CLINICAL *Pearl*

Asking the right questions helps determine the direction of treatment planning and implementation.

A multitude of questions are asked during an activity analysis; they might include questions such as "What are the sensory demands of the activity?" "What kind of visual, touch, pressure, kinesthetic, movement, and temperature feedback does the activity provide?" "How much strength or range of motion (ROM) is required?" "How complex are the bilateral integration (coordination of both sides of the body) or motor planning demands?" "What are the sequencing, visual, or auditory memory demands?" "What level of coping skills and self-control are required?" "What are the speed or rhythm requirements?" "What meaning does the activity have to the child?" "Is the activity purposeful?" "How will the activity help increase functional ability?" "What are the physical, social, and cultural environmental contexts?"

Grading activities

Grading activities involves changing one or more aspect of a task to make it easier or harder for the child. Each child's abilities and needs dictate the types and amount of grading to use for a specific activity. A seemingly small change in an activity can significantly increase a child's success.

One way to grade an activity is to sequence the steps. **Forward chaining** (teaching each step of an activity from beginning to end), **backward chaining** (teaching the last step of the activity first), or both can be used. During forward chaining, the child starts the activity and the occupational therapy practitioner finishes the steps the child has not yet learned. During backward chaining, the occupational therapy practitioner starts the activity, and the child performs the last step, allowing the child to feel an immediate sense of accomplishment and mastery. Eventually the child performs the last two steps independently and so on.

Depending on the child, the occupational therapy practitioner may choose to use both forward and backward chaining. Initially the child works only on the first and last steps of the sequence. The occupational therapy practitioner performs the steps in the middle. This technique can promote a positive learning experience because the child succeeds at the beginning and end. Gradually the child performs more steps until the entire sequence is learned.

Fading assistance is another means of grading an activity. For example, the practitioner may initially use hand-over-hand or maximum physical assistance but then gradually reduce the assistance level from maximum to moderate to minimal physical assistance to tactile assistance to verbal assistance and finally to visual and gestural cuing.

Another way to grade an activity is to move the bodily location at which physical assistance is provided. For example, as a child develops motor control of precise release and placement of objects, practitioners may move their hands from supporting the child's wrist to supporting the forearm, then the elbow, and then the upper arm.

Most daily living and work activities can be graded by increasing or decreasing one or more of the following elements: size, speed, duration, frequency, height, angle, number of steps, complexity, and sensation. As with activity analysis, asking the right questions can help determine the ways to grade an activity. The following are examples of the previously mentioned elements, common questions, and intervention methods for grading daily living and work activities.

- *Size.* Can a task be made easier by using larger or smaller than average materials? For example, starting or inserting a zipper is a complicated bimanual manipulation (two-handed) task; it may be most easily taught using the largest possible zipper. On the other hand, when teaching scissor skills, using small scissors that fit the size of the children's fingers often work best.
- *Speed, frequency, and duration.* Would working slower or faster or pairing a task with a rhythmic beat help the child learn better? Marching while singing helps some children walk and not run in hallways or on steps. Children with attention and hyperactivity problems may need fast and frequent activity changes to keep their interest. A kitchen timer or a dripping liquid toy used as a timer (found in novelty, new age, and some toy stores) can help prepare a child to start or stop an activity. Would shorter, more frequent practice sessions help? Olsen's "Handwriting without Tears" program recommends beginning with frequent 1- to 5-minute practice sessions and working on one letter at a time.[45] Monitoring the child's tolerance for an activity is an important strategy for deciding the length of a session. If the child fatigues or becomes too frustrated, training sessions could be shortened and occur more frequently.
- *Height and angle.* Would raising or lowering materials or equipment help? Raising a desk or lowering a chair may significantly help a child with postural control problems. Placing reading and writing materials on an angled or vertical surface can help children who have problems stabilizing their head and visual field.
- *Number of steps.* Would increasing or decreasing the number of steps in the task help? Breaking a task

BOX 13-1

Dealing with the Demands of a Child with Sensory Defensiveness

- The occupational therapy practitioner carefully gauges proximity (closeness) to the child. Hair or clothing may accidentally touch the child, causing an aversive response.
- The occupational therapy practitioner grades the volume of speech being used. A regular speaking voice may be too loud for the child.
- The occupational therapy practitioner watches for signs that the child may have trouble listening and working at the same time. Speaking while the child is working may be confusing or overwhelming for the child.

down into smaller steps facilitates success for some children. Reducing the number of steps to just three tasks can make the activity harder for some but less frustrating for others.

- *Complexity.* Would increased or decreased complexity enhance performance? A child with Asperger's syndrome, a type of autism in which intelligence is extremely high, may thrive on complex memory tasks but require simplified motor tasks.
- *Sensation.* In what ways can the sensory elements of the activity be changed to fit the needs of the child? In what ways can visual, auditory, tactile, pressure, kinesthetic, movement, and temperature input be increased or decreased? Reducing the volume of the occupational therapy practitioner's voice to a whisper may get a child's attention better than raising the voice. For a child with sensory defensiveness to tolerate or attend to an activity, background sensations like sound, lighting, visual complexity, or certain bright colors may need to be reduced. A child with low muscle tone and poor sensory discrimination may receive inadequate tactile and pressure feedback when working with flimsy items like cloth, shoelaces, or plastic spoons. Increasing the stiffness, thickness, texture, or weight of certain items may provide enough feedback for the child to feel the materials and then motor plan a response (Box 13-1).

Adapting activities

Adaptations involve activity modifications or the use of adaptive devices such as reachers, button hooks, zipper pulls, and pencil grips. **Adapting activities** makes them easier for the child to perform. Asking questions helps guide the process: (1) Would it help to change the loca-

tion or position of the materials? For a visually impaired child, storing self-care items in exactly the same place after each use is helpful. Feeding and many other activities may be accomplished using a "clock method." The placement of the meal on the table is compared to the hands on a clock. For example, the child is told that the water glass is at 2 o'clock and the peas on the plate are at 6 o'clock. (2) Could symmetrical motions be used instead of asymmetrical motions? Putting on a coat over the head instead of one arm at a time is a common symmetrical task taught to children with developmental delays and limited bilateral skills. (3) In what ways can the task be accomplished using different body parts? The child may be taught to stabilize or control objects with different parts of the body, such as the stomach, mouth, forehead, shoulder, hip, or foot. (4) Would the task be performed better with the child in a different position, such in a sitting or standing position? For example, a child with limited balance may perform toothbrushing tasks more effectively when seated; a hyperactive child may perform tabletop tasks better while standing.

Reading the Child in Context

Keen observational and analytical skills are vital to an effective therapeutic process. Stackhouse, Wilbarger, and Trunnell used the helpful expression, "reading the child."[47] They suggest that reading a child, or constantly analyzing what a child does in response to interactions with others, helps guide the planning and implementation of treatment for children with sensory problems.

The occupational therapy practitioner reads the child to "guide the child's interests and behaviors."[47] The child's responses reveal whether the activity is engaging and challenging; the responses provide a feedback loop. By reading the child, the occupational therapy practitioner decides when to intervene during a session and what to change for the next session.

The expression "reading the child" can be expanded to **reading the child in context.** "Reading the child in context" focuses attention on the relationship between the child and the current situation. It is a moment-to-moment observation and analysis of the child's relationship to social and physical environments and the child's responses to the therapeutic process. The best occupational therapy practitioners continuously read the child in context and modify their treatment plans and implementation accordingly.

To read a child in context, the occupational therapy practitioner monitors numerous factors before and during treatment. Following are some samples of questions a practitioner tries to answer during a hypothetical therapy session with a child. Does the child perform best in a quiet individual setting or with peer models nearby? Are competing background noises or tactile sensations interfering with the child's concentration? What happened to suddenly cause the child to switch from laughing to screaming? If the child becomes more oppositional than usual, would it help to increase calming activities or reduce task demands or both? Is the child oppositional because of a factor such as sickness, thirst, lack of sleep, a rough bus ride to school, or a family argument? Is the child's current facial expression a fear or pain response? Would it help to use slow handling movements or change the child's position? What are all the possible causes of the current change in behavior, and what can be done to improve it? If the child is truly engaged in a purposeful, meaningful activity, how long do I allow the activity to continue? When do I intervene again to keep the activity going?

The number of possible questions is endless. Asking the right questions is priceless. The following stories show the ways that careful reading of children in relationship to their contexts can lead to resolution of problems. The stories are examples of how reading a child in context can aid treatment planning and implementation as well as increase functional ability in a preschool classroom.

CRAIG'S CURSING STORY. *Craig, a 4-year-old boy who was exposed to drugs in the womb, displayed problems with oculomotor (eye) control, safety, motor planning, and spatial awareness. He was distracted, impulsive, oppositional, and sensory defensive, negatively overreacting to harmless input. While in the therapeutic nursery, Craig was first treated in a large treatment room with other staff and children present. He became distracted by the slightest sensation, such as the sight of a picture on the wall or the sound of another child in the room. He cursed at other children and adults without provocation, possibly to elicit a reaction or to keep them away. When Craig was treated in this large active area, his cursing hurt other children's feelings, and too much time was spent managing his behavior.*

Craig's treatment sessions were moved to a small room with reduced visual and auditory distractions. Craig was the only child in his treatment sessions; simple but firm rules such as "Be safe," "Use nice words," and "Follow directions" were reviewed at the beginning of each session. A matter-of-fact approach to his provocative behaviors was found to be effective, along with periodic reminders of the rules and frequent activity rewards.

Specific sensory activities were found to help Craig calm down, reduce impulsivity, increase focus of attention, and improve oculomotor skills. The sensory activities included the Wilbarger deep pressure and proprioceptive technique, (a deep pressure and joint compression technique that is performed with a special device)[55] as well as prolonged

spinning in a prone (face down) position while reaching for targets. These activities were used throughout each treatment session.

The OTR closely observed and analyzed Craig's responses to activities and interactions. The OTR also chose the right moments to pause and work on challenging self-care tasks, such as buttoning, and prehandwriting tasks, such as copying circles and crosses.

With the new structure and ongoing modifications that were made according to his emotional state, Craig steadily reduced the amount of cursing and increased participation in preschool activities. By closely reading Craig's responses in relation to different contexts, sensations, activities, and interactions, the OTR was able to plan and implement effective treatment.

FEAR OF THE BATHROOM STORY. *In a special preschool setting, a team of teachers, a COTA, and an educational supervisor became frustrated in their attempts to toilet train a classroom of children with pervasive developmental disorder. When approaching or entering the bathroom, four of the six children cried, screamed, pulled away, and threw a tantrum. The team identified both sensory defensive and fear responses, so they tried modifying numerous environmental factors, such as warming the toilet seat and not flushing the toilet. The children still refused to enter the bathroom.*

The educational supervisor and OTR soon determined the cause of the fear. The children could not tolerate the "sound of the lights" in the bathroom. Other team members assumed the lights were not a problem because the children tolerated the same level of fluorescent lighting in the classroom. The difference was that every time the bathroom lights were turned on, a faint, high-pitched whine was emitted and the children began to cry. The sound was barely noticeable to most people. When the bathroom lights were turned off, the children calmed down and entered the bathroom without resisting.

The educational supervisor's and OTR's careful observation, analysis and problem solving, and reading the children in context led to the discovery of the cause of the "sound of the lights" problem and an easy solution.

CLINICAL *Pearl*

Carefully reading changes in the child's behavioral and emotional state in relation to subtle environmental sensations and social interactions reveals the child's individual needs from moment to moment.

Practice versus Combined Treatment Approaches

Using practice and nothing else as an intervention approach is one of the most common mistakes made by occupational therapy practitioners. Although repetition and extra practice are especially important for many children with disabilities, repetitive practice may not resolve limitations. Results can be quicker and more permanent when combined treatment approaches are used.

For example, a child who has oral defensiveness (negative reactions to different sensations in the mouth) that interferes with toothbrushing cannot resolve the problem by toothbrushing practice only, even if the child is able to carry out all the steps under supervision. The occupational therapy practitioner may need to add intraoral (inside the mouth) and resistive oral-motor-respiratory techniques, such as chewing, sucking, and blowing, to address the defensiveness.

A child who has spasticity (muscle tightness) and limited ROM that interfere with dressing may become frustrated and fail if forced to simply practice the task over and over. The occupational therapy practitioner may need to perform inhibitory (slowing and calming) techniques to reduce tightness and increase flexibility before dressing practice and use adapted clothing and dressing methods.

CLINICAL *Pearl*

If practice alone could resolve deficits, teachers or other professionals could address problems without an occupational therapist's help. Although repetition is necessary for learning, practicing a skill should not be the only treatment approach.

Another example of a combined treatment approach is performing the Wilbarger deep pressure and proprioceptive technique for sensory defensiveness (a 2-minute procedure designed to reduce defensiveness) immediately before practicing dressing, bathing, toileting or going to bed.[55] The technique can make these experiences less stressful for both the child and the caregivers.

The Actual Treatment Session

In some settings, treatment sessions are highly structured for the COTA by the OTR. In others the COTA plans activities according to goals written by the OTR. A new COTA may need frequent, daily supervision. An experienced COTA may need little guidance in choosing therapeutic activities, structuring a session, or managing behavior.

COTAs ask OTRs and other professionals for guidance as needed. COTAs may ask an OTR for direction when they need new treatment ideas or want to try a different treatment approach. They often ask for assistance with a child's behavior problems or medical management. COTAs offer the OTR recommendations for goals and implementation and share new information with the OTR that is based on experience with a child, contacts with caregivers or team members, or information from other sources. In a special school setting, the following sequence of events could occur for a child who has a prescription for individual occupational therapy.

1. *Chart review.* When a new child is assigned to a COTA for treatment, the COTA reviews occupational therapy evaluations and goals as well as any other available reports. Medical and psychosocial histories, as well as educational and speech and language reports, can reveal food allergies, early traumatic experiences, learning styles, progress, and limitations.
2. *Interview.* Whenever possible the COTA speaks to the OTR, parents, caregivers, family members, and involved staff; these individuals can relay concerns and share effective strategies. For example, finding out from a parent that a child adores and imitates an older sibling is useful information for treatment. The COTA may mention the sibling's name to help improve the child's mood, or the COTA may ask the sibling to demonstrate a specific activity to the child at home.
3. *Observing and establishing trust.* The first treatment session may seem more social and casual than later sessions; however, the COTA is observing, analyzing, and problem solving during the entire session. For example, the COTA may sit next to the child, establish eye contact, smile, talk to the child, and assist with classroom participation if the child allows. The first contact with the child is noninvasive (that is, involves minimal physical contact). The COTA concentrates on establishing a trusting relationship with the child and reading the child in context. The COTA closely observes every aspect of the child's performance components and the ways they interact with the performance contexts to influence ADLs and work and performance areas. If trust and rapport are quickly established and the child appears emotionally and physically ready, the COTA may touch the child to perform a therapeutic technique, hold hands with the child, or take the child to the treatment area. This may or may not happen during the first session.

   Careful listening, observation, and analysis continue until the end of the session. The COTA then tells the child what the next session may involve and when and where it will occur. A sense of humor and casual tone puts many children at ease and reduces their fear of being with a stranger in a new environment. Read the children's cues to determine which types of approaches seem to elicit the most positive response.

4. *Documentation and problem solving.* Soon after the session the COTA documents important observations. Examples include the child's (1) postural control, effort used to move different body parts, and excessive use of certain postures or avoidance of others; (2) facial expressions and social interactions related to different activities, people, and environments; (3) enthusiasm for or resistance to certain activities; (4) spatial orientation and motor planning skills; (5) adaptive equipment needs (for example, measurements for seating); and (6) pencil grasp described in detail.

5. *Planning.* The OTR may be consulted before the next session to discuss any unexpected concerns or observations. The next sessions focus on systematically working toward the child's goals. The child's existing skills are used to work toward achieving independence.

6. *Implementation.* Treatment sessions often follow a developmental progression, which means working in a sequence such as the following:

   - Use specific sensations to calm or alert the child's senses as needed or engage in therapeutic handling and positioning preparatory tasks. The purpose of this step is to (1) promote an optimum **level of arousal** (that is, the amount of alertness and attention needed for an activity), (2) reduce sensory defensiveness and subsequent resistance to participation in challenging tasks, (3) reduce spasticity and abnormal movement patterns while promoting more normal muscle tone and movement patterns, and (4) increase joint mobility or stability.

   - A specific physical intervention or exercises to increase ROM, strength, or active movement patterns could follow the sensory and postural adjustments. Gross motor (large muscle) tasks usually precede fine motor (small muscle) tasks. For example, the COTA and child may perform stretching exercises and play a physical game (such as "Simon Says") to increase active ROM (AROM) in shoulders and hips. The COTA may ask the child to perform modified pushups against a wall or desk to strengthen back, shoulder, arm, and wrist muscles.

   - Integrated sensory, gross, fine, visual, and motor activities might take place here. For example, a child could swing in a prone (face down) position while reaching for toys at different heights. The prone position promotes hip, back, shoulder, and neck strength and stability. Reaching at different heights while swinging requires controlled head, arm, hand, and eye movements while using sensory feedback to precisely time all actions while grasping the toy.

   - Refined visual-motor (such as handwriting), visual-perceptual (such as sequencing pictures that tell a story), and self-care (such as shoe tying) activities are often the last skills practiced. The first three steps enhance concentration and the postural, head, and oculomotor (eye movement) control needed to perform higher level skills.

   - The session should end on a positive note if possible. In schools, occupational therapy practitioners should try to return children to their classrooms ready to pay attention and learn academic skills. After a successful session, children are calm and content and have better posture, focus, and eye-hand coordination.

The previous sequence does not fit the needs of all children. The COTA may discover that the child fatigues too quickly to do difficult refined tasks at the end of the session. The child may have such severe behavior problems that more time is spent on the first three areas. The first step may become a routine review of rules that must to be followed to earn a few minutes of free time. Some children, especially those with learning disabilities, may begin a session by choosing a sequence of activities and then carry out the sequence of combined sensory, visual, and motor tasks.

Although the COTA begins each treatment session with a plan for the session and the child's eventual goals in mind, reading the child's emotional and physical state in relation to the context is an ongoing process. Making mistakes is okay; occupational therapy practitioners use their mistakes to learn more effective strategies. Throwing out or drastically modifying the day's plan after realizing that a child is unusually emotional or after an unexpected event occurs is also okay.

CLINICAL *Pearl*

No technique works for every child. Although the OTR and COTA may plan a logical intervention, it may not work. This is all part of the problem-solving and implementation process.

ACTIVITIES OF DAILY LIVING
Feeding and Eating
Suck-swallow-breathe synchrony

At birth the infant begins coordinating sucking, swallowing, and breathing to survive. When the newborn begins to suckle the mother's breast or nipple of a bottle, the actions of sucking, swallowing, and breathing become rhythmically synchronized so that the infant can receive adequate nutrition. This **suck-swallow-breathe synchrony** (s-s-b synchrony) is a skill used continuously throughout life.[20] S-s-b synchrony allows individuals to breathe while simultaneously and unconsciously sucking in and swallowing food, drink, and saliva. Infants' strong sucking action develops the sensory discrimination and muscle control needed later for eating solid foods and talking without concentrating, suffocating, or drooling. A disruption in s-s-b synchrony can interfere profoundly with development.

Any noticeable problems with the s-s-b synchrony are addressed in a multidisciplinary manner. The COTA consults the OTR, speech and language pathologist, doctor, nurse, and caregivers. The goal automatic, smooth, and rhythmic sucking, swallowing, and breathing (Box 13-2).

The three following signs are common indicators of inefficient s-s-b synchrony:

1. *Inadequate lip seal while sucking.* Typically, no air or liquid escapes through the sides of the mouth while sucking. The lips should fit tightly around a nipple or straw, creating suction. Children usually easily establish a lip seal on whistles, balloons, and other blowing toys. If a break in lip seal is repeatedly observed or heard, intervention is recommended. Many children with low muscle tone have trouble with lip seal. These children also often have speech problems.

BOX 13-2

OTR Supervision of Oral-Motor Intervention

- The OTR recommends and specifically directs oral-motor intervention by the COTA.
- Medical personnel are consulted if the OTR suspects the child's oral-motor limitations could be caused by physical problems. Specific tests or other interventions may be requested before oral-motor intervention begins.
- Certain techniques may be contraindicated for a child who is medically fragile or feeding through a tube.

---

2. *Gasping for air while sucking or eating.* An infant who has s-s-b synchrony displays smooth, rhythmic breathing through the nose during feeding. Gasping for air indicates that breathing, sucking, and swallowing are not synchronized, and the child is probably uncomfortable. This problem naturally occurs when an individual has a bad head cold and must breathe through the mouth instead of the nose. A child who gasps for air but does not have a cold requires treatment.

3. *Excessive drooling when not being fed.* Typically, drooling is seen when an infant is teething or a toddler is concentrating on learning new activities. By about 2 years of age, drooling usually subsides. Initiate intervention if drooling is excessive.

The COTA addresses oral-motor problems only under the direction of the OTR and only after medical problems have been ruled out. If the OTR asks the COTA to work on s-s-b synchrony, the COTA can use the following techniques:

- To facilitate efficient swallowing while breathing, keep the child's head and neck vertical or somewhat flexed (bent forward). If the child's head is hyperextended (pulled back), the child may aspirate (inhale food into the esophagus) and choke. In the past, many children with physical disabilities and mental retardation were institutionalized, and feeding was often done in the fastest, cleanest way possible. Abnormal head hyperextension allowed quick meals and little spilling. This method was used so often, it was called *birdfeeding* (Figure 13-1, Box 13-3).

- In some clients, swallowing can be facilitated by slowly stroking upward on the lateral muscles of the throat; avoid touching the trachea. In theory, when swallowing muscles sense they are being gently pulled upward, they will react by resisting with a downward swallow.

- Sour tastes often improve lip pursing and swallowing in children.[43] Children indicate whether they like this approach by avoiding or seeking the taste. Try using tiny amounts of lemonade powder, frozen lemonade or limeade concentrate, or slices of fresh lemon. Children should never be forced to taste anything.

- Proper breathing can be enhanced using prone activities in which the stomach is in contact with soft, elastic surfaces.[39,43] These activities open the airway and activate and strengthen the diaphragm, leading to deeper breathing. With the child on the belly, try swinging the child on an inner tube swing or rocking the child over a therapy ball.

- To promote deep breathing for toddlers and children, use a variety of blowing toys and activities, such as bubbles, pinwheels, or whistles.[43] These activities will also increase lip seal by developing strength and sensation in the lips, oral musculature, and diaphragm. Older children may prefer to play harmonicas or other wind instruments, blow up balloons, or blow bubbles with bubble gum. Singing is beneficial for all ages.
- A partial supine (face up) posture makes it somewhat easier to work the diaphragm. Therefore sitting in a beanbag chair, or leaning on a pile of pillows can help the child gain enough force to breathe deeply and blow (Box 13-4).[20]

Transitioning from bottle to cup

The strong sucking actions of an infant prepare the muscles of the jaw, tongue, and throat for drinking from a cup, chewing, and talking. The actual transition from sucking on a nipple to drinking from a cup can be problematic and stressful for some children and parents. The child may resist the change for a variety of reasons:

- Sucking is a calming, nurturing sensation. The child may prefer to perform this familiar, relaxing action rather than allow any change to occur. Drinking from a cup introduces unfamiliar sensations that the child may not initially find satisfying.
- Abnormal muscle tone, whether it is hypertonicity (high muscle tone or tight muscles) or hypotonicity (low muscle tone or loose muscles), in the face and body can prevent proper lip and mouth control. Other neuromotor or physical problems can also interfere with muscle control that is needed to drink from a cup. Inhibition (calming or slowing) techniques for high tone or facilitation (exciting or speeding) techniques for low tone are used before addressing lip and mouth control. These techniques promote the proper tone in the trunk, upper extremities, and neck, which makes all feeding skills easier for the child.[39]

The COTA working with children who have physical problems require special training. Specific prefeeding postural techniques are learned directly from an experienced OTR, physical therapist (PT), or speech and language pathologist. Strategies can also be learned by attending workshops (see Chapter 13 Appendix D) on handling and positioning techniques for children.

The promotion of oral-motor control requires comfortable positioning for both therapist and child. The

---

BOX 13-3

Proper Feeding Positions

- Do not use the birdfeeding method. Birdfeeding is dangerous and can cause a child to inhale food into the windpipe.
- Swallowing is easiest with the head in a slightly flexed position.
- Even if a child constantly spits or drips food out of the mouth, maintain the head and neck in safe neutral or slightly flexed positions at all times to facilitate proper breathing and prevent aspiration (that is, food going down the windpipe into the lungs).

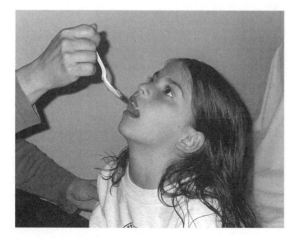

FIGURE 13-1   "Birdfeeding," in which the head is abnormally hyperextended, is dangerous and can cause choking.

BOX 13-4

Oral-Motor Activities

- CAUTION: Do *not* force oral-motor activities. Search for activities that the child finds rewarding.
- As with all eating and feeding activities, take extreme care to prevent discomfort and injury.
- If an infant or child resists participating in an activity, the child may be trying to tell the practitioner that it is not the right activity. Consult the OTR.
- If a child has a head cold and a runny nose, limit blowing activities until the cold has subsided. Forceful blowing can cause fluids or air to back up in the Eustachian tube, resulting in excess pressure behind the ear drum; the child could possibly burst an ear drum.

child's postural stability and alignment are essential for proper oral-motor function.[10,18,39]

One particular position is commonly used for oral-motor work with children who have physical limitations (Figure 13-2). The child is seated in a chair or on the practitioner's lap with equal weight on the hips; the trunk and the head are centered in midline. The shoulders are not too retracted (pulled back) or too protracted (rounded forward). The head is in a neutral (straight up) position or is slightly flexed (and never hyperextended). To keep the head and shoulders positioned properly, the occupational therapy practitioner's nondominant arm is placed around the child's shoulders and neck for support. The nondominant hand helps control the jaw, lips, and cheeks, whereas the dominant hand introduces food or drink into the child's mouth.

Efficient lip closure is an underlying skill needed for a successful transition from bottle to cup. Intervention strategies include the following:

- To promote lip closure around a bottle, cup, or spoon, use the positioning described previously (see Figure 13-2). With the practitioner's nondominant arm around the child, the occupational therapy practitioner uses ulnar side (same side as the little finger) of the hand to stabilize the child's jaw (see Figure 13-2). Using the index and middle fingers, gentle but firm pressure is applied just above the upper lip and just below the lower lip. The occupational therapy practitioner's dominant hand is free to control the bottle, cup, straw, spoon, or fork.
- Different sizes of nipples or spout, straw, or cutout cups may increase lip seal.[43] Finding the right nipple or spout may make the difference between inefficient lip closure and sucking (with its accompanying frustration and inadequate nutrition) and functional feeding.
- Lip closure can sometimes be facilitated by applying two, light downward strokes to the sensitive area of skin between the nose and upper lip.[30] The lip closure response may be delayed, occurring several seconds later. If this stroking method is used too frequently within a short period, the child may stop responding for a while. The occupational therapy practitioner can wait a minute and try again. If the child has many physical problems, this light stroking may cause the opposite effect and cause the mouth to open.

The transition from bottle to cup is a carefully negotiated process. The COTA consults frequently with the OTR for guidelines and coordinates activities with the child, caregivers, and other team members. Team members determine the developmental and physical

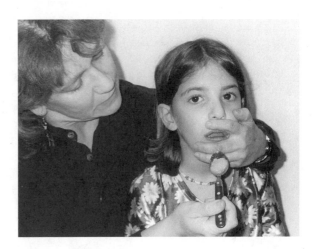

FIGURE 13-2   Therapist supports child's head, shoulders, jaw, and lips in proper position to aid oral-motor control.

BOX 13-5

Requirements for Drinking from a Cup

- Drinking from a cup is a completely new type of task for a child. It requires adequate postural control, jaw stability, and tongue and lip control.
- Biting the cup while drinking (at more than 24 months of age) may be a sign of inadequate jaw stability.
- Adequate discrimination of tactile and proprioceptive (deep-pressure) feedback by the mouth and lips as well as muscle control are important for learning to drink from a cup.

---

readiness of the child, the proper time and place for the transition, and the way spout cups will be used to aid the transition. Most importantly, parents' concerns are addressed (Box 13-5).

If the team determines the child is ready for the transition from bottle to cup, the COTA can assist in a number of ways (with the direction of the OTR). A variety of attractive transition, straw, or spout cups can be obtained through catalogs or stores (Figure 13-3). Some cups have two handles and some have weighted bottoms that prevent tipping. Certain transition cups have detachable nipples that can be replaced with either a spout or straw when the child is ready. Simply being able to choose between several appealing cups may ease the transition. Morris and Klein[39] discuss a wide variety of cups and their uses.

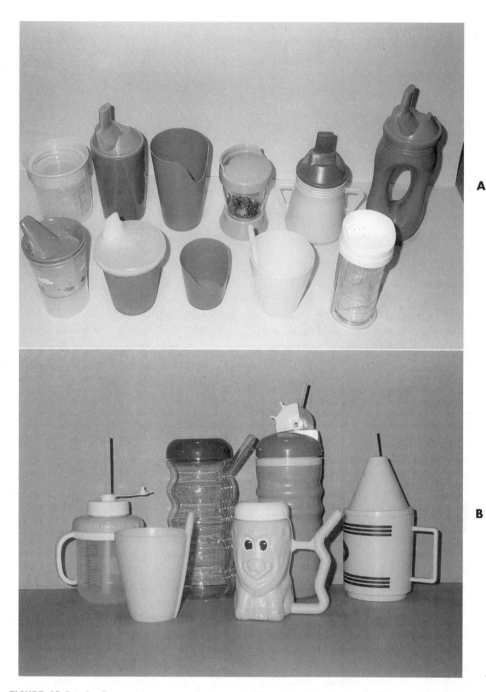

FIGURE 13-3 A, Cups with spouts, cutouts, and different hand holds can facilitate transition from bottle to cup. **B,** Numerous straw cups that are available.

Cutout cups are helpful for children with mild to moderate motor problems (Figure 13-3, A). One side is cut out in a U shape. As the cup is placed on the child's lower lip and tipped for drinking, the cutout portion fits around the child's nose. The child drinks more easily because the head does not have to tip backward.

A child's resistance to using a cup may be partially caused by oral defensiveness (that is, an aversion to harm-less oral sensations). Several techniques may help increase a child's tolerance to different tastes, textures, and temperatures. The Wilbarger intraoral (inside the mouth) technique for oral defensiveness can be learned at a continuing education course or from a person who has attended a course.[55] Incorrect performance of the technique may increase defensiveness and resistance to drinking from a cup. When performed correctly, it can quickly increase tolerance for different textures, temperatures, and shapes in the mouth. The jaw tug[43] involves placing a thumb or two fingers on lower teeth and gently but firmly tugging downward on the lower jaw 10 times. Some young children can be taught to perform this technique on themselves before drinking.

Other deep pressure techniques used in and around the mouth can increase tolerance for oral sensations as well as sensory awareness and motor control. An occupational therapy practitioner who is involved in feeding programs should attend continuing education classes in oral-motor techniques and read in depth material about therapeutic techniques and positioning and handling for feeding (see Recommended Reading and Chapter 13 Appendix D).

Chewing: transitioning from liquids to solids

Many useful techniques for facilitating chewing can be obtained from resources listed in the References and Recommended Reading. For children with mild oral-motor planning problems or jaw instability, several strategies are recommended.

1. Add small amounts of a thick-textured substance, such as pudding, wheat germ, or Thicket (a commercial product available from Milani Foods) to liquids. Gradually increase the liquid's consistency as the child becomes accustomed to the texture.
2. Add small amounts of chewable foods, such as chunks of cooked, skinned apple, to a pureed food, such as applesauce. Put a few noodles or cooked carrots into a vegetable puree.
3. Use foods that dissolve easily in the child's saliva, such as different types of oat, corn, or rice cereals. Adding milk causes the cereal soon to become a lumpy mixture that has texture and is chewable yet is also easy to swallow.
4. Place foods that dissolve easily in saliva such as a cracker, graham cracker, or sugar cookie between the child's upper and lower molars in the side of the mouth. Place fingers or a thumb under the lower jaw, and press straight up with firm, steady pressure (Figure 13-4). In theory the child will first close the molars on the food and then resist the fingers' upward pressure by opening the jaw. As the occupational therapy practitioner maintains pressure, rhythmic chewing often results.[18]
5. Put a tasty, juicy item such as a piece of meat or fruit inside a piece of cheesecloth (which is available in kitchen or housewares stores). Place the wrapped food between the molars, and apply steady upward pressure to the lower jaw as explained in strategy 4.[18]
6. Use a "bite and tug" game immediately before eating.[43] (CAUTION: The practitioner must be very careful to

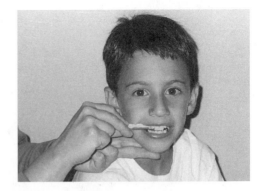

FIGURE 13-4 To facilitate chewing, a cracker is placed between molars while steady upward pressure is applied under lower jaw.

prevent fingers from being bitten.) The practitioner wraps a thick wash cloth or dish rag around the fingers. The cloth is dipped in a liquid the child likes such as juice or broth and inserted between the child's molars. A child who is ready for this strategy will bite the cloth, sucking out the juice. The therapist quickly and rhythmically tugs the cloth, allowing the child to simulate a chewing motion with the molars. This technique should not be used with children who have a tonic bite reflex (involuntary forceful clamping of teeth that is triggered by touch to the lips, gums, or teeth, and results in abnormal prolonged jaw muscle contraction).

Managing tongue thrust

Tongue control with rhythmic tongue retraction (pulling the tongue back into the mouth) is necessary to control liquids and solids. Excessive tongue protrusion (sticking the tongue out) and **tongue thrust** (extending the tongue outside the lips) are involuntary movements often seen in children with cerebral palsy and Down syndrome. Both problems interfere with swallowing and can cause food to be pushed out of the mouth in spite of the child's attempts to keep it in. Promotion of mature tongue retraction can help the child with excessive tongue protrusion or tongue thrust; however, excessive tongue retraction can also be an obstacle to efficient feeding.[39]

Proper positioning is vital for tongue control. The trunk, head, neck, and shoulders need to be stable and aligned. Abnormal tongue movements tend to occur more frequently when the head is hyperextended. After the child is positioned, tongue retraction can sometimes be initiated by placing a thumb or fingers on the soft part of skin directly under the chin, behind the jaw, and in front of the neck. The practitioner presses upward, being careful to avoid touching the trachea. This facilitates contraction of the muscles at the base of the tongue, which pulls the tongue back into the mouth.

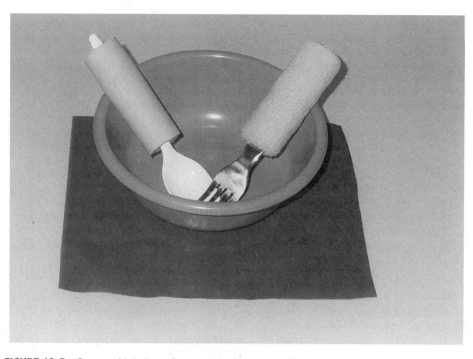

FIGURE 13-5 Spoon with built-up foam handle, fork with built-up Coban handle, and bowl stabilized by Dycem nonslip mat.

The occupational therapy practitioner can help a child retract the tongue several times before feeding. Tongue thrust can also be inhibited during feeding. Each time the child takes a bite, the occupational therapy practitioner presses the spoon down firmly on the center of the tongue and holds this pressure for about 3 seconds. The tongue usually relaxes and retracts.

CLINICAL *Pearl*

To inhibit tongue thrust, the spoon must be pressed downward in exactly the center of the tongue. If the spoon is too far forward, pressure on the tip of the tongue stimulates a stronger tongue thrust. If the spoon is too far back, a gag reflex may occur.

Transitioning from fingers to utensils

Learning to feed with utensils instead of fingers is a major developmental task for most children. This process is extremely difficult for children with incoordination, high or low muscle tone, weakness, or limited discrimination of touch-pressure feedback in the hands. The flimsy, lightweight plastic utensils commonly used in schools, hospitals, and even on family picnics can be especially prob-

lematic. Following are strategies and examples of adapted holders and utensils for helping children with a variety of limitations, including motor incoordination, weakness, and limited sensory discrimination:

1. Attach a universal weighted handle to a plastic utensil. Pediatric weighted universal grips and pediatric weighted spoons and forks are available from several equipment companies. (NOTE: These may not work for a child with severe weakness.)
2. Slide foam tubing or foam from a new hair curler onto any utensil to make the handle larger and easier to grip (Figure 13-5).
3. Wrap Coban, a textured elastic material that sticks to itself, around handles to increase the size of the handle and slightly increase the weight of the item (see Figure 13-5). A small, heavy object or small weight can also be attached to the handle with Coban.
4. Curved utensils can help children who are able bring their hands close to their mouths, but cannot orient utensils properly. Curved utensils are made for right or left handed use.
5. Children who have a strong tonic bite reflex can use rubber coated, plastic, or rubber spoons.
6. Small, flat spoons can be used by children with a strong tongue thrust.

7. Children with tremors or incoordination can use swivel utensils.
8. Children who are unable to grasp utensils can use long-handled, bendable, wrap-around spoons and forks.
9. Pediatric universal holders can be attached to children's hands with a spoon or fork inserted into the sleeve.
10. Visual cues can be used to make spreading and cutting with a knife easier. A piece of tape or a red dot on the edge of a knife shows the proper placement of the index finger.

ALEX'S SPOON STORY. *Alex is a nonverbal 5-year-old boy with pervasive developmental disorder, severe mental retardation, low muscle tone, severe sensory defensiveness, poor sensory discrimination, excessive self-stimulatory finger flicking, and severe delays in all areas of function. He actively resisted holding any utensil, even after engaging in sensory modulation and resistive hand and arm activities. When encouraged to hold a spoon, he either pushed it away or flicked it back and forth while watching it from the corner of his eye.*

His COTA worked hard to analyze his behavior and its possible causes. The COTA reasoned that if (1) his sensory defensiveness caused discomfort in holding the spoon and (2) his poor discrimination did not allow him to feel the spoon, then (3) maybe using a deep pressure technique would address both problems.

After consulting with the OTR supervisor, the COTA ordered pediatric weighted hand patches. The small neoprene fingerless gloves were placed on Alex's hands. Tiny ounce weights slid into a pocket on the dorsum of the hand. After a minute of apparent annoyance at the new feeling, and to everyone's delight, Alex stopped flicking his fingers and tolerated holding the spoon. Within a few days, with ongoing therapy, he began bringing the spoon to his mouth, after assistance to scoop.

CLINICAL *Pearl*

Deep pressure techniques can be calming and increase proprioceptive (deep pressure) feedback from muscles and joints. Accurate sensory feedback is needed for body awareness and motor planning.

Using tableware

Many types of adapted plates and bowls are available for children with limited motor coordination, limited vision, or the use of only one hand. Functional independence may increase by using one or more of the following items:

1. A bowl with a suction attachment on the bottom
2. Scoop plate, or a plate with a high rim around the edge against which to push food
3. For travel, a plastic or metal plate guard that can be attached to most plates at restaurants
4. Dycem, a nonslip material that prevents tableware from sliding (see Figure 13-5) can be used as a placemat. Dycem comes in a variety of forms, including thick precut rectangles and circles, a long, thin roll that can be cut into different sizes, and a lightweight mesh.
5. Holders for scoop bowls and plates, which can be created by carving out a block of firm foam[48]
6. Milk or juice carton holders and cup holders, which can be created by molding splinting material to fit the desired size and shape[48]

Managing special food and eating problems
Opening packages and containers

The ability to open packages and containers is a skill that is often overlooked in the development of independent feeding. The child may have mastered oral-motor skills and the use of tableware but still need help to open a juice carton, straw or ketchup package, plastic food container, or plastic-wrapped sandwich. The child can encounter these challenges in school, hospital, and community settings.

The occupational therapy practitioner helps children develop the underlying hand and finger skills needed to open packages, including tactile discrimination, strength, and dexterity. In addition, the occupational therapy practitioner helps children, parents, and involved adults problem solve in this area. For example, the practitioner may schedule a weekly treatment session at lunchtime to work on opening packages with the child or may ask parents to wrap the child's sandwich in aluminum foil or in plastic bags, which can be easier to manage than plastic wrap. The practitioner may work with teachers to design intervention strategies. The child may need adaptive equipment like a sandwich holder, which stabilizes the sandwich while freeing both hands for unwrapping. The child may need a small pair of scissors to use only on food packages or may need instructions to ask the teacher for help.

Gastrostomy tube

For medical conditions, such as a constricted esophagus, some children must be fed through a gastrostomy tube, which fits directly into the stomach. If the child's tube feeding is temporary, the COTA may be asked to carry out goals to help the child develop intraoral sensory awareness and motor control in preparation for future feeding by mouth. In some cases the COTA may be allowed to give

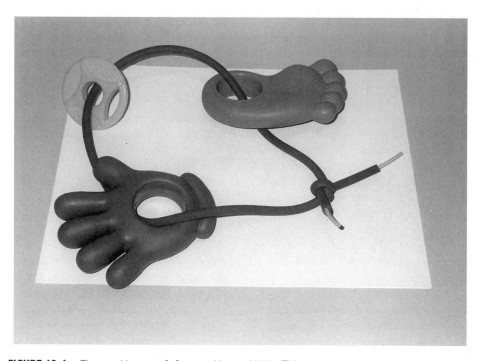

FIGURE 13-6 Chewy with toys safe for mouthing and biting. This chewy is designed for a child who bites people. Narrow tubing is threaded inside wider tubing to simulate feeling of skin sliding over muscle.

the child a teaspoon of water or other liquid through the mouth. Methods described previously for reducing oral defensiveness may also help prepare a child who is being fed through a gastrostomy tube for feeding by mouth.

Biting

Excessive biting of inedible objects is a problem often encountered in children with developmental disabilities or other impairments. These children may bite objects because they (1) are attempting to calm themselves to reduce anxiety, (2) are exploring the environment using the mouth because of an inability to discriminate objects with the hands, or (3) have inadequate jaw stability. These children may bite people to (1) express anger or frustration, (2) attempt to communicate, (3) physically explore the person with their mouth, or (4) to calm themselves.

A "chewy" can be extremely helpful for children who bite excessively (Figure 13-6). A chewy is a string or piece of tubing laced with chewable objects such as thick rubber toys, teethers, or oversized beads.[43] The chewy can be worn as a necklace, attached to a belt, or even put in a pocket so that it is always available. Adults use consistent teaching strategies to redirect unsafe biting of objects and people; they praise the child for biting the chewy when the urge to bite occurs. In severe cases the chew toys need to be especially durable so that the child cannot bite through them. Chew toys made for animals are usually very durable.

If the practitioner determines that a child bites objects to explore them because the child has decreased touch-pressure feedback from the hands, the COTA may implement additional approaches. The child should be allowed to bite and explore safe objects so that learning about shape, size, texture, and temperature still occurs. The child should also be taught which objects should not be bitten. Simultaneously the COTA addresses use of the hands. Deep pressure applied to the hands can increase proprioceptive (deep pressure) awareness, so the COTA could implement weightbearing activities such as crawling on textured surfaces. Squeeze toys can be used to increase sensory awareness in the hands and improve fine motor control needed for manipulating objects.

The sensation of biting skin and muscle can feel very satisfying to some children. Once biting skin becomes a habit, it can become dangerous and hard to stop. Children who persist in biting people can be given a special chewy made of two widths of Theratubing (see Figure 13-6). A piece of narrow tubing is threaded inside a piece of wider tubing, which simulates the feeling of skin sliding over muscle and provides a safe alternative to biting people.[32]

Spitting

Some children spit excessively or play with their own saliva. In these cases the team and a doctor are consulted to determine possible causes for the behavior. Some children may truly have excess saliva, and they can often be taught to handle it in an acceptable way.

RICKY'S SPITTING STORY. *Ricky, a nonverbal 4 year old, spit excessively on floors and tables. After ruling out medical and s-s-b problems, the team decided to show Ricky that spitting into a sink or waste basket was an acceptable way to get rid of his excess saliva. Ricky was encouraged to practice spitting in these places in school. When he spit on the table or floor, he was assisted with getting paper towels to clean it up. After Ricky learned the cleaning sequence, he was asked to clean up his spit independently when necessary. He was instructed in a matter-of-fact way. Even though Ricky could not ask for a place to spit, he soon learned to use only the sink or wastebasket for spitting in school.*

Ricky's spitting behavior was under control in the school environment. The team did not anticipate that he would have any problems outside of school. While on a field trip, the teachers noticed Ricky scanning an unfamiliar room and becoming increasingly agitated as he searched for a sink or wastebasket. He needed to spit and had learned not to do so on floors or tables. With urgency, Ricky darted to his teacher's large open pocketbook, the object looking most like a wastebasket to him, and spit into it. Ricky had solved his dilemma, and the teacher praised him for not spitting on the floor. The staff regarded the incident with a good sense of humor but also learned an important lesson: when teaching a new behavior, all potential factors that could affect the behavior, such as different settings, should be considered.

Regurgitation and pica behavior

Certain children with special needs regurgitate food and display pica behavior (crave inedible items such as plaster or dirt). Both behaviors are unsafe and socially unacceptable. Regurgitated stomach acids can destroy teeth, and ingestion of certain substances can be physically harmful. In the following stories, the occupational therapy practitioner is instrumental in providing alternative activities for the adolescents involved. She chooses activities for their behavior plans that fit the adolescents' severe cognitive, social, and visual impairments.

ERNIE'S REGURGITATION STORY. *Ernie was an adolescent in an institution. He was nonverbal, had mental retardation, was blind, had few remaining teeth, and regurgitated food after every meal. He then kept the regurgitated food in his mouth for some time before finally swallowing it. The treatment team determined that Ernie had developed this behavior because he was bored and still hungry after eating his meals.*

To address his boredom, the team increased Ernie's activity program, emphasizing his favorite activities and social interactions with staff and peers. Physical activities were increased and included going through an obstacle course that the occupational therapy practitioner had designed for the residents with visual impairments.

To address his hunger, the nurse and psychologist on the team devised an unusual strategy that proved quite successful. After each meal, Ernie was allowed to eat as much bread as he wanted. At first he ate more than half a loaf. With so much food in his stomach, he felt satiated. The bread was also too bulky for Ernie to regurgitate. As his activity program continued, Ernie began to realize he could eat as much as he wanted. Regurgitation stopped, and smiling increased. After a few weeks, Ernie reduced the amount of bread he ate to two or three slices.

MELVIN'S PICA BEHAVIOR STORY. *Melvin was also in an institution, had mental retardation, and was nonverbal and blind. He played with pieces of lint from the floor or tiny pieces of regurgitated food, alternately playing with them in his mouth or rolling and flicking them between his fingers. In addition, Melvin was self-abusive (banged his head on objects), became aggressive when frustrated or pushed to perform, and weighed more than 250 lb.*

While considering possible causes for his maladaptive pica behavior, the team determined the behavior had developed to help Melvin cope with growing up blind in an unstimulating institutional environment. He was bored and needed to play with something. Because he was so emotionally fragile and dangerous to himself and others, his intervention was carried out slowly and cautiously in phases.

- *Melvin was given one-on-one staffing using gentle primary caretakers who liked him and were able to calm him.*
- *Melvin was given a variety of small tactile and auditory toys. He developed a strong attachment to one toy in particular, a small plastic cube with a tiny marble inside. He kept the cube and took it with him everywhere.*
- *Melvin was given additional nurturing social contacts.*
- *Melvin participated in an enhanced, calming activity program, which involved rocking in a rocking chair, handling vibrating toys, listening to music, playing in water, and other activities that soothed him. With input from educational, recreational, and music therapy staff members, the occupational therapy practitioner developed this program.*
- *When he displayed pica behavior, Melvin's primary caregiver gently redirected him into a calming, desirable activity.*
- *When Melvin appeared agitated and resisted redirection, the staff avoided getting involved in any dangerous power struggles. Melvin was soothed until he was calm enough to give his primary caretaker the piece of lint or regurgitated food.*

After about 3 months of using this nurturing and socially and environmentally enriched program, Melvin's pica behavior disappeared.

Dressing

Learning to dress and undress are developmental accomplishments. Adaptive techniques are necessary for children with physical limitations, mental retardation, sensory or motor planning problems, and in some cases for those with emotional problems and attention deficit or learning disabilities. Two primary issues need to be addressed to help children achieve independence in dressing and undressing.

The occupational therapy practitioner first chooses the type of clothing and fasteners best suited to the child's capabilities and living situation. Sleeve style, neck openings, fabric qualities (that is, stretchy, soft, nonslipping), fastener style, and location should all be addressed. The occupational therapy practitioner then decides on the teaching method that is most likely to lead the child to dressing independence.

To address these two issues, the occupational therapist may need to find out the answers to questions such as the following: What is the cognitive level of the child, and how does the child learn best? Does a verbal explanation help or cause confusion? Would a picture sequence help? How much ROM and coordination are required? Does the child perform symmetrical tasks (tasks that are the same on both sides of the body) more easily than asymmetrical ones (tasks that are different on each side of the body)? Does the child have enough active wrist extension (straightening) and finger flexion (bending) for grasping? What are the realistic time and endurance factors involved with learning the tasks? For example, although a child may be able to learn to use a button hook and zipper pull, the effort and time it may take to actually carry out the task may be impractical. Struggling to dress

for an hour could reduce the child's energy to perform academic tasks in school later that day. The child and parents could use more adapted clothing instead (see Chapter 13 Appendix A) and ask the occupational therapy practitioner to help with their chosen methods.

The task of teaching dressing and undressing is broken down into a sequence of steps. Each step is analyzed according to its sensory, cognitive, spatial, postural, and fine and gross motor planning demands. The child's strengths are used, and the child's limitations are accommodated. Forward or backward chaining methods can be used (see Grading Activities section in this chapter).

Because undressing is easier than dressing, it is generally taught first. Adapted equipment should be used on a trial basis and shown to be effective before the items are purchased for home use. In the following sections, selecting adapted clothing and fasteners is addressed simultaneously with teaching methods.

Shirts and dresses

For children with weakness, abnormal movement patterns, or limited ROM, loose, oversized shirts and dresses are easiest to put on and remove. Use shirts or dresses with neck openings that are easy to handle, such as horizontal crossover neck, V-neck, or boat neck openings.

To prevent a shirt from becoming untucked by an active child, add buttons to the waistband of the pants. Shirts can then be buttoned to pants as they are in some infant clothing. To prevent fingers from getting caught while pushing hands through sleeves, have the child hold a small object or wear mittens while dressing. In addition, Dolman sleeves can be helpful because they have larger arm openings than set-in sleeves.

Many adapted methods have been developed to put on and take off shirts (Figures 13-7 through 13-16). Adapted methods of removing shirts include the over-the-head method, duck-the-head and sit-up method, and arms-in-front method.

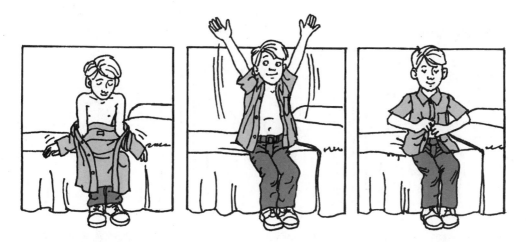

FIGURE 13-7 Adapted method of putting on a shirt: lap and over-the-head method.

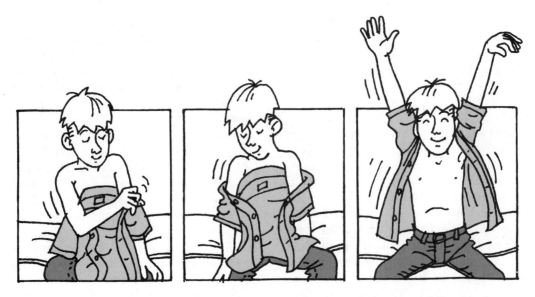

FIGURE 13-8 Adapted method of putting on a shirt: lap and over-the-head hemiplegic method.

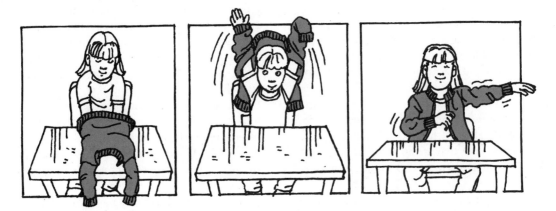

FIGURE 13-9 Adapted method of putting on a shirt: front lap and facing down method.

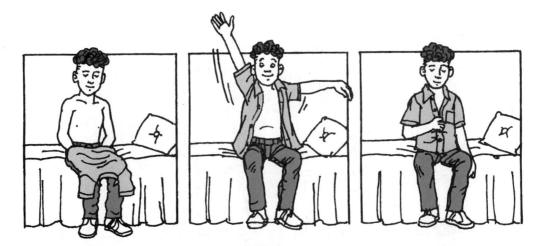

FIGURE 13-10 Adapted method of putting on a shirt: front lap and facing down hemiplegic method.

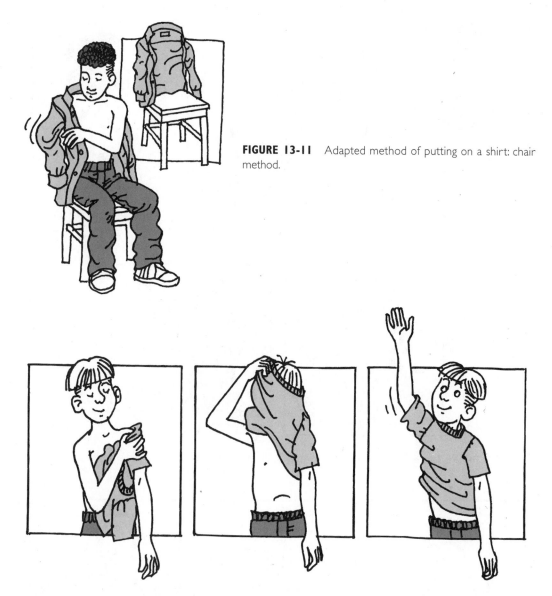

FIGURE 13-11 Adapted method of putting on a shirt: chair method.

FIGURE 13-12 Adapted method of putting on a shirt: arm-head-arm method.

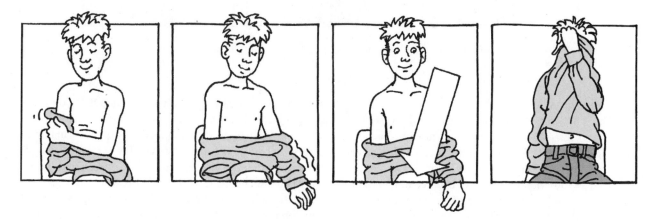

FIGURE 13-13 Adapted method of putting on a shirt: lap-arm-arm-neck method.

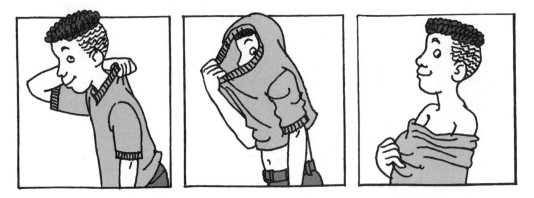

FIGURE 13-14   Adapted method of taking off a shirt: over-the-head method.

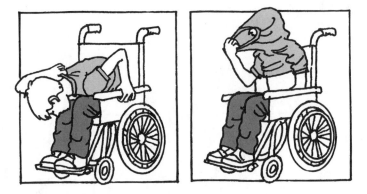

FIGURE 13-15   Adapted method of taking off a shirt: duck-the-head and sit up method.

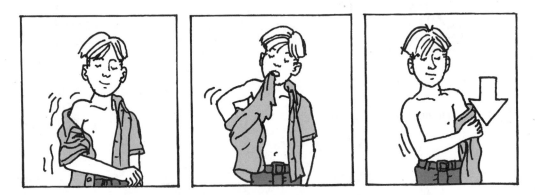

FIGURE 13-16   Adapted method of taking off a shirt: arms-in-front method.

Pants and skirts

Pants or skirts with elastic waistbands are the easiest to put on and remove. Waistbands may need to be fairly loose for children with severe weakness, abnormal movement patterns, or incoordination. Children with limited ROM, incoordination or impaired balance may use one or more clothes hooks, attached to the walls at various heights in their bedroom. These can stabilize clothing while dressing or undressing.

There are many adapted methods of putting on pants (Figures 13-17 through 13-21). All of the these methods can be reversed to undress pants. Children with physical limitations on one side of the body should remember to remove clothing from the affected side first. Children with spinal cord injuries, limited grasping ability, reaching ability, or hip flexion could benefit from using the quad-quip trouser pull method (see Figure 13-21). The trouser pull is attached to the waist of the pants before the feet are placed in the pants.

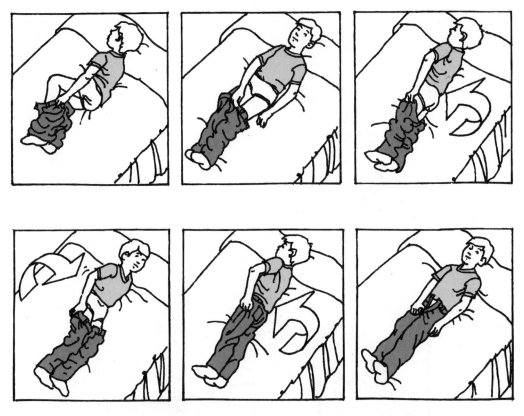

FIGURE 13-17 Adapted method of putting on pants: supine-roll method.

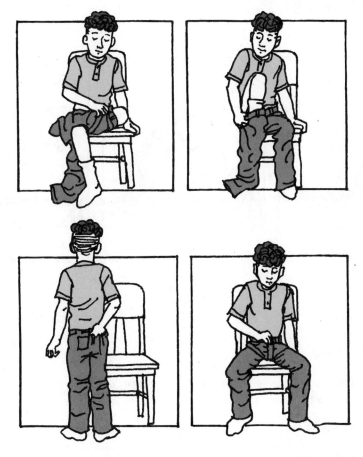

FIGURE 13-18 Adapted method of putting on pants: sit-stand-sit method.

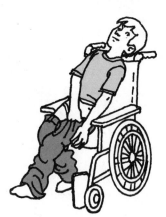

FIGURE 13-19 Adapted method of putting on pants: one-side-bridge sitting method.

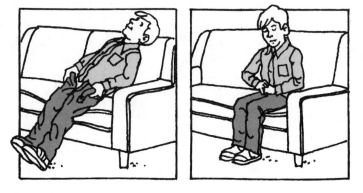

FIGURE 13-20 Adapted method of putting on pants: sitting bridge method.

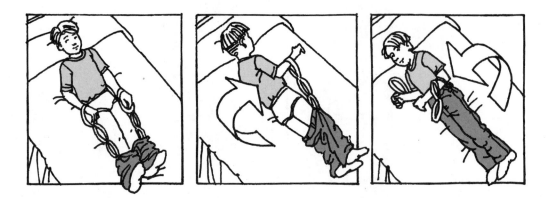

FIGURE 13-21 Adapted method of putting on pants: quad-quip trouser pull method.

Capes, jackets, and rain gear

Capes are usually easier to put on and take off than jackets. Certain adapted clothing companies make raingear designed to fit over an individual in a wheelchair (see Chapter 13 Appendix A). The individual is not required to get in or out of the chair to dress or undress the raingear. An inexpensive, hooded plastic rain poncho may prove equally functional.

MARK'S COAT STORY. *Mark was a 7-year-old-boy who was born with several bones and tendons missing in his left arm and hand. Because his ROM and coordination were moderately to severely limited in all his shoulder, forearm, wrist, and finger movements on his left side, putting on a jacket was a problem. Mark had developed his own compensatory but inefficient method of putting on his jacket.*

He put his right arm in the sleeve first and then twirled quickly around so that the jacket would flip over toward his left arm. Occasionally the jacket flew close enough to his left arm for him to catch it after only one or two twirls. However, usually Mark twirled and twirled and kept his class, the school bus, or his family waiting; he would eventually ask for help.

Because Mark was embarrassed by his limitations, the practitioner made sure to engage his curiosity and be respectful of his situation. The occupational therapy practitioner told him she had a new idea for him and needed his opinion about it.

Mark was taught to put on his jacket more efficiently. The practitioner used a forward chaining method accompanied by a demonstration and clear, slow verbal explanation to teach Mark to use the following sequence: (1) find the collar by looking for the label; (2) hold the collar in your right hand; (3) reach across your body to pull the left sleeve onto your left arm; (4) while still holding the collar, bring your right arm around your head, pulling the jacket around your right shoulder; (5) slide your right hand toward and down and into the right sleeve.

It took Mark only a few tries to succeed. In spite of memory, attention, and sequencing problems, he never forgot this skill. He put on his jacket quickly and independently from that day on.

CLINICAL *Pearl*

Dress and undress the affected or weak side first.

SUSAN'S JACKET STORY. *Susan was an 8-year-old girl with mild spasticity, severe mental retardation, severe sensory defensiveness, severely limited discrimination of tactile-proprioceptive feedback, severely limited motor planning, bilateral incoordination, and autism. She could not understand verbal explanations. Visual demonstrations involving simple, symmetrical movements were the most meaningful methods to teach her to put on her jacket.*

After using calming and focusing sensory activities, Susan's occupational therapy practitioner had Susan use the lap and over-the-head method (see Figure 13-7) to put on her jacket. The jacket was placed upside down on the table in front of Susan, with the collar closest to Susan's midline. Demonstrations and physical assistance were used to help her slap both hands onto the armholes. Susan was assisted with flinging both arms forcefully over her head and bringing her arms through the sleeves at the same time. By learning the slapping and flinging steps first, Susan learned them

within a few months. She was later taught to place the jacket on the table in the proper position independently.

Socks

For a child with hemiplegia or limited balance, sitting with back support may be the best starting position for putting on and removing socks. The child lifts the affected leg onto a box or step to bring the foot closer to the unaffected hand. A wide sock opening can prevent frustration during the most difficult part of putting on socks, which is inserting the toes.

To take off socks, children often use the pull-the-toe method. Using a thumb or one or two fingers, children can push the sock down and around the heel. The toe of the sock is grasped and pulled off. New types of sock and stocking dressing aids are available through equipment catalogs. They help keep the sock or stocking openings wide while children slide their feet in. They may benefit children with limited reaching, coordination, and lower extremity function. Sock and stocking aids are usually inserted into and attached to the sock or stockings before the items are pulled on. While seated, children place their toes into the sock or stocking and then pull the straps or sticks on the dressing aid to pull them on completely. These aids can be difficult to use, so children should try to use several different types before purchasing one.

Putting on nylon stockings or tights can be one of the most challenging dressing tasks. Stockings and tights are difficult to grasp and provide little feedback for children and adolescents with coordination or sensory problems. Some dressing aids are designed specifically for stockings but can be difficult to use. If possible, try to use stockings made of thicker fabrics, which provide more feedback. Choose a size that is one or two times larger than the child normally wears so that they are easier to put on and require less adjustment.

Adjusting and fastening clothing
Adjusting clothing
Adjusting clothing is sometimes more problematic than putting it on or fastening it. A child may lack the tactile discrimination needed to determine whether pants are on straight or a shirt is tucked in. Visual cues can help, such as lining up the top button or front seam of pants with the child's belly button. Checking the appearance of the clothing in a mirror (front and back) before leaving the house and after using the bathroom can be taught as part of dressing and toileting routines.

Fastening
For individuals who only have the use of one hand or who have limited strength, ROM, or coordination, a variety of fastening aids that are available through equipment

catalogs may be helpful. These aids include buttonhooks, bow ties, Velcro shoe closures, and zipper pulls. A dressing stick with a hook or clasp at the end can be used to reach back fasteners. Velcro fasteners may make dressing and undressing easier and quicker; they can be sewn into clothing in place of buttons, snaps, zippers, or ties. Some clothes with Velcro closures, such as shoes, are commonly sold in stores or through catalogs.

Fastening boards and cubes provide stable surfaces for children who are developing beginning fastening skills. Playing "dress up" is a valuable learning activity. Children can put on costumes with fasteners to act out scenes such as playing house or going shopping. Dress up dolls, which come with a variety of fasteners, are also fun and useful learning tools. Some child-size pop-up tents found in equipment catalogs are made with four entrances operated by four different fasteners and can also be used for fastening practice.

Buttoning

Buttoning is a bimanual task that requires refined touch-pressure discrimination and fine motor skills. An in-hand manipulation skill called *shift*, which allows objects to slide across fingers, is also needed (see Handwriting section in this chapter). Buttonhooks may help some children with limited ROM or orthopedic conditions button more efficiently; however, they can make tasks more difficult for children with abnormal muscle tone and subsequent incoordination, such as children with cerebral palsy. The following examples present two methods of resolving buttoning problems.

EVAN'S ADAPTED BUTTONING STORY. *Evan, a 19 year old with quadriplegia, struggled with learning to use a variety of buttoning aids. Although he eventually succeeded, the task required much time and energy. Evan asked the occupational therapy practitioner about adapted clothing (see Chapter 13 Appendix A) and eventually requested Velcro closures. He brought in several of his own shirts, and the occupational therapy practitioner sewed buttons over the buttonholes and Velcro closures inside the front opening. Evan could then fasten and unfasten his favorite shirts easily, and the shirts still appeared as if they were buttoned.*

CARL'S BUTTONING STORY. *Carl was a 3½-year-old boy with severely low muscle tone, weakness, and limited body awareness, but he had excellent visual discrimination and normal to above normal intelligence. He could not determine what sensations he felt when using his fingertips, which kept him from establishing a motor plan for a sequence of actions. He had no idea how to begin dressing or fastening tasks and actively avoided them. The flimsy texture of cloth was confusing to him because he could not properly interpret or respond to the sensation.*

The buttoning task was graded for Carl to help him with his problem. He began each session by engaging in many resistive upper extremity hand and finger tasks to increase strength and discrimination. He was then taught an activity similar to buttoning, which provided firm touch-pressure feedback that allowed Carl to discriminate the sensations with his fingertips. The occupational therapy practitioner provided a plastic lid with a slot. The practitioner held the lid vertically for Carl, and he was shown the way to push a penny through the slot with one hand and remove it with the other hand (Figure 13-22). Because Carl tended to push the penny in but forget to pull it out, the occupational therapy practitioner prompted him in a playful voice and said, "Don't let the penny fall! Get the penny!" Carl laughed each time the occupational therapy practitioner repeated the prompts. He repeated the activity to hear her say them over again. The activity simulated the bimanual sequence of buttoning, while giving Carl increased sensory feedback that he could interpret.

After a few weeks, the penny activity was followed immediately by a task that involved buttoning and unbuttoning large buttons on a vest that was on the floor. The floor provided a firm support, and the occupational therapy practitioner provided physical assistance. A backward chaining method was used to give Carl a feeling of immediate success. At first Carl was prompted to watch the occupational therapy practitioner push the button into the buttonhole. Carl was then asked to pull the button out, allowing him to feel he successfully completed a buttoning or unbuttoning activity. Soon, with physical assistance, Carl began to (1) pinch the vest in one hand, (2) pinch the button in the other hand, (3) pull the button hole open, (4) push the button through the hole, (5) feel and pinch the button with his opposite hand, and (6) pull it through.

Within 3 months Carl was holding the practice vest on his lap while buttoning and unbuttoning it himself. He was then able to button and unbutton the vest on his own body. Eventually, Carl began practicing with his own clothing.

Zipping

The motor skills required to simply pull a zipper up or down involve being able to (1) grasp the zipper in one hand, preferably with a pincer grasp (using the tips or pads of the thumb and index finger) or fine lateral pinch (with the thumb and thumb side of index finger), (2) stabilize the fabric with the other hand or another body part, and (3) pull the hands in opposite directions. A large key ring or a piece of fishing line make inexpensive zipping aids for children with limited grasping ability, ROM, strength, or coordination. They can be threaded onto a

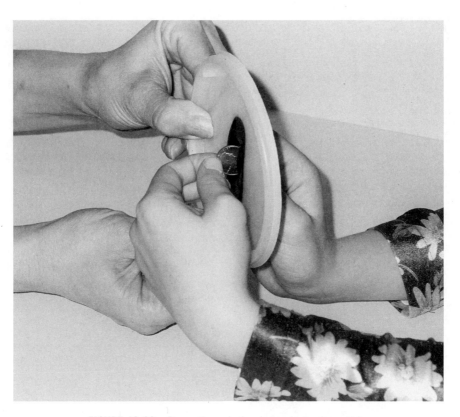

FIGURE 13-22 Penny-through-the-slot prebuttoning activity.

zipper so that the children can simply hook a finger or thumb into the key ring or loop of fishing line to pull the zipper up or down.

Engaging, or inserting, a zipper is much more complicated than pulling the zipper up or down. The occupational therapy practitioner generally teaches a child to unzip first and then to zip (after the zipper has already been inserted for the child). A child is taught to insert a zipper only after learning to pull a zipper up and down and usually after mastery of buttoning and unbuttoning.

An oversized easy zipper is helpful for teaching zipping activities. It may be helpful to first insert the zipper on a garment or board that is laying on a firm surface (such as a table) in front of the child. Whether through verbal, physical, or visual means, the child must learn the zipper has three parts that are tightly connected in a specific sequence. The three parts are labeled as follows for the purpose of explanation: (1) part one, or the pull; (2) part two, or the stop; and (3) part three, or the post (Figure 13-23). Children with average verbal and cognitive skills often benefit from these concrete distinctions among each part.

Part one, or the zipper pull, is the moving handle that is grasped and pulled up and down. The following sequence is used for zipping: (1) part one is pulled down

tightly against part two, or the zipper stop (the tiny bar that stops the pull from coming off) at the bottom of the same side of fabric; (2) parts one and two, the zipper pull and stop, are pinched and held snugly together while (3) part three, or the post, from the other side of fabric is oriented and inserted into the slot; (4) hand placement is reversed, and while (5) one hand pinches the fabric on the post side and pulls it down, (6) the other hand pulls up part one, the zipper pull.

Many children need extra help to properly orient the post to the slot, to hold the pull and stop in place during insertion, to get extra fabric out of the way and to straighten fabric. Strategies of jiggling the closure, pinching, pulling tight, and starting over can also be taught.

Once children are inserting a zipper on clothing or a dressing board on a stable surface, the children should practice zipping a vest or jacket they are wearing. New demands such as reaching, adjusting fabric, and accommodating visual focus significantly increase the challenge.

Snapping

Oversized fasteners are useful tools for teaching the task of snapping. Because of the increased proprioceptive feedback inherent in snapping, many children learn to snap before inserting a zipper and sometimes before buttoning. However, if a child has weakness, poor discrimination of

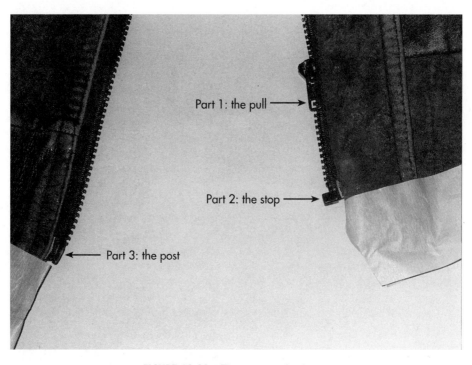

Part 1: the pull →

Part 2: the stop →

← Part 3: the post

FIGURE 13-23 Three parts of a zipper.

tactile-proprioceptive feedback, and relies primarily on visual guidance to learn (as many children with low muscle tone do), snapping may prove quite challenging.

To teach children to snap, have them use their visual skills to line up the top half of the snap over the bottom half. When the top is placed over the bottom, the children should rely on touch-pressure feedback to be sure the parts stay together and do not slide apart. They need adequate proprioceptive (deep pressure) discrimination and strength to properly gauge the amount of force needed to push the two parts together.

Buckling

Buckling can be broken down into a five-step sequence: (1) straighten both sides of the belt and orient the ends properly; (2) slide the end of the belt under the first bar of the buckle; (3) tighten the belt so it is snug but comfortable; (4) insert the prong into the closest hole; and (5) slide the end of the belt under the second bar.

Buckling can often be accomplished using only one hand. It becomes more challenging if the buckle is small or located on a shoe or sandal. Buckling can be practiced on a doll, on a dressing cube, or on the item of clothing on a table. Once mastered in one of these scenarios, it is practiced while the clothing is on the child. When buckling belted pants, skirts, or dresses, it may be most efficient to thread the belt through the belt loops before pulling on the clothing.

Tying shoelaces

Tying a bow is a complicated bimanual task that requires functional visual-motor skills and discrimination of tactile-proprioceptive (touch-pressure) feedback. The child detects the location and movement of the lightweight texture of shoelaces primarily through tactile and proprioceptive discrimination. The sequencing, adjusting, and tightening aspects of tying a bow require visual perception, directionality concepts, visual and motor memory, fine motor planning, and problem solving.

Shoelaces provide little physical feedback to a child with poor sensory discrimination. The child may be completely unable to manipulate the laces and simply twist them around. Laces may feel unpleasant to child with sensory defensiveness. This child may become overstimulated by the tickly touch of the laces and act silly or oppositional and lose focus. Use wide, thick, stiff laces to provide increased touch-pressure feedback, which facilitates both motor planning and a calmer response.

There are other ways to grade materials for bow tying. Using extra long laces can reduce frustration. Children often tie loose bows at first. Long laces prevent them from pulling out during the last step of tightening. Black laces on a black shoe can be confusing for the child with learning disabilities or visual perceptual problems. To increase visual cues, two laces of different colors are tied together before lacing the shoe, so each side of the bow is a different color. The shoe is a third color, increasing visual contrast.

Before working on bow tying, stimulate the child's hand muscles and improve sensory processing by performing resistive finger activities. Using squeeze toys, pulling pennies or pegs out of putty, picking up small objects with tweezers, and pulling ropes are a few examples. Bunny Bow Tie (OT Ideas; see Appendix C), is a popular beginning bow tie device. This sturdy 8-inch by 8-inch wooden square has a picture of a bunny on it with one large blue ear and one large red ear. Two long laces, one red and one blue, are attached to the center of the square between the bunny's ears. Bunny Bow Tie can be used in a variety of ways. Repeating the same motor sequence and using the same cuing phrases during each trial can aid a child's memory. The following 10-step sequence of instructions can be modified according to each child's abilities and each occupational therapy practitioner's style:

1. Place the blue lace on the blue ear and the red lace on the red ear to make an X.
2. Pinch the middle of the X where the laces cross. Look for a tunnel below your fingers.
3. Find the lace on top and fold it behind the bottom lace. Push it through the tunnel so that it comes out in front. Pull it all the way out.
4. Pull both laces tight.
5. Now pinch one lace close to the bunny's face, and fold a little piece (2 to 3 inches) over to make a bunny ear (a loop). The loop is about the size of the bunny ear in the picture. Pinch the bottom of that loop tightly so that a long piece of lace is left over at the end.
6. With your other hand, wind the second lace snugly one time around the finger and thumb that are pinching the loop. Look for your pinching thumb or finger peeking out of a new tunnel. (If the new tunnel keeps slipping off, you may need to hold it in place by pinching it together with the first loop.) Leave the new tunnel large enough so that you can see it.
7. Still pinching the bottom of the first loop, push a small fold of the second string through the tunnel. This turns into the second loop.
8. Switch hands so you can hold a loop in each hand to pull them bigger. Keep fingers outside the loops (not inside).
9. To tighten the bow, start with your hands palm up. Grab each loop in a fist (with the fingers on the outside) and pull out to the sides three times, as tightly as you can.
10. Check to see whether the bow is tight by pinching the center. Do you think it is a little, medium or very tight?

CLINICAL *Pearl*

While teaching shoe tying or any challenging activity, use positive words. For example, instead of saying "The bow is not tight," say, "Well, that seems medium tight to me," or "Wow, that is pretty tight, but I bet you could make it *super* tight." By phrasing it in this way, the child may feel successful and motivated to try for "very tight" instead of giving up.

Children have special cuing needs based on particular problems. Some may need extra demonstrations and reminders to keep the laces snug or to tighten them. Self-checking (evaluating their own performance) is a key to problem solving and taking responsibility.

Adjusting laces can be taught as part of the initial bow tie sequence or later, depending on the child. Tying and untying double knots and lacing shoes are often taught separately. Some children master the sequence of tying a bow but continue to have problems adjusting, retightening, self-checking, or untying knots. Laces may come untied repeatedly throughout the day, and children may still need adult assistance to keep the shoes tied.

Adjusting laces requires either visual or tactile self-checking to determine whether any loop or lace is touching the ground when shoes are flat on the ground. If any piece touches the ground, the child gently pulls on the opposite lace or loop until no part is touching the ground. The child always retightens the laces after adjusting them.

Tying a double knot can be broken down into the following four-step sequence of instructions:

1. Pretend the loops are single strings, and hold each loop in a fist.
2. Make an X with the loops and pinch the center of the X, being sure to leave a big tunnel below your fingers.
3. Fold the top loop behind the bottom loop, and push it all the way through the tunnel so that it comes out the front.
4. Pull both loops gently. Keep the double knot a little loose so that it will be easy to untie with your fingertips.

Untying a double knot or any knot can be frustrating. If the knot is too tight, the occupational therapy practitioner can start the process by loosening it; the child finishes untying it. At these frustrating times, a sense of humor is helpful. Singing a silly song about the ways fingertips help to loosen and untie knots may lighten the mood while encouraging a child to persist.

All lacing activities are useful training exercises for learning to tie shoes. Lacing shoes can also be broken down into a sequence and taught step by step. The child should always be encouraged to self-check, either visually or using a touch-pressure method. Numerous shoe-tying aids are available in equipment catalogs. Many involve one-handed manipulations. Some have laces made of elastic so that once shoes are tied, they can be slipped on and off without tying and untying.

CHUCK'S SHOE-TYING STORY. *Chuck was an 11-year-old boy who was overweight, had poor abdominal muscle strength, and had limited hip flexion (bending ability). He could not balance to squat or kneel on one knee. Even when sitting on a chair with his foot on a step stool, he needed to internally rotate his hip and stretch with effort to reach the side of his shoe. His strength and ROM were so limited that he could not reach the middle of his shoe where the bow is typically tied.*

Using the occupational therapy tools of activity analysis, grading and adapting activities, and reading the child were essential in helping Chuck learn to tie his own shoes. The key questions addressed were (1) how much postural strength, flexibility, balance and control were needed for Chuck to tie his own shoes and (2) how the task could be modified so that Chuck could succeed.

The postural demands of shoe tying were much more problematic for Chuck than the bow-tying sequence. The occupational therapy practitioner adjusted the length of his laces so that a bow tied on the side of his shoe would hang evenly. His mother was notified of the new strategy so that she could help reinforce the procedure. Because Chuck was self-conscious about his weight, care was taken to reinforce his self-esteem by praising his bow-tying progress and using an accepting, matter-of-fact tone to address his postural problems.

ALISON'S SHOE-TYING STORY. *Alison was a 15 year old girl with moderate mental retardation, perceptual-motor problems, sensory defensiveness, extreme distractibility, impulsivity, poor sitting tolerance, and poor judgment. She attended a special school that provided extra structure and emphasized functional and prevocational skills. Because Alison could not tie her shoes, they came untied repeatedly every day. A staff person always had to take time away from teaching to retie Alison's shoes.*

To address this problem, Alison's COTA began each session with intensive sensory modulation activities to increase sitting tolerance, focus of attention, and tolerance for physical cuing and the tickly feeling of shoelaces. Frequent, short practice sessions involving forward and backward chaining with color-coded laces began. Alison first practiced tying on a board, then on an oversized wooden shoe, then on a regular shoe placed on a table, and

*eventually on her own sneakers. In spite of her lower developmental level, Alison learned the higher-level **splinter skill** of tying her own shoes, thereby increasing her independence and self-esteem at home and at school. A splinter skill is a specific, often complex task that is mastered by a child who lacks the underlying developmental capabilities. It is usually accomplished through compensatory methods and practice rather than by remediating underlying developmental components.*

Hygiene

Learning and remembering when and how often to perform hygiene skills is a challenge for many children, especially those with disabilities. Proper sequencing of steps and thorough performance can also be problematic. A primary role of the COTA is to help children learn the skills required to bathe adequately and stay clean.

The Attainment Company (see Appendix C) markets materials, such as videos, games and picture cards that teach independent living skills to children and adults with mild to moderate cognitive and motor impairments. Their picture sequences use clear drawings of individuals performing the steps of bathing, showering, toileting and toothbrushing as well as other daily living skills.

Bathing and showering

The COTA may assist children and their families in choosing and learning to use adapted methods of bathing or showering. Although many children can learn to get safely into the tub or shower and bathe themselves, others have more severe physical or cognitive disabilities that preclude independence.

Transferring a child with severe disabilities into the tub or shower is extremely demanding for the caregiver. Lifting and lowering an adolescent or large child into a tub on a regular basis could easily injure the caregiver's back. Families of children with severe physical disabilities may consider the following modifications:

1. Create a roll-in shower in the home. A roll-in shower is a large shower with a raised edge instead of a lip. It is designed to allow a wheeled bath chair to roll inside and turn around. The child is transferred into the chair before entering the shower. Using a seat belt and other postural supports, the child may be able to assist in the showering process. Roll-in showers can be attractive and convenient for all family members.
2. Children who depend on others for bathing and transferring may need adapted bath chairs with seat belts, a chest harness, knee abductors, and footrests or headrests. Chairs for these clients may feature netting that supports the child in a semireclined position.

Some wheeled shower chairs can be rolled into a roll-in shower or over a toilet for dual use.

3. Create a raised tub in the home, which eliminates the need to lower the child into and lift the child out of a deep tub and significantly reduces strain to the caregiver's back.

4. A Hoyer or other hydraulic lift with sling seat can be used to eliminate lifting for the caretaker.

5. Portable, inflatable tubs are also available. As the child is rolled from side to side on a bed, the deflated tub is laid underneath. It is then inflated with air and filled with water as the child lies on it. As with all inflatable equipment, these vinyl tubs can develop leaks and need to be repaired. In spite of this inconvenience, some families prefer using an inflatable tub to other bathing options.

Safety is the primary concern for the child with mild to moderate physical disabilities who is learning bath and shower skills. The COTA teaches transfers and bathing skills thoroughly to ensure that they are safely carried out in the home. Ideally, skills are taught and refined with the caregivers in the child's actual home. Transferring into and out of a tub or shower requires the motor skills of weight shifting without losing balance, standing, turning, flexing (bending) the abdomen (stomach), knees and hips, and usually weight bearing on hands. Washing body parts requires all of these skills as well as reaching, grasping and manipulating faucets, soap, sponge or washcloth, and often a hand held shower device.

Adapted equipment for bathing, showering, and transferring in and out of tubs and showers is available from equipment catalogs, medical supply stores, and some pharmacies. Examples of adapted equipment and their uses include the following:

1. A nonslip mat in the bathtub or shower is essential to prevent slipping.

2. Outside the tub or shower, a bath mat with nonslip coating on the bottom, low pile, and no fringe is the safest type of mat.

3. The simplest bath chair is a stool that can be easily placed into and removed from the tub or shower. If the child is susceptible to skin problems, a padded chair may help. Children with poor balance use a chair with a backrest. Those who need extra help in transferring use a chair that extends over the side of the tub.

4. A hand-held shower device is useful for most children. It can be found in hardware or houseware stores. For children who sit on bath chairs, a holder can be attached to the tub wall close to their dominant hand. One style of bath chair provides a slot for storing the shower device, as well as a soap holder. Foot-operated controls are available for the hand-held shower device.

5. Tub side grab bars that clamp onto the side of a tub are inexpensive, functional adaptations that do not require permanent installation. Permanently installed grab bars make bathing safer for everyone. They can usually be purchased from surgical supply stores, and the vendor can install them. The OTR can tell the COTA what types of bars are needed and where they should be placed. Make sure during installation that the American National Standards for accessibility are being followed. Bars must be installed securely into wall studs according to instructions. A plumber or carpenter may also install tub bars. Obtain permission from the landlord before installing wall-mounted grab bars in rented homes.

6. Many bathing aids are available, including the following: suction soap holders, which are attached to the wall; long-handled sponges and brushes; curved-handled sponges and brushes; small sponges on long handles to clean between toes; terry cloth bath mitts; "soap on a rope"; bath mitts with soap pockets, eliminating the need to hold soap or pick it up if dropped.

DONALD'S HYGIENE STORY. *Some children, especially those with sensory defensiveness, may not tolerate the slimy feeling of bar soap or the cold sensation of liquid soap. Paper towels may feel too scratchy or dry. This was the case for Donald, a 7 year old, who told the occupational therapy practitioner he never washed his hands. To determine his reasons, Donald was questioned about his feelings on each aspect of hand washing. Fortunately, he was able to explain the ways the texture and temperature of the soap and temperature of the water bothered him.*

Several modifications were made for Donald. After reviewing hand-washing rules, such as when and why hand washing is done, Donald was given a choice of using bar or liquid soap. He chose liquid soap because the texture was slightly less aversive than that of bar soap. At first the occupational therapy practitioner warmed the liquid soap in her hands. She helped Donald rub it on his hands and then helped him rub his hands together under warm (not hot) water. Donald was then taught how to adjust the water temperature and warm up the soap in his own hands. Because he continued to resist using bar soap, liquid soap was always provided. He was given the option of air drying his hands because disliked the feeling of paper towels.

The occupational therapy staff and Donald's parents continued to reinforce the reasons hand washing with soap was necessary after toileting and before and after eating. Soon Donald needed only periodic verbal cues to wash his hands and occasional reminders of how to regulate water and soap temperature.

Oral hygiene

A number of modified toothbrushes now on the market may ease the task of toothbrushing for children with limited coordination or motor planning. Large-handled brushes with small heads and soft bristles can be found in many pharmacies and health supply stores. Children with mild to moderate motor impairments can simplify brushing by using an electric toothbrush (Figure 13-24, A). The large, vibrating handle requires less sustained strength to hold and may facilitate muscle hand contractions, which improves grasp. Small or precise coordinated brushing actions are unnecessary when using an electric toothbrush, which is simply moved slowly across all tooth, gum, and tongue surfaces. Use caution when selecting an electric toothbrush. Some children are frightened by the vibrations, whereas others find the sound aversive, especially the sound of sonic electric toothbrushes.

The pleasing textured surface of Nuk brushes, which have rubber nubs instead of bristles, can be chewed on by children before being introduced for actual toothbrushing. Johnson and Johnson's small soft toothbrush with its oval handle can be independently grabbed and put in the mouth by children; it's wide handle prevents them from being gagged or poked (Figure 13-24, B). The fingertip training toothbrush (see Figure 13-24, B) has small, soft, molded plastic bristles and slides over the tip and first knuckle of a finger. The child or caregiver slips it on and uses it like a toothbrush to clean teeth and gums. Children with severe motor impairments need either hand-over-hand assistance to brush their own teeth or need their teeth cleaned for them. Toothettes, which are cardboard sticks with minty sponges on the end, can be used with some children (see Figure 13-24, B). Toothettes are not safe for children who have a strong tonic bite reflex or a tendency to chew or swallow inedible objects.

DARREN'S TOOTHBRUSHING STORY. *Eight-year-old Darren had resisted having his teeth cleaned since he was a baby. His mother said that he also refused to attempt many other self-care tasks. He allowed his mother or father to brush his teeth only once a day. His parents requested the occupational therapy practitioner's assistance in school.*

In Darren's first occupational therapy toothbrushing session no toothpaste was used. Darren was told it was more important to brush than to use toothpaste. His parents had found a toothpaste he tolerated, strawberry-flavored Tom's Toothpaste for Children, which was also purchased for Darren's occupational therapy sessions.

Darren tolerated the feeling of water on his hands and learned the way to adjust the water temperature and rate of flow. Although he tolerated the sticky feeling of toothpaste in his mouth, Darren became agitated when he felt toothpaste

and water dripping on his lips or chin. He also had a strong aversion to the smell of many toothpastes.

Considering Darren's tactile aversions, a gentle approach was taken. Darren used his strawberry-flavored toothpaste, an appealing two-piece travel toothbrush, and the preparatory jaw-tug technique[43] (See Transitioning from Bottle to Cup section in this chapter). Practice sessions were short and included demonstrations, humor, and verbal prompting. Before starting a toothbrushing activity, Darren was given a paper towel to wipe drips from his mouth and chin.

A mirror also proved helpful for Darren (although some children find mirrors perceptually confusing). Darren was given slow, verbal instructions and repeated visual cues to remind him to reach all teeth on the inside and outside. Humor was easily incorporated as the occupational therapy practitioner tried to give clear verbal instructions and demonstrate toothbrushing at the same time. To reinforce the skills Darren had learned, the occupational therapy practitioner periodically asked Darren to explain the sequence of toothbrushing and how often and why people need to brush their teeth. With his parents' gentle encouragement, Darren began brushing his teeth at home within several months.

Nose blowing

Many children with special needs have problems learning to blow their noses when necessary. Limited facial sensory awareness can prevent a child from feeling the sensation of a runny nose. If the child already knows the sequence of nose blowing, the COTA may simply provide reminders about when it should be and instruction in how to check in a mirror to see if nostrils are clean.

Other children have significant problems developing the skill of nose blowing. Limited respiratory control, motor planning, or touch-pressure discrimination may prevent them from sequencing or carrying out the task. Sensory defensiveness may cause aversive reactions to tissues. Caregivers and team members may need to work together to develop creative, individualized strategies for learning this difficult skill.

Demonstrating nose blowing is almost impossible because a tissue hides the nose during the task. Even when the tissue is removed and the occupational therapy practitioner forces air through the nostrils, the action can only be heard, not seen.

Several techniques may prove helpful. First, while demonstrating how to blow air through the nostrils while the lips are tightly closed, the occupational therapy practitioner places the child's hand under the practitioner's nose so that the child can feel the blowing air. Second, the practitioner shows the child how tissue flutters when it is held in front of the face and air is blown on it through the nostrils with the lips closed. Third, powder

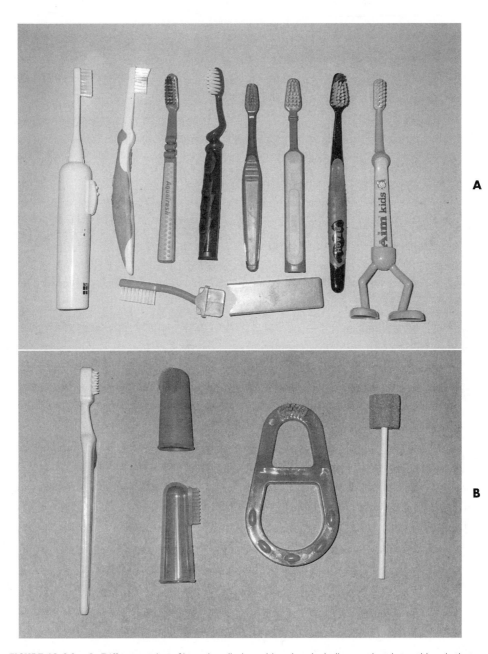

FIGURE 13-24 **A,** Different styles of large-handled toothbrushes, including an electric toothbrush, that can make toothbrushing easier. **B,** Modified toothbrushes *(left to right):* Nuk training brush, fingertip toothbrushes, rounded toothbrush (which is safe for infants), toothette.

is sprinkled on a piece of dark paper or cardboard and placed under the occupational therapy practitioner's nose. A child who learns visually can benefit from seeing the powder fly away as the occupational therapy practitioner forcefully blows air through the nostrils. The powder-covered paper is then placed under the child's nose to encourage the same response. When successful, the child receives immediate visual feedback. The occupational therapy practitioner may need to spend extra time help-

ing the child keep the lips closed while blowing out through the nose.

Extra care should be taken to help children with sensory defensiveness tolerate the sensation of the tissues. Clean their noses gently, and avoid vigorous wiping. A tissue dampened with warm water can make it feel less scratchy, and some children may tolerate a soft, cloth handkerchief more easily than paper. Lotion or petroleum jelly may be applied after nose wiping to prevent skin from becoming chapped. Some children with sensory defensiveness choose to wipe their own noses, even if they are unable to blow them. The occupational therapy practitioner should give them tissues or handkerchiefs as needed. Being given control over the task often reduces aversive responses.

Toilet hygiene

Skills needed for proper toilet hygiene include visual and tactile recognition of cleanliness, adequate sitting balance, trunk rotation, shoulder extension and rotation (for reaching), and sufficient strength and proprioceptive (deep pressure) discrimination to apply pressure for wiping. These skills can be addressed separately in addition to being used during actual daily toileting routines.

One problem related to toileting that is often overlooked is washing hands with soap and water after each use of the toilet. Although this is almost always taught to young children, once children are independently eliminating and wiping, the hand-washing aspect can easily be forgotten. Anyone who works with children knows how frequently children and staff get sick with colds or the flu. One of the most common causes of bacterial and viral transmission is insufficient hand washing.

Each time a child uses the toilet, the COTA may either assist with hand washing, or ask the child if hands were washed with soap and water. Answers may be surprising. Frequent responses are, "Yes, but I just used water," "My mom says I don't have to," "I already washed my hands before lunch," or "Oh, I forgot again." To prevent the spread of contagion, always check on handwashing. A response of, "Yes, I used soap and water," provides an opportunity to praise the child.

Toilet training

In school settings, teachers may be the primary trainers of toileting skills. Schedule training programs are often effective in helping students learn to use the toilet at regular intervals. Children learning toileting skills should be taken to the bathroom about every half hour to every hour. The toileting routine, including pulling pants up and down and washing hands, is learned by this type of repetition. With so many opportunities to use the toilet, many children begin to eliminate in the toilet successfully. They begin wearing underwear instead of diapers during the day. The praise they receive and their new self-control can increase their self-esteem, leading to further independence.

Children may resist using a toilet for several reasons. Diapers feel warm, snug, supportive, and comforting. The feeling of underwear is unfamiliar and does not provide the same comfort or support. The toilet may be too high and therefore frightening. Sitting on a toilet can feel cold and hard. The sound or sight of the toilet flushing may be scary. Some children even believe that part of their body is falling into and disappearing in the toilet. Consider the following solutions:

1. Provide underwear that is extra thick and snug. Some children may benefit from Neoprene shorts, which are warm and provide external support (Benik; Silverdale, Washington) (see Chapter 13 Appendix C).
2. Use a padded toilet seat or warm the seat with a hair dryer or heat lamp. Make the bathroom environment comfortable.
3. Use a "potty seat" that is close to the ground. If this is not possible, provide a footrest and a potty insert to make the opening of the regular toilet smaller.
4. Temporarily omit flushing from practice sessions to determine whether this helps the child tolerate the toilet better. Once the child masters eliminating in the toilet, develop strategies to address the fear of flushing (for example, use a quieter toilet).
5. Help young children deal with their fear of losing part of the body in the toilet by placing a diaper in the bottom of the potty seat. The child sees the urine or feces go into the diaper, just like it did before the potty was used.[53]

Adapted equipment for toileting

Various adapted toilet seats are available. Pediatric toilet safety armrests (Achievement Products; Canton, Ohio) (see Chapter 13 Appendix C) are often adult-style armrests that can be attached to child-size toilets. They are relatively inexpensive, useful for most children and adults, and easy to attach. The armrests curve under the toilet seat, and the child's weight stabilizes them. These armrests are safer and easier to use than toilet armrests with legs. One disadvantage to the leg-style type of toilet armrest is that people trip over the legs. In addition, some children with disabilities tend to pull up on the armrests instead of push down. If a child pulls up on the leg-style of armrest, it comes off the ground and can throw the child off balance. In contrast, when a child pulls up on the under-the-seat armrest, it tends to stay in place and provide support.

Although under-the-seat pediatric toilet safety armrests are more useful, the armrests themselves are most often at an adult height of about 7 to 8 inches above the seat. For very small children, armrests are at or near the underarms. Children with mild incoordination or low muscle tone often adapt to these armrests. Other children may need more specialized equipment with a seat belt, back and trunk supports, footrests, and a headrest. For children with cerebral palsy, moderate motor incoordination, paralysis, weakness, or the use of only one hand, try the following possibilities:

1. Search equipment catalogs (see Chapter 13 Appendix C), the *American Journal of Occupational Therapy*, Oc-

cupational Therapy Week, and other journals for information about adapted toilet seats and positioning aids.

2. Consult with the supervising OTR and other occupational therapy practitioners about toilet seats that they have found to be effective.

3. Use your activity analysis skills to determine which adapted toilet seat will restrict the child's movement the least, fit in the existing space in the home, be most cost effective, and be most convenient for the child, caregivers, and family members.

All factors should be considered when choosing a toileting device. The caregiver's concerns are extremely important. If a device is too cumbersome or too messy to clean, even the most capable caregiver may revert to putting their child in diapers. If the family only has one toilet, a mobile toilet seat that rolls over the toilet and locks into place for the child's use often provides an ideal solution.

Menstrual care

Adolescence brings a new toileting challenge for all girls— menstrual care. Menstrual care tasks become even more challenging for girls with physical or cognitive disabilities.

KELLY'S MENSTRUAL CARE STORY. *Kelly is a 12-year-old girl with severe mental retardation, severe sensory defensiveness, decreased ability to interpret touch-pressure feedback, weakness, incoordination, motor planning problems, and limited ROM including decreased trunk rotation; she was assisted in several ways.*

During occupational therapy sessions Kelly regularly practiced trunk rotation activities to help her develop the skill of reaching behind her back during toileting. To increase her awareness of how hard she was pressing while wiping, she performed many resistive finger and hand tasks, performed weightbearing tasks on her hands, and wiped tables and blackboards. She also practiced regular toileting routines, including wiping in a front-to-back motion (to prevent urinary tract infections), adjusting clothing, and pressing hard enough during handwashing to wash and dry hands thoroughly.

When she was menstruating, Kelly brought her own pad to occupational therapy sessions. Kelly's parents provided large pads with adhesive tabs and side wings because they were the easiest for her to manage. She also brought pictures that her COTA and speech therapist had created as cues to remind her of her bathroom sequence. Combined with the COTA's verbal and gestural guidance, the picture cues reminded Kelly to look and see whether her pad needed changing and to fold up the dirty pad, roll it in toilet paper, and discard it in a special container, as well as open and attach a new pad to her underwear.

When her underwear had blood on it, the COTA used verbal and visual cues to help Kelly change her underwear.

While wearing latex gloves, the COTA assisted Kelly with washing out the dirty underwear with cold water and soap. The wet underwear was then placed in a plastic bag, which Kelly brought home for laundering.

Grooming

Hair care

Having hair shampooed, cut, and groomed can be a trying experience for a child and caregiver. The child may scream and cry during shampooing no matter how gentle the process. Just one memory of getting soap in the eyes can cause an unreasonable fear response in a toddler. Children with sensory defensiveness commonly resist hair care, and being unable to see or control the process increases anxiety. During shampooing the multiple texture and temperature changes (dry hair, wet hair, soapy hair, watery hair, warm air, cool air) and actions such as towel drying may cause the child to feel bombarded with attacks to the head.

When hair is brushed, combed, braided, or put into hair bands or barrettes, the child receives multiple alternating sensations, from tickly to tugging and sometimes pinching, especially if hair is tangled. Sensations may seem completely unpredictable and therefore more painful to a child with sensory defensiveness. Getting a haircut is one of the most traumatic events for a child with sensory defensiveness, especially if an electric trimmer is being used. The tickly vibration on the back of the head or neck, combined with the intense buzzing beside the ears and prickly, newly cut hairs, may be more than the child can handle. Some of the following interventions for hair care may help:

1. Johnson and Johnson baby shampoo causes little or no stinging when it get in the eyes. (Other companies also make shampoos that do not sting.)

2. Even if the child does not yet understand language, each time hair is shampooed and dried, use a soothing voice to repeat what will happen next. The rhythmic repetition of words can be calming. If the child understands the words, knowing what is going to happen can lessen anxiety.

3. Carry out each hair care step with a smooth, firm touch. Sometimes in their well-meaning attempts to be careful with a sensitive child, caregivers are too gentle, resulting in tickly sensations instead of firm deep pressure. Light, moving touches are the most uncomfortable for this type of child.

4. Be sure water and room temperatures are warm but not too hot. Keep a towel handy in case the eyes or face need to be wiped quickly.

5. Whenever possible, allow the child to control the hair-care procedure. Even if attempts are unsuccessful and the caregiver must take over, the child may

begin to become accustomed to the sensations by controlling part of the procedure.

6. A spray detangler works well on dry hair. Look for products that are alcohol-free because alcohol dries out hair.

7. Make the hair-cutting experience fun by providing special treats. Many barbers know that giving a child a lollipop during a haircut can be soothing and distracting. Some children need multiple distractions, such as a favorite story along with a toy and lollipop.

8. Use the Wilbarger deep pressure and proprioceptive technique 2 or 3 times before giving a child a haircut.[55] If possible, spend an hour in the park and sing songs or play with blowing toys right before the haircut. These activities help modulate the child's nervous system. Applying deep pressure to the head before the haircut, as during a head massage, may also help.

9. If an electric trimmer is not necessary, ask the barber not to use one.

10. Consider asking a trusted family member to cut the child's hair in the home. The secure feeling provided by a familiar relative and the home environment can help a child tolerate a haircut. A child who screams and throws a tantrum at a barbershop may sit quietly for an uncle who cuts the child's hair at home, even when an electric trimmer is used.

Independent hair care is taught on different levels depending on children's needs. Some children need to gain knowledge about how often to wash and comb their hair and have it cut. Others need to learn step-by-step procedures for each skill. Some children need to attain a positive attitude in regards to taking responsibility for hair care, checking themselves, and evaluating the outcome of their efforts.

Some children benefit from using a mirror during hair grooming, whereas others are confused by the backward mirror image. Adaptive devices such as a long- or bent-handled hairbrush may be helpful. A heavy hairbrush with a large handle and indented finger and thumb holds provides extra physical feedback for the child with limited sensory awareness.

MARY'S HAIR CARE STORY. *Mary was a 13-year-old girl with severe mental retardation, sensory defensiveness, poor ability to reach across her midline, and an inability to accurately feel the hairbrush; she needed a special approach to hair care. Mary depended on visual feedback to guide her hand movements, so she practiced in front of a mirror. She used spray detangler and a large-handled hairbrush with a well-defined handhold. The brush had bristles on all sides, so it was effective no matter which way Mary turned it.*

Although Mary was right handed, she brushed more thoroughly on the left side of her head using her left hand. By using each hand to brush each side of her head, Mary did not have to struggle to rotate her trunk and reach across her midline. Mary alternated using each hand to brush the back of her head. If Mary were younger or had fewer physical disabilities, it might have been possible for her to develop trunk rotation and spontaneous midline crossing skills for more efficient hair brushing.

Shaving

Because of safety issues, make sure to obtain administrative approval, written permission from parents or guardians, and input from supervisors and team members when implementing a shaving program. Extra supervision is needed for girls and boys with emotional impairments; razors may need to be stored in a locked cabinet that they cannot access.

Shaving may not be necessary for girls. Unless a girl is highly invested in shaving her legs or underarms, shaving might not need to be part of a grooming program. For adolescent girls, shaving instructions should entail how often to shave, materials needed to shave, how to obtain materials, the cost of materials for shaving, the motor sequence of shaving, safety precautions, positioning methods, self-evaluation, cleanup, and how to change the razor.

A group-shaving program can be helpful for adolescent boys with limited coordination, cognition, sequencing abilities, sensory awareness, and strength. The camaraderie and pride associated with shaving independently can be shared.

EARL'S AND GREG'S SHAVING STORY. *At age 17, neither Earl nor Greg had the coordination to safely handle regular razors. Earl was diagnosed with fragile X syndrome, (a genetic disorder, which can result in autism, caused by a "fragile site" on the X chromosome), mental retardation, and attention deficit disorder (ADD). Greg had a history of lead poisoning, which causes mental retardation. Both boys had emotional problems. Their COTA used an activity analysis and knowledge of the boys' strengths and limitations to implement an effective training program for both of them.*

The COTA obtained permission from school administrators and the boys' parents. The COTA searched catalogs, local stores, and newspaper discount ads until she found a low-priced, good-quality, safe, wet-and-dry use electric razor.

Mirrors can help or hinder the shaving process, depending on the child. With Earl and Greg, tabletop mirrors proved helpful in carrying out the shaving sequence as well as checking their success. Because of Earl's severe sensory defensiveness, the COTA kept the water warm and allowed him to be in control of all touching on his face. The program included learning to clean the razors and change the blades.

Nail care

Being given the opportunity to choose from a variety of trimming and cleaning tools may help a reluctant child participate in nail care tasks. Although girls are often enticed by pretty nail polish and keeping nails long, boys may have little interest in nail care tasks.

Nail clippers can be dangerous or impossible to operate for children with limited coordination or weakness. The occupational therapy practitioner and child should explore different types of nail trimmers to find the most suitable one.

Some adapted nail clippers are attached to a board that has suction cups on the bottom, which eliminates the need to simultaneously hold, position, and pinch the clipper with one hand. Instead the child positions the finger to be trimmed on the device and pushes down on the clipper. This method can still be somewhat dangerous for some children. An oversized emery board may be easier and safer. Pharmacies and cosmetics stores sell many styles, including block-style, curved, round, oval, and extra-wide emery boards in many colors. Other children may prefer the sensation of a metal nail file. Some children can learn to use fingernail scissors. Scissors with a round tip are the safest, and they are often found in the baby section of the pharmacy. Children with limited motor planning skills, hand strength, and dexterity may benefit from preparatory resistive fingertip exercises, frequent and short practice sessions, and extra help in evaluating their performance by looking at and feeling their nails.

In addition to trimming nails, cleaning fingernails can be addressed in a nail care program. The COTA can help the child with nail cleaning and checking progress. The child can choose from a several different appealing nail-brushes. Allow the child to choose the style and texture of the nailbrush, because some are too stiff and scratchy for certain children.

Skin care

Children with spinal cord injuries, limited mobility, or limited sensory awareness can be taught to check their skin for bedsores. Different sizes of mirrors with various bed or wall attachments can be angled for this purpose. After training by a doctor, nurse, or OTR, the COTA teaches the child procedures for prevention and treatment of bedsores. Children who have intact cognitive skills but severely impaired mobility can be taught ways to inform a home attendant about skin care.

Children with developmental delays, emotional impairments, or physical disabilities often need extra help taking care of their skin. In dry or cold climates, they may need to learn ways to check their skin to see whether it is rough, red, dry, or chapped and when and how to use skin lotion and lip moisturizer.

TERRI'S SKIN CARE STORY. *Terri was a 7-year-old girl with Turner's syndrome (a genetic disorder in which the individual has only one X chromosome), attention deficit hyperactivity disorder (ADHD), learning disabilities, and severe sensory defensiveness. She was extremely distracted by tactile, visual, and auditory input, so much so that she could not screen out background stimulation without help. Every winter her lips became so chapped that she could not stop touching and picking at them. This behavior not only caused her lips to bleed, but it also repeatedly interfered with her focus on classroom activities.*

Terri's intervention focused on three areas: (1) finding a tolerable lip moisturizer, (2) creating a schedule for the application of lip moisturizer, and (3) creating a plan to help Terri cope with her sensory defensiveness.

Finding a lip moisturizer that Terri tolerated was not easy. Her olfactory and oral sensory defensiveness were severe. Terri's mother and the occupational therapy practitioner found two kinds of lip balm that Terri inconsistently tolerated. One day she would choose one kind, but the next day she would change her mind and chose the other one. Both were made available to her at all times.

Terri needed a schedule to apply the lip moisturizer frequently so that her lips would heal and stop distracting her. As a reminder to apply the moisturizer, a drawing of lip balm was taped to her school desk. School staff members also verbally reminded her to use her moisturizer.

Terri also needed a program to help regulate her sensory defensiveness. The Wilbarger deep pressure and proprioceptive technique,[55] blowing bubbles, and rhythmic bouncing were used regularly in occupational therapy. Terri stopped picking her lips during these activities. The Wilbarger intraoral technique[55] and the jaw-tug technique[43] were also used. When all the techniques were used consistently throughout the day and Terri used her lip balm frequently, she picked at her lips significantly less. She was able to pay attention more consistently in school.

Using deodorant

Children with disabilities may find spray deodorants easier to use than roll-on deodorants. Children with limited coordination or strength may use adapters for spray cans, which are available from many adaptive equipment companies. Children with sensitive skin may be unable to use antiperspirants. A spray made from natural crystal deodorant may be a gentler yet just as effective alternative.

COTAs can instruct children in deodorant use as well as practice the technique with them. Practice is frequently necessary for adolescent girls and boys. Deodorant use should be taught in a matter-of-fact way so that children are not embarrassed.

EARL'S AND GREG'S DEODORANT STORY. *Earl and Greg, the previously mentioned 17 year olds who had difficulties shaving, also had trouble using deodorant regularly. They had cognitive, sensory, motor planning, and emotional problems. Earl could not read, and Greg could only read at a third-grade level. At home, they were given the responsibility for their own daily hygiene and dressing tasks.*

Figure 13-25 is a daily living skills checklist that can be used to help children take responsibility for their own hygiene, grooming, and functional interactions. It has simple statements so that children who are able to read can use it; it also has drawings for children who are not able to read.

Earl and Greg completed their own individual checklist daily, which reminded them to carry out their own daily living skills. For example, after reviewing his checklist, Greg often reported that he had forgotten to use deodorant. He was then given deodorant and asked to go to the men's room to put it on. His privacy was respected and he was trusted to complete the job by himself.

Health Maintenance

Nutrition

Many factors present obstacles to proper nutrition, such as poor oral-motor skills, oral defensiveness, emotional problems, limited access to nutritious foods (which is common in some institutions and certain low-income families), limited knowledge of nutrition, food allergies, gastrointestinal problems, and limited food preferences. Although many children may simply be classified as being "picky eaters," the following techniques may help increase children's desire to eat:

1. Provide a clean, attractive eating environment with tableware and utensils children like. For example, serve milk in a special cup with a straw or peas in a child's favorite sports bowl. Even some adolescents appreciate these personal touches.
2. Children with sensory defensiveness may need to eat in a quiet place or before or after other children have eaten so that they can concentrate on eating rather than on competing environmental sensations. Plastic plates and bowls make less noise when utensils knock against them than metal and ceramic dishes.

3. Communication board placemats are helpful and easy to make out of stiff paper or cardboard covered with clear contact paper. Placemats can include pictures of a plate and utensils in the proper position or may list educational or meal time rules and reminders. They could include communication symbols or key words from the child's regular communication book or board, which may be too large to place beside the food. Children who do not speak can use the placemats to request things such as juice or milk by pointing to their pictures on the mat or to engage in social interactions. If the placemat has shapes, letters, mazes, or appealing pictures, the occupational therapy practitioner can use it to distract and soothe an anxious child.
4. A calm, accepting, positive social atmosphere is essential for stimulating children to eat. Children will be unable to eat properly if they are not relaxed and content. If possible, allow children to see adults enjoying food and hear them talking about it.[34]
5. Give children extra time to eat. Although children with cerebral palsy or other motor problems may be difficult to feed, patience and nurturing are key aspects of the process.
6. Making foods more interesting usually helps. Some children like to eat raw vegetables only when they are dipped into dressing. Melted cheese or tasty sauces can make cooked vegetables more enticing. Some children enjoy eating frozen peas or raw vegetables as snacks.
7. Try to pay attention to children's requests for food. If they say they are hungry, take the opportunity to give them nutritious food. If their request for food is ignored or denied too many times, they may become unable to recognize their bodies' own needs. Poor eating habits, such as gorging at every eating opportunity, can result.
8. Children with poor discrimination and interpretation of touch-pressure feedback in the mouth or stomach may not sense when their mouths or stomachs are full. Children who frequently use food to calm themselves also need assistance so that they do not overeat and with choosing different mouth-related activities to satisfy their oral needs.

In their attempts to be the best possible caregivers, some parents become overly concerned with feeding their child. They may believe that their picky child is not receiving proper nutrition. In some cases, making a list of all the foods the child eats reveals that the child is eating a balanced diet and reassures parents.[22] In other situations, caregivers use food to manage their child's behavior, but this technique can result in overfeeding. Childhood obesity coupled with inactivity can result in joint problems and lead to an impaired social life. In these cases,

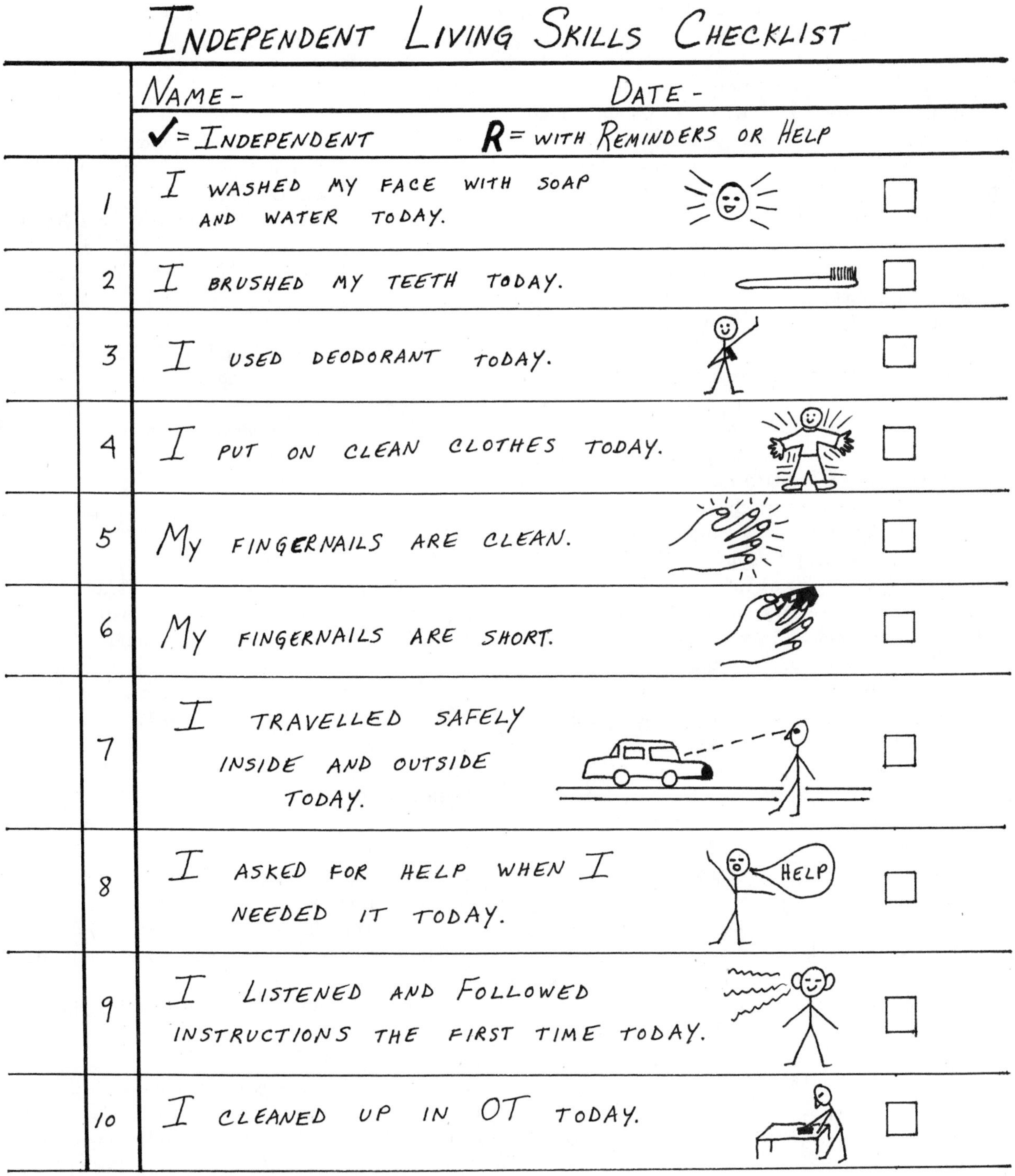

INDEPENDENT LIVING SKILLS CHECKLIST

NAME -   DATE -

✓ = INDEPENDENT   **R** = WITH REMINDERS OR HELP

1	I WASHED MY FACE WITH SOAP AND WATER TODAY.		☐
2	I BRUSHED MY TEETH TODAY.		☐
3	I USED DEODORANT TODAY.		☐
4	I PUT ON CLEAN CLOTHES TODAY.		☐
5	MY FINGERNAILS ARE CLEAN.		☐
6	MY FINGERNAILS ARE SHORT.		☐
7	I TRAVELLED SAFELY INSIDE AND OUTSIDE TODAY.		☐
8	I ASKED FOR HELP WHEN I NEEDED IT TODAY.		☐
9	I LISTENED AND FOLLOWED INSTRUCTIONS THE FIRST TIME TODAY.		☐
10	I CLEANED UP IN OT TODAY.		☐

FIGURE 13-25   Greg's and Earl's independent living skills checklist.

family workers and other team members, including the COTA, help caregivers learn to use alternative behavior management techniques.

Occupational therapy practitioners frequently use resistive oral-motor treats to provide deep pressure sensations inside the mouth. The treats can be calming and nutritious. Small resistive oral-motor treats are best used at the beginning of a treatment session to help the child focus on a challenging task or to calm a child in transition between activities, rooms, or buildings. A few examples of resistive oral-motor treats are popcorn without butter, pretzels, carrot sticks dipped in low-fat salad dressing, dried fruit, and water or juice in a cup with a straw. Avoid snacks with food coloring and food additives because they may cause unusual behavioral reactions.

Food rewards are sometimes given after task performance and are called *primary reinforcers*. Use primary reinforcers when more interactive motivational strategies have been exhausted. Food rewards that are given often to a child may interfere with the child's ability to recognize the sensation of hunger and can decrease the child's interest in participating in the task. Before giving a child a food or drink, carefully consider whether a small food item is needed to reward the child or the child is truly hungry or thirsty. "Choice time" or "free time" incorporating the use of therapeutic equipment is a reward that promotes creativity, cognitive problem solving, spatial and motor planning, and environmental interactions.

JERRY'S FOOD REINFORCER STORY. *Jerry was an 18-year-old boy in an institution who had normal intelligence but was totally deaf and blind and had severe behavioral problems partly resulting from overuse of primary food reinforcers. Jerry had been taught that he would receive a piece of candy each time he performed a requested activity. Jerry learned to expect the reward, so when he was not given a piece of candy after performing a requested activity, he would go into a rage, becoming destructive and aggressive, throwing furniture, and attacking people. Overuse of primary reinforcers limited his curiosity and exploratory skills and restricted his development. Jerry needed activity rewards that were suited to his normal level of intelligence and would stimulate further exploration of materials and the environment.*

Food allergies

Many children with special needs, such as those with ADHD, learning disabilities, minimal brain dysfunction, or autism, have food allergies, so nutritional programs may be necessary. Behavioral, cognitive, and muscular deficits may indicate a sensitivity to particular foods or foods that contain certain products.[15,16] Examples of foods and certain chemicals to be aware of include the following:

- Synthetic or artificial colors that are listed as "U.S. certified color" or in a numerical form such FD&C yellow No 5 or FD&C red No 40
- Synthetic or artificial flavors that are listed as "flavoring" or "artifical flavoring"; additives and salicylates that are found in the child's daily diet
- Antioxidant preservatives that are listed as "BHT, BHA" and "TBHQ."
- Natural salicylates found in apples, all berries, cucumbers, tomatoes, raisins, oranges, plums and peaches
- Aspirin and medications that contain aspirin
- Milk and lactose products
- Wheat and gluten products
- Nuts

When certain foods and synthetic chemicals are eliminated from the diet of food-sensitive children, dramatic improvements may be seen in children with various diagnoses.[15,16] The COTA may discuss food-related concerns with the OTR and other staff involved with children. With proper consent from administration and the OTR, the COTA may explore the possibility of food sensitivities with parents.

Physical fitness

COTAs are often involved in helping children with disabilities choose and learn activities that increase endurance, strength, and flexibility. Examples of fun and realistic activities include swimming, playing in a park, roller skating or riding a bike with assistance, dancing or stretching to music, playing catch, horseback riding, or modified sports activities.

To maintain cardiovascular fitness, a child should engage in a physical activity 3 times a week for at least 20 minutes. In a school, hospital, or clinic setting the COTA could lead a movement group for children with special needs. Numerous books and cassette tapes contain practical and fun physical activities for children with disabilities (see Chapter 13 Appendix C). Yoga, which promotes flexibility and postural and respiratory control, can also be adapted for children with special needs.[50]

Too few after-school and physical fitness programs exist for children with disabilities, regardless of whether the school is in a rural or urban setting. COTAs can contribute significantly by developing and managing fitness programs for children with special needs. Many community sports or after-school programs now enroll children who have mild or moderate disabilities. Some parents are able to hire an adolescent or young adult to assist the child during class. Although children may express interest in karate or lifting weights, carefully consider all factors before enrolling them in a class. Adolescents who have mild or moderate mental retardation, head injuries, or emotional impairments might not have the judgment to use these skills safely. For example they may try to protect a person who is being mugged and be seriously hurt, or they may use the skills to hurt someone else.

Hippotherapy

In hippotherapy, an occupational therapy practitioner, physical therapist, or speech therapist trained in hippotherapy uses a horse's movement to promote therapeutic goals.[28] Children are placed on a horse's back in a variety of positions that facilitate postural control, speech, breathing, and other functional skills. An aid walks on one side of the horse with the therapist on the other side. The therapist directs a horse trainer to lead the horse in different movements.

The wide base of support provided by the horse's back increases the child's balance while sitting. The vestibular (that is, movement) input helps coordinate postural and head control with visual focus and hand movements. Feeling the strong rhythm of the horse's gait may help improve a child's unsteady gait. Leg, trunk, and neck strength may be increased for a child with weakness. High muscle tone may be reduced through gentle stretching of hips and legs.

Numerous benefits can result from hippotherapy and therapeutic riding, which teaches horseback riding to children with special needs. Sitting high up on a horse increases the child's sense of well being and self-esteem. Learning to care for and guide a horse can help an adolescent who has behavioral problems. Even a child who is unable to walk may learn to ride a horse. A child who learns to control the reins gains a functional recreational and physical fitness skill that can be used throughout life.

Personal device care

Personal devices include hearing aids, glasses, splints, orthotics, braces, prosthetic limbs, artificial eyes, and aids to mobility. An OTR, a nurse, a hearing specialist, a physical therapist, or another professional initially gives the COTA all pertinent information about the device and trains the COTA in why, when, where, and how the device is used.

After learning the way to apply and remove the device, the COTA may have responsibility for teaching the child to apply and remove it, as well as for routinely reinforcing the child's performance. In some cases, such as one involving a child who uses a hand splint, the COTA may be in charge of instructing the parents, teachers, or other involved persons. Drawing pictures or writing down the

(1) sequence of putting on the device, (2) device's proper fit, (3) frequency and duration of the device's use, and (4) precautions to take with the device can all be helpful.

The COTA's role may include instructing the child in the following: cleaning personal devices (especially glasses), storing devices when they are not in use; replacing parts, or scheduling a doctor's appointment for a new device. Once trained, the COTA may also instruct caregivers or other staff about these issues. Hearing aids need periodic adjustment and battery replacement. A speech therapist or audiologist can instruct a COTA in adjusting the level of the hearing aid and recognizing when batteries should be replaced.

Depending on the level of expertise, the COTA may create splints for a child with a doctor's prescription and OTR supervision. The COTA may design a variety of accessories for personal devices, making them more attractive to the child. For example, the COTA can help a child create a beaded necklace that is used to hold glasses or to carry a hearing aid and battery case. Some devices can be personalized by letting a child add stickers or drawings. The COTA can be instrumental in identifying problems associated with the personal devices; for example, observation of the child's appearance and behavior may reveal skin irritation or asymmetrical placement of the device. The COTA may ask the parent or family worker whether the item can be refitted.

The COTA often develops creative solutions to the numerous problems that arise regarding personal devices. For example, many children resist wearing their devices. Analyzing the problem and reading the child in context are important tools for resolving these issues. Some children lose or break their glasses, hearing aids, or other personal devices repeatedly so that they do not have to wear them. The COTA can request a team meeting to explore causes of and solve personal device problems. The team may recommend reducing the amount of time the device is worn. For example, a child who wears glasses may only have to wear them at school or while doing homework; a child born with anophthalmia (no eyeballs) may only have to wear the prosthetic eyeballs during the day and not at night.

Some children need extra instruction and experience in applying, removing, cleaning, storing, and maintaining the device. Feeling more adept at handling and taking care of the device may reduce their discomfort and subsequently increase use. COTAs should use an accepting attitude when dealing with children who are wearing devices and reinforce the children's pride in wearing and caring for them.

WEARING GLASSES STORY. *After gently questioning an adolescent, an occupational therapy practitioner discovered the boy did not bring his glasses to school because he did not have a glasses case. This was remedied by asking a staff member to donate an old glasses case. Another child refused to wear his glasses because he did not like the way they looked or felt; fortunately, he also needed a new prescription. His parents were able to afford a new pair of glasses that fit him better. All the staff members complimented him on his new glasses, which seemed to help his self-esteem. Combined with the improved fit and prescription, the praise increased his tolerance for wearing glasses.*

Medication routine

Caregivers, nurses, teachers, or other team members collaborate to give children their medication according to a prescribed schedule. Through team meetings and chart reviews, COTAs learn the type and purpose of medications prescribed. If asked to do so, COTAs take children to the nurse to receive scheduled medication.

Unusual sleepiness, silliness, inattention, crying, complaints of stomachaches or headache, tics (that is, repetitive involuntary movements), and other atypical behaviors may be related to increases, decreases, or changes in medication. The COTA reports significant behavioral changes to the child's OTR as well as the child's doctor, nurse, team, and caregivers. This type of information can be invaluable to doctors, who may use team members' anecdotal observations to recommend changes in medication.

Socialization

Socialization involves a wide range of interactions with other people. Individuals meet their emotional and physical needs by finding opportunities to engage with others in different environmental and cultural contexts.[1] Functional skills in the psychosocial performance components of role performance, social conduct, interpersonal skills, and self-expression provide the building blocks of socialization (see Chapter 6).

Role performance

Examples of early socialization include an infant responding to parents and family members with a social smile or babbling to elicit a response. Later in life, a child may begin peer interactions by imitating other children. In school, children are taught to interact in different ways than they are at home.

The child's social role changes in different contexts and as the child grows. In school the child interacts by watching and listening to the teacher, asking and responding to questions, and following directions. The social role in school is more structured than in the family or during play with peers. Social roles are generally more flexible with peers. The child may be a leader one mo-

ment and a follower the next. Verbal interactions are less formal with peers than they are at school. The COTA can be instrumental in helping a child learn the social roles for different settings.

Social conduct

Basic interactions facilitate socialization in any context. Basic social interactions include using polite greetings, responding when spoken to, and saying, "good-bye," "thank you," or "excuse me" when necessary. Caregivers and team members should model polite interactions and provide opportunities for the child to use them in different contexts.

Many polite phrases needed for proper social conduct can be learned through the rote method of learning. **Rote learning** refers to the acquisition of routine behaviors that may not be completely understood or performed with sincerity by the individual using them. Rote learning usually occurs through memorization or repetition. While all involved adults try to convey the meaning and importance of phrases needed for proper social conduct, it is thought to be more critical that the child use them regularly. If social phrases are used correctly, the child may be treated more kindly. If social phrases are not used, the child may be considered rude. Whether they are used in a rote manner or with true understanding, basic social conduct interactions ease the child's ability to move in and out of different social contexts.

Interpersonal skills and self-expression

More complex socialization requires the child to continuously adapt to varying situations and modify behavioral responses. Unlike basic social conduct, which may be learned and practiced in a rote manner, interpersonal skills and self-expression require flexibility and quick interpretation of changing conditions. These more complex behaviors involve smooth reciprocal exchanges such as conversations, resolving disagreements, expressing anger in acceptable ways, making and keeping friends, and dating.

Products, programs, and games that promote development of underlying psychosocial skill components are available in catalogs, bookstores, and toy stores (see Chapter 13 Appendix C). A.P. Goldstein, has developed a social skills curriculum called "Skillstreaming" for both elementary school and adolescent children.[23,37,38]

Depending on the child's goals as determined by the OTR, parents, or other team members, COTA's can play an important part in aiding socialization. Role playing specific problem areas is a fun and useful strategy. Making and reviewing videotapes with children also enhances learning.

Wheelchair and eye contact survey

A common mistake made by well meaning adults is failing to speak to children at eye level. In a survey of five group homes for children in wheelchairs, only 3 of 12 children observed were spoken to at eye level.[31] For children in wheelchairs and small children, interactions at eye level help them feel respected and safe. In contrast, interactions above eye level can cause children to feel controlled, intimidated, and unimportant.

In the same survey, different types of social interactions were observed. The majority comprised two types of interactions: (1) staff giving physical assistance or verbal instructions to children and (2) children conveying needs to staff through speech, gestures, or facial expressions. Study of the children's interactions with each other revealed a pronounced deficiency in peer interactions.

Promoting peer interactions

Numerous children with special needs have problems with daily social or peer interactions in which typical children spontaneously engage. These include planning, creating, and carrying out play sequences, problem solving and negotiating, and sincerely listening to each other. The poor peer interactions are not easily understood, but many methods can be used to promote peer interactions across many contexts.

Use of developmental groups may promote peer interactions in any context. Children are paired or grouped according to their social developmental levels. For example, in parallel groups younger, lower-functioning children simply share materials while performing similar activities. Few social interactions may been seen in parallel groups, although practitioners hope that more will evolve. Older, higher-functioning children work together on a project and try to mutually achieve a certain outcome.[40]

As revealed by the previously mentioned wheelchair survey, a predominance of helping and supervisory interactions are seen among staff and dependent children in group homes. This fact can be explained in part by the inherent role of the staff members in group homes. Their jobs require them to supervise and help children. In many cases, no goals are written for enhancement of peer interactions. However, simple solutions may facilitate socialization, such as moving two children so that they can sit side by side or face to face.

Dyadic (that is, two-person) and group treatment sessions provide unique opportunities to work on socialization and peer interactions. The occupational therapy practitioner sets up activities in which the children need to work together. Many opportunities can be provided for children to work things out for themselves. They can be asked to decide who goes first in a relay, what free-time activity to do together, how to set up an obstacle course together, or who should explain the activities. When treating children in a group, review concrete rules about teamwork and helping one another.

Reduce or eliminate competitive interaction when treating children with low self-esteem that is caused by emotional, sensory, learning, or physical limitations. Pairing an older child who has a moderate impairment with a younger child who has a mild impairment can improve self-esteem for both, improving the development of skills, teamwork, and mutual respect.

AN UNUSUAL FRIENDSHIP STORY. *In a school for children with special needs, an unusual peer pairing proved beneficial in occupational therapy. Vaughn was a 12-year-old boy with pervasive developmental disorder, learned helplessness (see description that follows), low muscle tone, sensory defensiveness, limited gross and fine motor skills, and a history of severe, prolonged tantrums brought on by minor events. Because he was dependent and defensive and complained a lot, his classmates often picked on him and refused to play with him. He was paired with Wayne, an 8 year old with Asperger's syndrome, a type of autism associated with very high intelligence. Wayne also had underlying low muscle tone. He often displayed provocative and dangerous behaviors, testing limits frequently. Wayne was often impatient and irritated with his classmates, partly because of his better academic skills but also because of his confusion about social relationships.*

Some suspected that Vaughn and Wayne would fight or become impossible to control. Surprisingly, Wayne admired Vaughn because he was bigger and older. Vaughn seemed happy to have a partner who did not make fun of him. They had a common interest in computer games. The two boys began having meaningful, sincere conversations that included proper use of questioning and listening skills and expansion on themes. A friendship emerged. Although power struggles occurred, they were rare and often resolved without outside help. The boys helped each other when social problems developed.

Learned helplessness

Children with severe handicaps frequently receive attention when they are assisted with accomplishing daily activities. They may learn that one way to obtain more attention is to ask for more help or become needy and dependent. In their attempts to be the best caregivers possible, some adults do everything for their child and do not encourage or expect the child to perform independently. This relationship may produce **learned helplessness.** Even though the caregiver's aim is to help the child as efficiently as possible, the child then cannot independently perform daily living activities.

The occupational therapy practitioner's role is to facilitate children's independence. Part of this role includes helping others understand the importance of encouraging independence. Mastery of any daily living task enhances a child's self-esteem and allows freer movement in various environments.

Functional Communication

Handwriting skills

Handwriting is one of the most challenging occupations for children. Occupational therapy practitioners are commonly asked to help children improve drawing, prehandwriting, and handwriting skills, which are sometimes grouped under the category of *graphomotor skills* and include the skills needed to make any types of drawn or written marks.

Prehandwriting skills

Prehandwriting skills include scribbling, coloring inside shapes, tracing, imitating and copying shapes, as well as learning to hold and control drawing utensils. At about 12 months old or before an infant learns to bang a crayon or marker using a fisted grasp. Soon after this, the infant learns to scribble back and forth using large movements controlled by the shoulder. At this point, scribbling is enjoyed more for its kinesthetic (limb movement) feedback rather than its visual interest.

Imitation skills emerge next, followed by copying skills. Imitation skills are less complex than copying skills. Imitation refers to the fact that the child watches a person demonstrate drawing a pattern and then attempts to do the same. Copying refers to the fact that the child looks only a picture or a predrawn pattern and does not watch a demonstration before attempting to draw the same picture.

After scribbling spontaneously, children learn to control their scribbles by imitating vertical, then horizontal, and then circular scribbles. By about 18 to 24 months of age, most children have learned to imitate drawing a vertical line. This skill is soon followed by imitation of drawing a horizontal line. By about 30 to 36 months of age, most children are able to imitate drawing a closed circle.

The ability to copy shapes develops next. The child usually copies vertical lines first, then horizontal lines, and then neat, closed circles.[19] (Although this is the general sequence for children, some variation may occur.) The occupational therapy practitioner carefully observes and analyzes children's unique abilities to aid their development.

After learning to copy a circle, the child learns to imitate and then copy a cross. Imitating and copying a right-to-left diagonal line usually occurs next, followed by imitating and copying a square.

Imitating and then copying a left-to-right diagonal line often occurs next. Imitating and copying an X, a triangle, and a diamond, which all consist of multiple diag-

onal lines, are the last major prewriting skills to emerge. Some children with special needs require extra help in developing the skill to draw diagonal lines.

The occupational therapy practitioner can use numerous techniques to promote the development of prehandwriting skills. One method that captures the interest of many children with severely limited cognitive skills is using sounds during prewriting activities. For example, for a child who shows no interest in drawing or holding a drawing utensil, the occupational therapy practitioner could begin banging a pen against paper to make dots while saying something like "bing, bing, bing" as she makes three dots. Then the practitioner could draw vertical lines while saying something like "zhoomp, zhoomp, zhoomp." As soon as the child begins to watch the activity, the occupational therapy practitioner should gently place the drawing utensil in the child's hand. The practitioner should use hand-over-hand assistance to help the child draw dots and lines while making the same noises. Many children eventually show less resistance to performing the task or actually become truly interested in prehandwriting activities.

Tracing is another helpful technique to promote prehandwriting skills; use a plastic or cardboard stencil. Use of a stencil increases kinesthetic (limb movement) feedback and reinforces learning a motor plan. The child may also trace over a predrawn shape or dotted lines. Coloring inside a square, triangle, or diamond also helps the child learn how to draw these shapes.

Foundation skills for prehandwriting and handwriting

The COTA should utilize the many resources that deal extensively with prehandwriting and handwriting skills (see References and Suggested Reading). The following skills and activities provide a strong foundation for the development of an efficient pencil grasp and functional prehandwriting and handwriting skills. Note that hand dexterity is essential for most self-care tasks. Most of the skills and activities mentioned in this section help to improve self-care performance as well as prehandwriting and handwriting.

Trunk and neck control

The principles used for proper handling and positioning are based on the premise that stability is necessary for mobility.[6] A stable base of support in the hips and lower extremities is necessary to position and move the trunk correctly. Strong trunk and neck muscles allow the child to sustain an upright posture and hold up the head and shoulders against gravity. A comfortable upright posture frees the arms for reaching activities and the hands for other tasks.

A child with low muscle tone, weakness, or poor sensory discrimination skills often benefits from strengthening the large muscles of the trunk and neck. A balance between extensor (straightening) and flexor (bending) strength provides a foundation for trunk and neck control. The prone (face-down) extension and supine (face-up) flexion positions are two postures that are commonly used to increase trunk and neck strength.

PRONE EXTENSION. In a prone extension posture the child supports the body on the abdomen (stomach) in a prone position. The back, hips, neck, head, and arms are lifted against gravity, strengthening all the muscles used.

Numerous activities can be used to strengthen extensor muscles. The child may be positioned in a prone position on a scooter board, a swing, a spinning board, or the floor (Figure 13-26). While in a prone extension posture on a scooter board, the child may go down ramps, push off walls, or negotiate obstacle courses.

Coloring, looking at books, or playing board games can be performed in partial prone extension positions while lying on a mat, a rug, or pillows. The child may be asked to shift weight or rotate the trunk to reach for, place, or toss objects from this position. A small pillow or wedge placed under the chest can help children with cerebral palsy, weakness, or other physical disabilities perform the task. Some children tolerate prone positioning for only a few minutes. The occupational therapy practitioner watches for signs of discomfort or fatigue and modifies activities accordingly.

SUPINE FLEXION. Supine flexion involves lying on the back in a supine position. The whole body is then flexed upward against gravity (Figure 13-27). Supine flexion activities strengthen flexor muscles of the abdomen, neck, hips, and arms. Children with developmental disabilities often have weakness in these muscles.

Modified supine flexion activities also strengthen flexor muscles. These activities can be performed while children lie on a wedge, in a bean bag chair, or even while leaning back in a sitting position. From supine and modified supine positions, children can reach high with their hands for objects such as balls, balloons, bean bags, or items suspended above them. They can kick, touch, or lift objects with their feet. Older children and adolescents can perform abdominal crunches and other stomach exercises to work the flexor muscles against gravity.

A fun activity that promotes flexor strength involves a flexion swing. Children wrap their arms and legs around a rope while sitting on a small disk or other seat. Flexion swings require significant strength; however, they eliminate the demand of having to work against gravity from a full supine position.

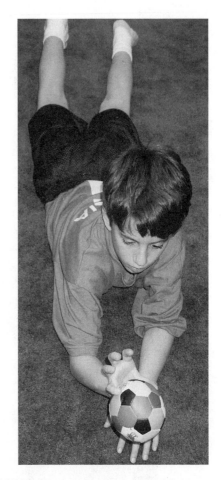

FIGURE 13-26   Prone extension activities develop control of extensor (straightening) muscles against gravity.

TRUNK ROTATION. Trunk rotation requires use of trunk extensor and flexor muscles. Smooth trunk rotation sometimes affects the development of hand preference (see Bimanual Coordination section in this chapter). Trunk rotation activities often involve reaching at arm's length across midline. Watch for signs that the child is compensating, such as the child turning the whole body as a unit instead of rotating the trunk. To facilitate trunk rotation, practitioners can try to stabilize the child's hips with their hands before the child reaches for an item. Promoting trunk rotation may be easier while the child side sits on the floor or straddles a barrel or rocking-riding toy.

Shoulder and arm stability

Another foundation skill for prehandwriting and handwriting is shoulder and arm stability. The stability adds to the trunk's base of support, which is needed for hand mobility. Common problems in children with special needs are shoulder instability (looseness), fixing the shoulders (holding the shoulders tightly) in an elevated posi-

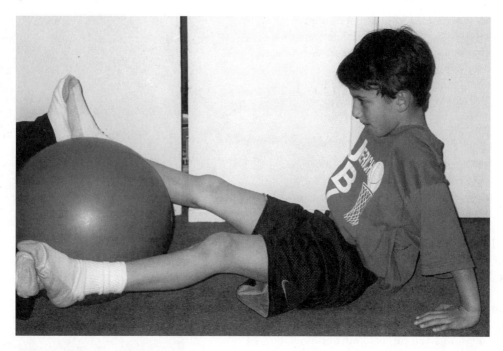

FIGURE 13-27 Modified supine flexion activities develop control of flexor (bending) muscles against gravity.

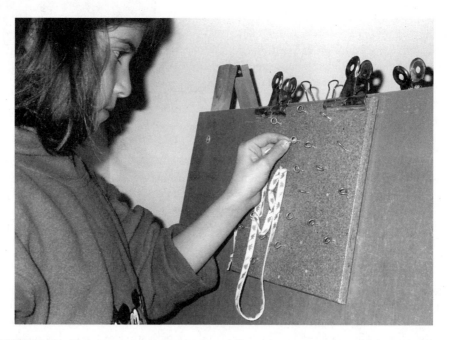

FIGURE 13-28 To increase shoulder and wrist stability and promote wrist extension, girl laces eye screws on board attached to inclined surface.

tion, and shoulder tightness caused by high muscle tone. Children may fix the shoulders tightly in one position to help hold up the entire body. Shoulder fixing restricts reaching and limits arm positioning for handwriting.[6]

Glenohumeral tightness (that is, tightness between the glenoid area of the shoulder blade and the humerus of the upper arm) occurs when the upper arm cannot move without pulling the shoulder blade completely out of place. It occurs with shoulder tightness, whether caused by fixing or high muscle tone. The occupational therapy practitioner should search for signs of glenohumeral tightness by palpating (feeling) and watching the shoulder

BOX 13-6

Reducing Fixing and Tightness While Increasing Stability in the Arms and Shoulders

STRATEGY ONE: WORKING ON AN INCLINED OR VERTICAL SURFACE

Have the child try some of the following activities:

- Use a Lite Brite or other angled toys.
- Attach push pins to a cork board on a wall. Loop colorful rubber bands around the push pins to make patterns.
- Paint or draw on paper attached to an angled board or wall.
- Use an easel to position activities, such as putting magnets or pegs on boards. Place a lacing board with eye screws on an easel (see Figure 13-28).
- Apply firm downward pressure to the child's shoulders using a gentle shaking motion to help separate shoulder and upper arm movements.
- Insert pennies into a bank that has a vertical opening.

If an activity is too challenging, lower the height at which the activity is being performed, reduce the strength required for the activity, reduce the duration of the activity, or use larger objects in the activity.

STRATEGY TWO: WEIGHTBEARING ON THE HANDS

Have the child try some of the following activities:

- Creep on hands and knees; go through barrels, tunnels, and hideouts.
- Push toy cars or hold small objects in the hands while creeping.
- Reach from a hands and knees (quadruped) position.
- From a sitting position, push up with both hands to lift the entire body.
- Wheelbarrow walk (that is, walk on the hands while another child or the occupational therapy practitioner holds the legs).
- Crab walk (that is, from a sitting position, place hands on floor behind body, lift body off the floor, and walk using hands and feet).
- Perform pushups and modified pushups on an incline. For modified pushups, lean hands on a wall, ledge, or table edge and then perform a pushup.
- Stand and place hands on a table or desk; try to lift the body off the floor.

blade as the child raises the arm all the way overhead. The child raises the arm overhead twice, first flexing the shoulder (lifting the arm forward) and then abducting the shoulder (lifting the arm out to the side with the palm up). The shoulder blade may pull out tightly toward the raised arm. The skin and connective tissue between the upper arm and shoulder blade may stick out and feel taut like a rope. Various techniques can help reduce fixing and tightness in the shoulders and increase shoulder and arm stability (Figure 13-28 and Box 13-6).

Bimanual coordination

Both hands must be used smoothly together for handwriting. Children use one hand to write and the other hand to position and stabilize paper. Although hand preference is often well established by 3 years of age, it may not develop until 5 or 6 years of age. The following story shows the way that failure to develop hand preference can interfere with the development of handwriting skills.

TAMARA'S HAND PREFERENCE STORY. *Tamara was a 7-year-old girl with sensory defensiveness, learning disabilities, ADHD, oculomotor (eye control) problems, impulsivity, extreme distractibility, and motor planning problems. She avoided trunk rotation and reaching across midline and constantly switched the hand she used for writing. When given any writing or drawing task, she usually started on the left with the left hand and switched hands at midline to finish on the right with the right hand. Her handwriting skills seemed to be fairly equal in both hands.*

Tamara's failure to establish a hand preference began to interfere with development of handwriting skills. She became confused during any printing or number-writing tasks. She had no consistent way of forming letters or numbers. To help Tamara's hand preference emerge naturally, the OTR emphasized trunk rotation and reaching across midline during treatment. For several days, Tamara's teacher systematically counted the number of times Tamara picked up an object with each hand. The teacher found that Tamara used her right hand for about 65% to 75% of the tasks.

The teacher and OTR used their problem-solving skills to develop a plan of intervention for handwriting. Tamara needed to choose a hand preference on her own. When she picked up a pencil, chalk, or marker with one hand, she was asked to at least complete the line she was writing with the same hand. Soon she was asked to complete the whole page using the same hand. Within several months, she was consistently using her right hand. After seeing Tamara's quick response to intervention, her teacher and occupational therapy practitioner agreed that her right hand was her naturally preferred hand, and she had been ready to make this choice.

Functional grasp

A functional, mature grasp helps increase legibility and endurance while handwriting. Functional grasp patterns for handwriting include the tripod grasp (which involves the thumb, index, and middle finger), quadripod grasp (which involves four fingers), and a modified tripod grasp (in which the pencil rests between the index and middle fingers, with the thumb opposing the pencil). (See Chapter 4 for discussion of mature grasp patterns.) Following are the necessary components of a functional grasp.

FOREARM SUPINATION. In an efficient pencil grasp the forearm is neither palm down nor palm up. Partial supination (that is, a partial palm-up position) is required. Some children tend to pronate their forearms (that is, turn their arms palm down) excessively. They can benefit from activities that promote forearm supination.

Examples of activities that promote forearm supination include using oversized nuts and bolts, playing imitation games such as slapping hands on the legs palm up and palm down in rhythmic patterns, flipping cards over, and using a toy screwdriver. Reaching for objects that are presented in a vertical position requires partial forearm supination (Figure 13-29).

WRIST STABILITY. An efficient pencil grasp requires stability and 30 degrees of wrist extension.[4] Many children compensate for poor stability by flexing the wrist (bending it down). Extending the wrist to 30 degrees promotes positioning of the thumb in opposition to the index, which is the position used in a functional pencil grasp. The activities described in Box 13-6 may be used to help extend the wrist and increase stability.

ARCH DEVELOPMENT. Strong arches in the palm of the hand help facilitate skilled finger movements in prehandwriting and handwriting tasks.[4] The hand has transverse (side-to-side), longitudinal (fingertip-to-wrist), and oblique (diagonal) arches. Muscles at the base of the thumb and little finger need to be strong enough to cup the palm into a hollow at the center. Proper arch development enables the fingers to wrap around objects of varying sizes and helps the fingers gauge strength needed for grasping.

Activities promoting proper arch development include manipulating pegs of varying sizes, cupping round objects in the palm, and using cupped hands to shake dice or scoop up beans, rice, marbles, paper clips, or other small objects,

The oblique, or diagonal, arch is developed using opposition of the thumb to any finger (often the little finger). Pulling tiny objects with the thumb and little finger, like a coffee stirrer, increases the oblique arch. Using tools such as a plastic knife, screwdriver, or pizza cutter also require use of the oblique arch.

RADIAL-ULNAR DISSOCIATION. A mature grasp does not emerge unless the child has developed independent control of the thumb (that is, radial) side and little finger (that is, ulnar) side of the writing hand. In other words the child learns to control the muscles of the two sides of the hands separately; occupational therapy practitioners call this process **radial-ulnar dissociation.** This process can be described more simply to parents, administrators, and other staff members as "separation of skill and stability sides of the hand."

Stability on the ulnar side of the hand supports the skilled movements on the radial side of the hand. Ulnar stability allows the child to rest the side of the hand on the writing surface and curl the ring and little finger into the palm. Insufficient separation of two sides of the hand results in an immature fisted grasp or an abnormal grasp in which the fingers are hooked around a pencil (Figure 13-30). Activities that promote separation of the skill side and stability side of the hands include the following:

1. Using tools, such as hairbrushes, toothbrushes, play hammers, drum sticks, or play screwdrivers
2. Pulling ropes; tubing; hoops; and round, thick objects to strengthen the ulnar (stability) side of the hand;
3. Using scissors while trapping a small sponge in the palm with the ring and little fingers
4. Operating any squeeze or pump spray bottle or squirt gun (for example, using a spray bottle to help clean the school blackboard or desk)
5. Holding a small object in the palm (such as a cotton ball, triangular cosmetic sponge, or tiny rubber spiny ball) while performing any activity with hands (such as creeping on hands and knees, placing pegs in a pegboard, stringing beads, or completing a puzzle while keeping a cotton ball in the palm)

OPEN WEB SPACE. An open **web space** (the loose skin between index finger and thumb) in a pencil grasp al-

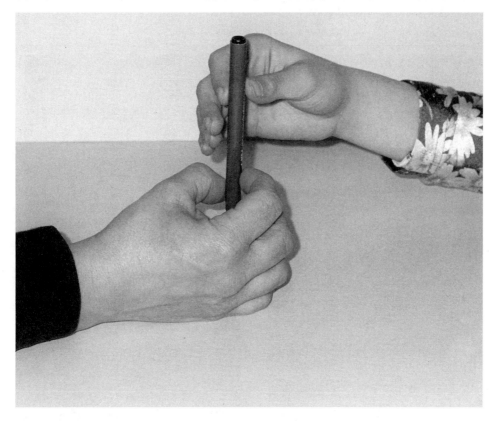

FIGURE 13-29 Reaching for items presented vertically promotes partial forearm supination.

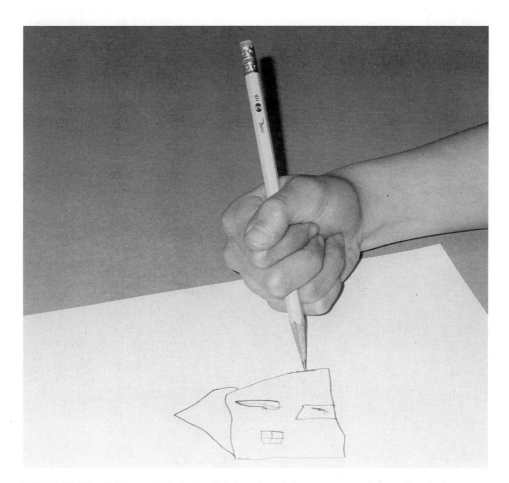

FIGURE 13-30 Children with limited radial-ulnar dissociation may use an abnormal hooked grasp.

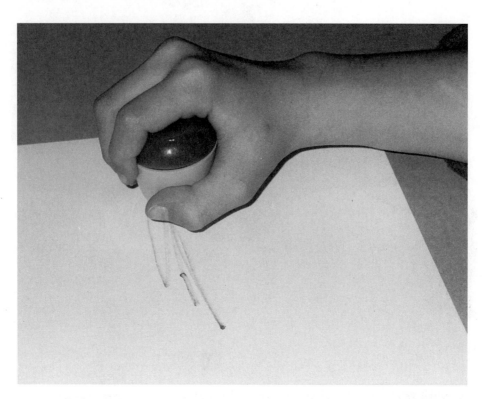

FIGURE 13-31 Palm-size markers help children maintain an open web space.

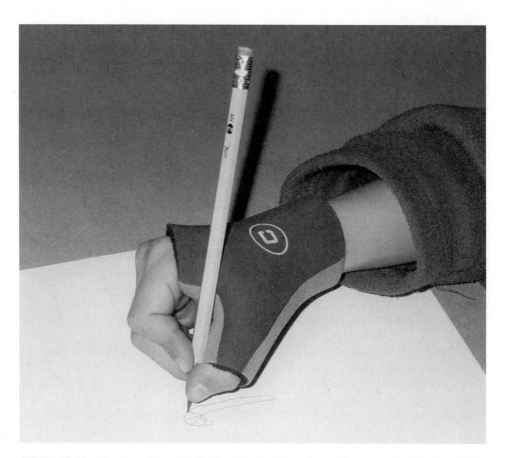

FIGURE 13-32 Fingerless gloves (Benik; Silverdale, Washington) provide support for thumb and help children maintain an open web space.

lows nerves to send accurate sensory-motor information between the tips of thumb, index finger, and middle fingers, and the brain.[4] Children with weakness, low muscle tone, or limited sensory discrimination often have cramped web spaces. They may hold the pencil tightly in an attempt to increase motor control or sensory feedback or both. Helping a child develop an open web space can be a challenging task. Activities that help a child maintain an open web space include the following:

1. Weightbearing on an open hand
2. Gripping or holding wide, hand-sized objects such as a cup, large block, or foam football
3. Using large, palm-sized markers (Figure 13-31)
4. Performing myofascial release (techniques to release the overlaying fascia from muscle), passive range of motion (PROM) exercises, and other inhibitory (that is, calming and loosening) techniques (that are learned directly from trained professionals or at workshops) immediately before handwriting activities (see Chapter 13 Appendix D)
5. Using special fingerless gloves or soft thumb splints to open the web space and allow the child to concentrate on other areas of handwriting; for example, using gloves distributed by Benik (Figure 13-32) that are made of Neoprene and contain a seam on both sides of the thumb (can be worn by some children for only 5-minute intervals during their most challenging writing tasks before causing irritation but can be comfortably worn by other children)

THUMB OPPOSITION. In an efficient pencil grasp the thumb rotates toward the little finger resulting in the tip of the thumb moving opposite the tip index finger. A common problem interfering with an efficient pencil grasp is the use of excessive thumb lateralization (that is, pressing the thumb against the side of the index finger) (Figure 13-33). This grasp is fatiguing and can cause pain in the thumb and index finger; it also prevents accurate sensory feedback from the thumb pad, which is needed to gauge force and direction of pressure. An inefficient lateralized pencil grasp often develops when stability in the wrist, hand, and thumb are inadequate, as in children with low muscle tone or weakness.

Activities that promote thumb opposition include the following:

1. Using a toy requiring the thumb to push a button opposite the index and middle fingers, such as a spinning sparkling wheel or small three-point grabber (such as the one typically used to grasp pickles or olives) (Figure 13-34)

2. Retrieving objects such as pennies, pegs, or Cheerios from a small opening (that is, approximately 1 to 2 inches wide) to prevent the use of a less mature lateral grasp[3]
3. Pulling tiny objects out of putty or clay
4. Using a tiny (that is, approximately ½-inch) piece of chalk to write on a blackboard
5. Manipulating tiny objects, such as stringing ⅜-inch beads or making a collage with beans
6. Painting with half of a Q-tip

IN-HAND MANIPULATION. In-hand manipulation consists of actions performed entirely by and within one hand. In-hand manipulation increases efficiency in handwriting. Numerous minute pencil adjustments are achieved using in-hand manipulation skills: translation, shift, and rotation. Translation and shift are required to position a pencil properly. Translation actions involve moving an item between the fingers and the palm. Shift involves alternating finger and thumb movements on an object; it is often used to adjust or refine a grasp on an object.[13] When picking up a pencil, the typical child moves it from the fingertips to the palm (which is translation) and then quickly slides it into the correct position with the alternating thumb, index, and middle finger movements (which is shift). Poor translation or shifting skills cause the child to use the opposite hand to position the pencil or fail to position the pencil altogether. The following activities are helpful in developing and improving translation and shift:

1. To improve translation skills, children use one hand to pick up about 10 small objects one at a time, holding all of them in the palm. To help children with this task, suggest that they use the ring and little fingers to hold the objects in place. When the hand is full, the children then try to insert the objects one by one into a slot without dropping any or helping with the other hand.
2. To improve shifting skills, use the "finger-thumb race." Children hold a pencil in a tripod grasp near the eraser end. They then alternate moving the thumb and fingers forward on the pencil as fast as they can until they reach the point end. Then the occupational therapy practitioner asks which finger won the race. (This is a modified version of Benbow's Inchworm activity.[4])

Rotating actions are often used to turn a pencil in two ways: (1) rotating the pencil from end to end to erase efficiently—children who lack rotation skills use the opposite hand to turn the pencil to the eraser end; and (2) twisting the pencil slightly to reposition it toward the sharpest side of the point—children with limited rotation

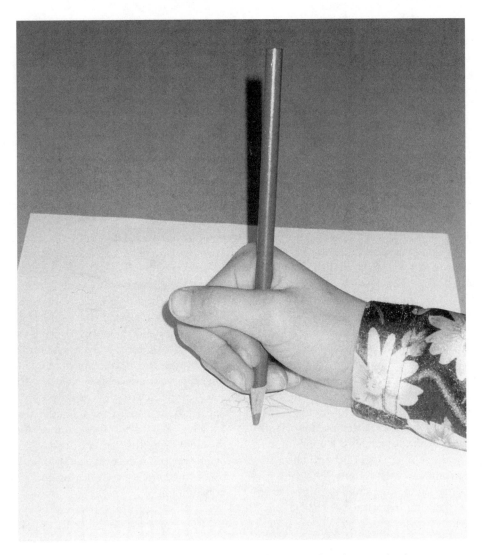

FIGURE 13-33   Inefficient pencil grasp with lateralized thumb and cramped web space.

skills usually fail to make tiny positioning adjustments during writing or drawing tasks. Activities facilitating rotation are performed with many materials, including coins, small balls, knobs, small sponges, clay, small bits of paper, or a dish of water. Objects are rotated clockwise and counterclockwise.[4]

DELICATE TOUCH.   A delicate touch is also necessary for efficient handwriting.[4] A delicate touch requires that the web space of the hand be open and the thumb opposed. Activities that promote use of delicate, controlled touch include the following:

1. Lining up dominoes by standing them on their narrow edge and then knocking them down[4]

2. Playing pick-up sticks[4]
3. Using tweezers to pick up fragile objects, such as marshmallows, pieces of foam, or pieces of cereal without denting them[4]
4. Writing carefully on tissue paper without tearing it

Methods and materials for handwriting

The OTR or teacher usually chooses the handwriting curriculum. Different handwriting approaches work better with certain students. For example, children with severe learning disabilities, mental retardation, or head injuries may find that Handwriting without Tears[45] is the easiest method to follow.

Children with greater language and sequencing capabilities may enjoy Loops and Other Groups for creative

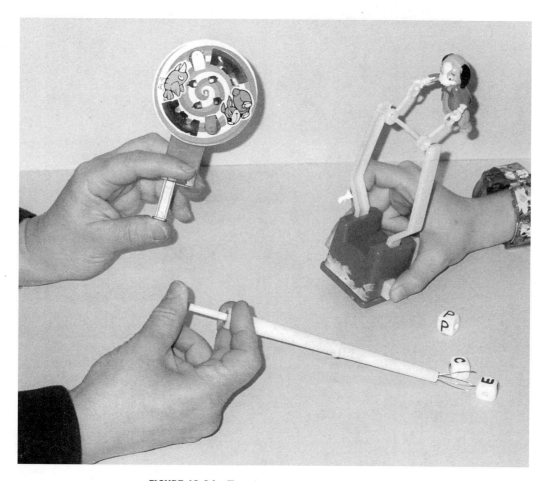

FIGURE 13-34 Toys that promote thumb opposition.

handwriting.[4] Before any prehandwriting or handwriting activity, have the child perform activities requiring hand and finger strength, coordination, and sensory awareness. Strategies that may help children learn to form letters correctly include the following:

1. Using large arm movements to form shapes in the air
2. Using the fingertips to finger-paint or make shapes in chocolate syrup on a plate or pudding on a mirror
3. Using the fingertips to trace sandpaper or textured shapes
4. Tracing stencils of shapes
5. Using sticks to make shapes in sand, gravel, or dirt
6. Using a popsicle stick, tongue depressor, or chop stick to draw shapes in clay (Figure 13-35) (because the resistance created by the clay increases

feedback to muscles and joints, reinforcing learning of the proper motor sequence)

Strategies that may help children write their letters and numbers in neat lines while writing on a piece of paper include the following:

1. Position paper at about a 30-degree angle, with the right corner higher for right-handed children and the left corner higher for left-handed children.
2. Use special paper with red and green lines (available from Therapro and other equipment companies; see Chapter 13 Appendix C) to help children see where to start and stop letters.
3. Highlight the bottom line with markers.
4. Use paper with raised lines to help children who need tactile cues or have limited vision.
5. Turn lined paper on its side to help children line up math problems.

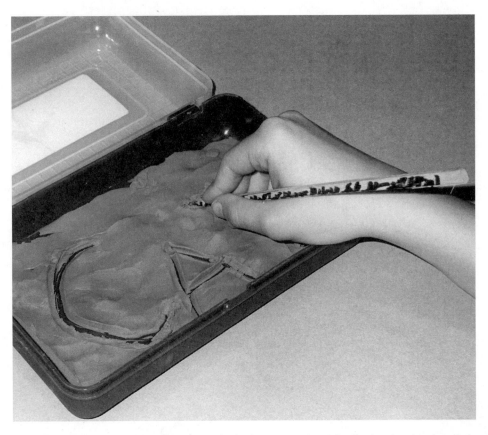

FIGURE 13-35   Using a stick to form letters in clay increases sensory feedback to hand and can help children learn to write.

Two strategies that may help children space letters and words more evenly include the following:

1. Use graph paper; each box can be used for a letter.
2. Place a popsicle stick or finger between each word.

Certain techniques requiring specialized training have been shown to help some children with learning disabilities or spatial problems improve the legibility of their handwriting. Cranial electrical stimulation (that is, 10 to 20 minutes of mild electrical stimulation of specific areas of the head) is one method that has helped some children increase their handwriting control and legibility.[44]

Pencil grips and adaptations

Pencil grips (Figure 13-36, A), and modified pens and pencils (Figure 13-36, B) may promote a more efficient handwriting grasp. Even with grips and modified writing tools, some children still use inefficient grasp patterns. The occupational therapy practitioner can intervene in several ways: (1) position children's fingers correctly on the grip, (2) remind children to their check finger positioning before writing each word, and (3) and ask teach-

ers to periodically correct children's grips. A few examples of pencil grips and adapted holders follow:

1. The Pencil Grip is a wide rubber grip often useful for children with a cramped web space and a tendency to lateralize the thumb (see Chapter 13 Appendix C).
2. The Stetro Grip may be best for children who have tiny fingers (available from OT Ideas and other catalogs; see Chapter 13 Appendix C).
3. The soft triangle grip by North Coast Medical can reduce fatigue and promote a functional grasp pattern for children with weakness or limited endurance for handwriting.
4. A pediatric weighted utensil holder (Figure 13-37) is available from Sammons Preston (see Chapter 13 Appendix C). Children who lack sensory discrimination skills in the hands (and who often also have low muscle tone, weakness, or poor motor planning skills) use the weighted holder. The weight increases proprioceptive (deep-pressure) feedback to the joints and muscles in the hand and wrist, adding to children's awareness of the position and movement of the hand, fingers, and wrist relative to the pencil and paper. This increased awareness often improves control of the motor sequence. The weighted utensil holder also helps children who have

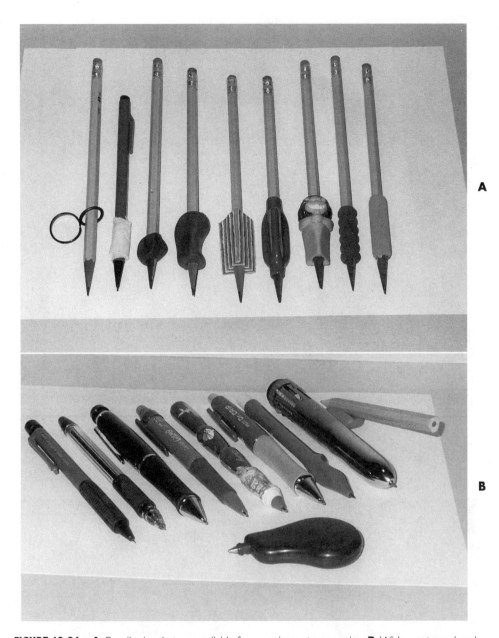

FIGURE 13-36 **A,** Pencil grips that are available from equipment companies. **B,** Wide, contoured, and triangle pens and pencils that are available in stores and from equipment companies.

tremors that interfere with controlled writing by stabilizing the grasp and steadying movements. It is used for 1- to 5-minute periods to prevent fatigue or injury to small finger or wrist joints.

5. Looping two rubber bands together may help children who can oppose their thumb but have trouble resting the pencil in the web space. Attach one band near the eraser and the other around the children's wrist, which pulls the pencil into the web space (Figure 13-38).

Vertical and inclined surfaces

Sitting at a desk to write requires children to hold their back in a vertical plane with their legs, head, and eyes in a horizontal plane. Many children are unable to maintain this complex posture.

Writing on a vertical surface (such as a blackboard or paper taped to a wall) or an inclined surface (such as an easel, inclined table top, or inclined board) allows the trunk, head, and eyes to be in the same plane as the writing surface. The reduced postural demand may allow the child to concentrate more on letter formation and legibility. Working on vertical or inclined surfaces is also beneficial because it facilitates wrist extension and helps the writing utensil fall into the proper position. Gravity literally pulls the utensil down into the web space.

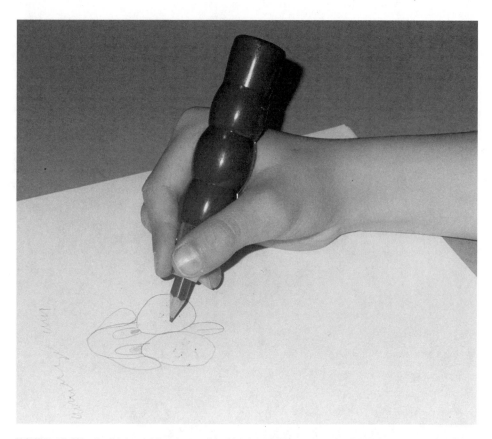

FIGURE 13-37 Pediatric weighted utensil holder increases sensory feedback and can increase fine motor control.

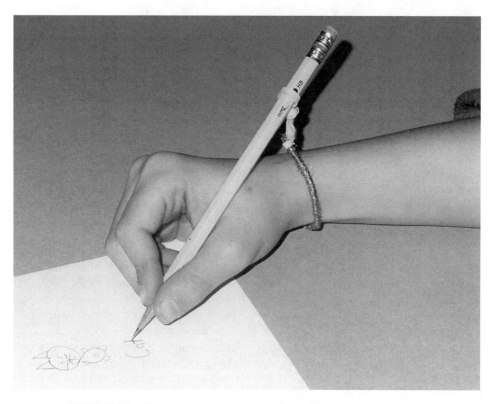

FIGURE 13-38 Elastic bands being used to pull pencil into web space of hand.

Telephone use

It may be the COTA's responsibility to find a suitable adapted phone system or teach children or adolescents the proper social skills for the phone. Phone companies offer adapted phone systems for children and adults who have various limitations. Some phones have extra large push buttons and enlarged print for those with incoordination or visual impairments. Phones can be hooked up to computers for those with hearing impairments. Other phone adaptations are available from equipment companies. Children or adults with limited hand use may benefit from using speaker phones, hands-free phones with headsets, or holders for phone receivers. Children may need instruction in what to say and not to say on the phone. For children who can read, use written scripts that they can use to answer the phone, start a conversation on the phone, or make an inquiry over the phone. Children can practice their phone conversations using disconnected phones. Children should be taught not to give personal information to strangers, tell strangers who is home, or tell strangers when the family will be on vacation.

Computers

Computers are now used in almost all schools as instructional tools as well as for recreation. Children who have significant problems with handwriting may find a computer or word processor to be the pathway to success in school. Learning the keyboard seems to be the biggest obstacle to efficiently writing with a computer. Numerous keyboard options are available, such as alphabetical keyboards, one-handed keyboards, and pointer (one-finger) keyboards.[2] Children of all ages can use the many computer programs that teach keyboard techniques (see Chapter 13 Appendix B and Chapter 16).

Communication boards and alternative systems

Children who are unable to speak use communication boards. Beginning communication boards have only two or three pictures or symbols on them. Children who have a large vocabulary may need a communication book that has several pages of words or symbols. Alternative communication systems include sign language and computer-generated speech programs.

A COTA who believes a child might benefit from using a communication board or alternative system should consult the other team members. The speech therapist may already know of a system that fits the child's needs and capabilities. Depending on the setting and the COTA's job responsibilities, the COTA may help identify the proper alternative communication method for a child (see Chapter 16).

Pointing

Pointing is an early fine motor skill as well as an early communication skill. Pointing is used with communication boards and computer keyboards. The occupational therapy practitioner can considerably improve a child's pointing skills.

Caregivers and team members rely on the occupational therapy practitioner to inform them about the child's fine motor capabilities and any obstacles to pointing, such as being unable to isolate the index finger and use it separately from the other fingers. During treatment the occupational therapy practitioner helps the child develop underlying hand skills or adapted techniques. The following strategies may be helpful:

1. To isolate the index finger for pointing, the child uses middle, ring, and little fingers to hold a pencil or the occupational therapy practitioner's finger.
2. To facilitate extensor (straightening) muscles, the occupational therapy practitioner strokes the back of the index finger.
3. To help develop isolated index finger movements, the child handles tiny objects such as pieces of cereal, raisins, or small beads.
4. To develop the radial-ulnar dissociation needed for pointing, see the Handwriting section on Radial-Ulnar Dissociation in this chapter.

If the child is completely unable to point with a finger, and the OTR determines that an alternate method should be used, consider having the child use the following strategies:

1. Use the fist.
2. Use a universal art holder that has a pointer.
3. Use a pediatric weighted utensil holder that has a pointer.
4. Use a universal cuff that has a pointer.
5. Use a head pointer.
6. Attach a pointer to another part of the body that has more precise control.
7. For children with severe incoordination or spasticity (that is, muscle tightness), the eyes can be used to focus on widely spaced pictures. (See the discussion of eye control in the Oculomotor Skills section of this chapter.)

Sign or reduced language

Although occupational therapy practitioners do not usually teach sign language, they may need to use it on a regular basis depending on their clients and the therapeutic setting. Sign language may be used with a child who has hearing impairment or does not speak. Depending on the approach of the parents and team members, the child may be taught to use speech or a communication board in combination with sign language. Sign language may also be used with a child who has vision impairments and a limited speech capacity. The child learns to interpret signs through touch; the occupational therapy practitioner makes the sign and then cups the child's hand over it. To facilitate this learning process, the occupational therapy practitioner assists the child with developing fine tactile discrimination skills such as stereognosis (that is, the ability to identify objects through touch).

The occupational therapy practitioner may use "reduced language" with a child if the team determines that it could be beneficial. Reduced language is used when a child has some verbal skills but becomes easily confused by rapid or verbose speech. The practitioner omits adjectives, prepositions, and extra phrases. For example, instead of saying, "Excuse me, Timmy. Would you mind putting the spider plant on the windowsill for me? My hands are full," the practitioner would say, "Timmy, take plant window, please." Although this technique can be quite effective, all team members and caregivers must use the same system. Gradually increase the complexity of the language that is used to prepare the child for community interactions, which do not involve reduced language.

Functional Mobility

Safe mobility

The COTA's responsibilities may include teaching safe mobility skills to children who use wheelchairs or are unable to walk. (For information on wheelchairs and other positioning devices, see Chapters 16 and 17.) Children who use manual or electric wheelchairs need to learn the following safe mobility skills: (1) locking and unlocking the wheelchair; (2) starting or stopping for obstacles such as walls or people; (3) going straight; (4) slowing or stopping on request; (5) timing, sequencing, and gauging force and direction of movements; (6) negotiating around corners and furniture; (7) moving through tight spaces such as doorways, bathrooms, and elevators; (8) moving over different surfaces such as ramps and carpets; and (9) refining actions such as opening and closing doors or going over thresholds. For children with manual wheelchairs, gloves may be used to increase friction on the wheels while protecting the hands and are available from several equipment companies (see Chapter 13 Appendix C).

Children who are able to walk may have problems mobilizing safely for several reasons. Limited head or eye control can interfere with environmental awareness. Limited postural control, body awareness, or motor planning can impair children's ability to control their bodies. Children with mobility problems may tend to run instead of walk and may bang into walls or doors, letting obstacles stop them instead of slowing and stopping on their own. They may have trouble estimating distance and knowing where to move. An inability to anticipate potential acci-

dents and time actions accordingly can result in collisions with people or furniture. The following strategies may help children improve safety while mobilizing:

1. To increase environmental awareness, improve eye control as needed.
2. To improve body awareness, move under, between, and through small spaces (such as between two chairs, under heavy pillows, or through tunnels or makeshift tents).
3. To improve body awareness, make a "mat sandwich." Have the child lie down between two mats or cushions. Press down firmly on the mats and child, and pretend to put on sandwich toppings.
4. To improve motor planning, use obstacle courses or relay races in which children must avoid touching certain items.
5. To learn what a normal moving speed is (not too slow and not too fast), move the wheelchair, or march in rhythm to music.
6. To increase awareness of the environment, play a game in which the child moves onto visually located targets such as shapes, letters, or numbers on the floor.
7. To improve attention to visual cues, play a game in which the child stops moving when the occupational therapy practitioner holds up a red sign, moves slowly in response to a yellow sign, and moves quickly in response to a green sign.
8. To increase attention to auditory cues and enhance postural and impulse control, play games in which the child "freezes" in place when music that is playing is turned off. The child may also be told to move very slowly, very quickly, or in a different direction on command.
9. To increase postural control, especially in a child who is able to walk but tends to run or bang into walls or people, have the child carry a weighted object such as a bucket of sand while moving from one room to another.
10. To help the child remember safe mobility skills, review concrete rules for safe mobility before each session. For example, have the child describe the proper speed for walking in the halls or up steps and what to do if a person is in the way.

SAFE HALLWAY TRANSITION STORY. *In a special school for children with pervasive developmental disorder and emotional impairments, classroom transitions (moving from classroom to classroom) were problematic. The children had poor body and environmental awareness, sensory defensiveness, and limited motor planning skills. During transitions from room to room, they swayed, repeatedly bumped into furniture or each other, and then overreacted by pushing or hitting, stumbling, running, or grabbed artwork from walls. They were unable to* coordinate their bodies long enough to follow the frequent, clear, verbal directions from the teachers.

To address the transition problems, the occupational therapy practitioner utilized the theory that deep-pressure (proprioceptive) feedback to the joints and muscles could enhance body awareness and initiate a calming response. The practitioner hypothesized that the children might improve their body control if they carried weighted objects during transitions from one room to another.

The practitioner purchased pumpkin-shaped pails (the ones commonly used for trick-or-treating on Halloween) for each child. A volunteer sewed about 2 lb of rice into terry cloth hand towels to make weights. The weighted towels were placed in the pumpkin pails, and each child carried the pails during room transitions.

The results were amazing. The children stopped swaying and bumping into furniture and each other during room transitions. They stopped grabbing artwork from the walls, walked using a steady pace with little stumbling, and were even able to follow verbal directions.[9]

Travel training in the community

Children with vision impairments are trained to travel by an orientation and mobility teacher. Children who are able to see are taught ways to travel in the community by a travel trainer, occupational therapy practitioner, or special educator trained in this area. Children who use wheelchairs benefit from occupational therapy intervention in travel skills.

Propelling a manual wheelchair down a sidewalk is not a simple task. Sidewalks are generally sloped toward the street for water drainage. To keep the wheelchair going straight, the child must push almost twice as hard on the street side of the chair. Children with electric wheelchairs also need to learn to adjust their steering to accommodate the slope of the sidewalk.

Moving around corners, people, and obstacles in the outdoors is similar to moving indoors; however, more vigilance and caution are required outdoors because of increased variability in terrain, high-speed automobiles, and unpredictable obstacles. Regardless of whether they use a wheelchair, children may encounter problems negotiating cracks or bumps in the sidewalk, gravel, hills, and grassy or rocky surfaces. Children who are able walk are often referred to a physical therapist for help with their gait and negotiating different types of surfaces. Children who have problems with vision, sensory processing, body awareness, coordination, or motor planning have particular difficulty accommodating terrain changes.

Crossing the street

Numerous individuals, including parents and older relatives, occupational therapy practitioners, and other adults involved with children, can teach children to cross the street. Although this is a common activity, even children and adults without disabilities get into accidents while crossing the street. Young children or those with cognitive problems may benefit from learning rules involving little or no problem-solving tasks such as the following:

1. Only cross the street with an adult.
2. Always cross at an intersection.
3. Even when with an adult, look both ways before stepping off the curb.
4. If you see a car coming toward you, wait until it passes, no matter how far away it is.
5. Watch for cars turning into your path from side streets.
6. Talk only about the current traffic situation when crossing a street.
7. Listen to the traffic noises around you; if you hear a siren, look for it.

Children with higher cognitive functioning who are attempting to become independent in the community need to practice crossing the street at different types of intersections—with traffic lights and stop signs and without any traffic signals at all. Children need to learn to estimate the speed of traffic that is far away to assess their ability to cross the street in a safe amount of time.

FEAR OF THE CURB STORY. *Sherry was a 14-year-old girl with incoordination, mental retardation, severe sensory defensiveness, and environmental awareness problems. Her teachers reported she was afraid to step off the curb, and her COTA was asked for help. Sherry's parents reported that as an infant she refused to walk on grass and became frightened when encouraged to walk on different surfaces.*

The COTA first ruled out the possibility that Sherry needed glasses. According to her eye doctor, Sherry did not have any visual acuity (that is, clarity or distinction) problems. To address Sherry's problem with curbs, her COTA started the therapy sessions with techniques to reduce sensory defensiveness. These calming techniques also helped decrease Sherry's anxiety and distractibility. The COTA then worked on indoor and outdoor mobility skills.

In Sherry's school, the COTA assisted Sherry with moving through obstacle courses involving numerous surface changes. To increase her environmental awareness, Sherry played with a ball and performed tasks that involved reaching for targets, especially with her feet. These activities were often combined with vestibular (movement) tasks to help Sherry time and coordinate her actions while moving. Sherry was sent on errands, such as delivering messages to classrooms on different floors, so that she could practice going up and down stairs.

The COTA also took Sherry outside regularly. After using calming techniques, the COTA and Sherry went behind the school to a safe, relatively private curb. The COTA and Sherry practiced stepping up to and down from the curb numerous times. Sherry was unable to look both ways for cars and step off the curb at the same time, so the task was broken down into smaller steps. She learned to (1) stop at the curb, (2) look both ways for cars, (3) look down at the street, (4) step down from the curb, and (5) look both ways again before walking across. The COTA accompanied Sherry on weekly class trips to the grocery store to help her master the curb task and learn other community travel skills.

Public transportation

Adolescents often begin travel training for a specific purpose, such as going to and from school, the store, or a prevocational program. They may be preparing to travel to a vocational program that does not provide transportation, which usually means that they must learn to use public transportation.

To help children and teenagers become familiar with travel routes, COTAs may incorporate subway, bus, or street maps into therapy sessions. Map activities may also be used for several other purposes, such as helping children improve their environmental awareness, sense of direction, eye movements, and sequencing and problem solving skills.

Children who use wheelchairs need to learn and practice the way to enter adapted buses and wheelchair-accessible commuter train stations. This task is commonly an occupational therapy practitioner's responsibility. Regardless of whether children have physical disabilities, they need to learn how to buy tickets, tokens, or transit cards and deposit change on a bus. They need to learn how to determine when their stop is approaching and how to prepare to exit. They need to learn when and how to signal a bus driver to stop a bus. As children become more proficient at performing the sequence of actions, the occupational therapy practitioner should reduce the level of assistance given to them and present problems for the children to solve. For example, the occupational therapy practitioner could allow children to miss a bus stop to see how they handle the situation and allow them to think of solutions.

Role of the shadow

Most community travel training programs designed for children who are able to walk use a "shadow" person. The shadow is usually someone other than the child's occupational therapy practitioner. Once a child is able to carry out a travel sequence consistently in the presence of a trainer, the child is allowed to travel semiindependently. The shadow follows the child at a distance, getting on and off buses or subways at the same stop as the child, and observing the situation for any problems that might arise. While using public transportation, some children engage in excessive self-stimulation, unknowingly push people, or talk to strangers. The shadow does not intervene unless a dangerous situation develops or the child has trouble solving a problem.

Public phones

Using public phones is an essential tool for independent community travel. This skill may be taught by an occupational therapy practitioner, special education teacher, caregiver, travel trainer, prevocational teacher, or a combination of these individuals. Children should always carry extra change for a phone call. The following techniques may be helpful for teaching children to use public phones:

1. Identify all the public phones along children's travel routes.
2. Have children practice using pay phones on the street to call school, home, or a vocational center.
3. Have children think of solutions to possible phone predicaments, such encountering a broken phone or having no money.
4. Have children handle coins and practice translation skills, which are required to remove coins from a wallet and insert them into a public phone (see In-Hand Manipulation section in this chapter).

Money

Money skills, which are taught by caregivers and various professionals, are often addressed in occupational therapy. Whenever possible, have a child use money skills during actual community interactions. For example, if during an occupational therapy session a child earns the long-term reward of going out for pizza and soda, the child should be allowed to buy the pizza and soda as independently as possible by standing in line, ordering the pizza, paying for the pizza, ensuring that the correct change has been provided, and finding straws and napkins.

Community interactions

Again, depending on the setting, funding agency, and agency purpose, the COTA may be responsible for teaching children to use community services such as a library, bank, post office, or grocery store. Learning these community skills may involve the assistance of several disciplines, such as occupational therapy, special education, and speech therapy. Whenever possible the occupational therapy practitioner participates in community interactions with children. Complex problems, such as being too friendly to strangers or an inability to count change correctly under pressure, can be identified and addressed during outings.

Emergency Response and Safety

Emergency response

Occupational therapy practitioners, caregivers, and teachers may be involved in teaching children how to take care of themselves in an emergency. The first skill children often need is being able to say, write, or otherwise indicate their name, address, and phone number. If children are unable to speak or write but able to understand the question, they can use a printed card with their name, address, and phone number to show to the proper individuals when they are lost.

Emergency responses may be somewhat different for children in wheelchairs, depending on the situation and their capabilities. In case they ever fall out of their chairs, the occupational therapy practitioner should make sure children know how to pull themselves to a phone, pull themselves back into their chairs from the floor, or operate an emergency call system (see Chapter 16).

In preparation for a fire emergency, practice the "stop, drop, and roll" sequence with children. In institutions such as schools, fire drills with full evacuations are practiced regularly. Staff should maintain a calm atmosphere while quickly and quietly helping children get out of the building and move to a safe location. Fire alarms frighten some children, causing them to cry, scream, or become aggressive. Occupational therapy practitioners should give assistance as needed. They could arrange in advance to help a certain child with whom they have a special relationship or at the request of a teacher.

In settings that have children in wheelchairs, a supply of evacuation chairs, also known as *evac chairs*, may be needed for evacuating the building in case of a fire or other disaster. Evac chairs are lightweight, small, and designed to go down steps more easily than standard wheelchairs or electric wheelchairs (which are extremely heavy because of the battery). In many facilities, nursing staff are responsible for acquiring evac chairs and training other personnel in their use. In other facilities, occupational therapy practitioners may have this responsibility. Some children can be trained in how to instruct a caregiver to use an evac chair.

Most children who are able to speak are taught to dial 9-1-1 in case of an emergency. Some children may not know what constitutes an actual emergency. In an occupational therapy session, it can be revealing, fun, and useful to work on solving problems that are related to emergencies. The occupational therapy practitioner could ask children to choose a card that describes or depicts an emergency, and the children could then explain or act out what they might do in the situation. Often more than one solution can solve the problem. If dialing 9-1-1 is the solution to one of the problems, have children practice dialing, reporting the emergency, and stating their name and address on an unplugged or toy phone.

In school, most children are taught to be wary of strangers. Children with special needs often need extra instruction. Children need concrete definitions of who is actually a stranger, such as "a stranger is someone who does not work at or go to your school." They also need specific strategies to use when approached by strangers, such as going to their teacher. COTAs who observe children interacting with strangers should (after ensuring the children's safety) alert the team so that they can address the problem together.

SAFETY SIGNS STORY. *A COTA who was working in a special school setting with adolescents who had pervasive developmental disorder, mental retardation, and emotional impairments became concerned about their ability to respond to an emergency. Many could not read, and they all depended on adults to tell them what to do.*

After discussing her plan with the OTR, the COTA ordered safety signs that included words such as STOP, EXIT, FIRE, POISON, and DANGER. For a few minutes of each occupational therapy session, students were quizzed on the meaning of each sign. Some students had the goal of distinguishing two or three signs, whereas others worked on differentiating between eight or more signs. Safety procedures were reviewed for various emergency situations, and students were asked to explain them. Eventually, they used role playing to act out emergency situations with the COTA and each other. While walking in the halls and during field trips, they practiced looking for and identifying safety signs. All students seemed to enjoy these activities and feel proud that they had learned this important information.

Safety

Limited safety skills can be the most serious element interfering with progress toward independence. Limited safety skills can lead to injury of the child or others, prevent movement to a less restrictive environment, and block improvements in areas such as social interactions and self-esteem. Some children try to play with peers by hitting them. Some children bite their own hands when frustrated. Whatever the cause, the occupational therapy practitioner and other team members should address safety issues immediately.

While planning and implementing treatment for safety problems, the occupational therapy practitioner should use methods that quickly resolve the issues. Prevent self-injurious and aggressive behaviors by reducing overstimulating sensory input and increasing pleasing sensory input. Methods such as using a helmet, using a consistent behavior management plan, reducing demands, or providing one-on-one supervision may help ensure the safety of the child and others. The occupational therapy practitioner also addresses underlying developmental factors and coping skills. With help from caregivers and other team members, the child may eventually be able to function without modified sensory input, adaptive equipment, strict limits, or constant supervision.

Sexual Expression

Sexual expression is an ADL. The COTA addresses sexual expression issues differently depending on the age and marital status of the client. (For example, a COTA would not use the same techniques with a 14-year-old boy and two 19-year-old married individuals who have suffered traumatic injuries.) Team members may ask the COTA to address issues such as positioning, adaptive equipment, or techniques related to sexual activity. (See Burton[8] for a discussion of the COTAs role in treating sexual expression issues of individuals with disabilities.)

Sexual expression can be quite important to adolescents. They may struggle with the proper way to sexually express themselves and to whom. The COTA should considers adolescents' unique issues and develop possible intervention strategies. A dyadic treatment session involving a boy and girl could help them learn to interact with the opposite sex. Team members can help adolescents set up lunch dates or attend dances or social events with their peers.

COTAs should prepare themselves for potential encounters involving boys or girls who are exploring their own sexuality. Adolescents with mental retardation or other developmental delays, head injuries, or emotional problems may flirt with or make sexual comments to COTAs. They may comment on or try to touch COTAs' genitals or breasts. Immediately report any incident of this nature to the OTR, family worker, psychologist, parent or caregiver, or on-site supervisor. Being matter of fact and setting firm limits against touching is often the best approach. Some adolescents may need to meet with counselors to discuss why their behavior is unacceptable and explore avenues for developing a romantic relationship with a peer.

Some children and adolescents may touch their genitals excessively. (Very young children may do this when they need to use the bathroom, and the COTA can help them learn what to do.) This socially unacceptable behavior can elicit negative reactions from peers and people in the community. Many children need to be reminded repeatedly about when it is and is not okay to touch their genitals. Establish concrete rules for children with limited cognitive skills such as, "It is okay to touch your private parts in the bathroom or the bedroom when no one else is there."

Use a team approach when this technique is not enough. Some children may need a medical evaluation to rule out infections. Anxiety may be a factor, so fidget toys such as squeeze toys or even hand-held video games can positively redirect the child. Reward children who have behaved in a socially acceptable way for short periods with their choice of toys.

SCOTT'S SEXUAL APPROACH STORY. *Scott was a 17 year old with fragile X syndrome (a type of autism caused by an abnormality in the X chromosome), mental retardation, and poor judgment. He frightened several young female staff members by lunging at them and trying to touch their legs when they wore skirts. A COTA reported this to the OTR supervisor who consulted the family worker. The family worker discussed the issue with Scott's mother, who greatly appreciated the feedback. She had never witnessed this behavior and was unaware that it was happening. She and her husband had always taught Scott to interact with everyone respectfully.*

Scott's mother and father also said that they did not think Scott was ready to handle intimacy, even though he often talked about imaginary girlfriends. His mother stated he was capable of satisfying himself at home by masturbating in his bedroom. She and her husband said they would address the problem at home. They asked school personnel to continue gently, but firmly enforcing limits with Scott. During supervision sessions the OTR supervisor and COTA discussed ways the COTA could redirect Scott's behavior in a matter-of-fact way and help him learn how to interact more positively with women.

TEDDY'S MASTURBATION STORY. *Teddy was a 16 year old with severe mental retardation and autism. Some days in school he could not stop touching his genitals. When encouraged to stop, he became agitated and aggressive. The multidisciplinary team and parents determined that Teddy's behavior could be caused by frustration resulting from being asked to stop what he was doing. Because the team knew he was capable of satisfying himself through masturbation, a behavior plan was devised that incorporated this behavior. When Teddy became so agitated by his need to touch genitals that he could not participate in classwork, he was asked to go to the bathroom. A male staff person respectfully monitored him and assisted Teddy with refocusing on his classwork when he was finished.*

WORK AND PRODUCTIVE ACTIVITIES

The work and productive activities of children involve educational activities such as going to school and managing assignments. Children are also usually expected to do chores at home such as making their beds, washing dishes, or preparing themselves a sandwich; this section addresses only educational activities.

Educational Activities

Many underlying performance components affect educational activities, including postural control, sensory processing, oculomotor (eye) control, visual-motor skills, visual perception, and fine motor skills. The occupational therapy practitioner often addresses these components.

Positioning for instruction

Proper positioning and postural control are key components affecting the ability to focus on instructions and succeed in performing table-top activities such as handwriting. One principle used during handling and positioning techniques is that mobility is supported by stability. To control motions of the head, eyes, arms, and hands, the trunk, hips, legs, and feet form a stable base of support (see Chapter 17).

CLINICAL *Pearl*

Proper positioning benefits all children regardless of whether they have motor, attention, sensory, learning, or cognitive problems.

The occupational therapy practitioner working on educational activities typically assesses the child's positioning during one of the first treatment sessions. The practitioner uses a tape measure to measure the child and furniture.

Determining table-top height

The occupational therapy practitioner measures the distance between the floor and the child's elbows while the elbows are hanging at the child's side; the most functional table-top height is about 2 inches higher than this distance. When working at a table, the shoulders tend to slightly round and flex (bend) forward, which raises the elbows somewhat.

Determining seat height

A new occupational therapy practitioner may need to measure the hip angle with a goniometer (a tool for measuring joint angles), whereas an experienced practitioner may be able to visually assess this angle successfully. The hips should be at a 90-degree angle or more flexed (bent). Slightly increased hip flexion of 70 or 80 degrees may provide more stability and comfort. Slightly increased hip flexion also reduces extensor tone in a child with spasticity.[5]

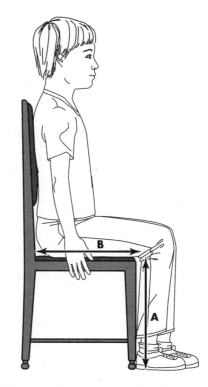

FIGURE 13-39 Positioning for instruction. *A,* Seat height: 1 to 2 inches less than distance between heel (with shoes on) and inside knee. *B,* Seat depth: 1 to 2 inches less than distance between back of hip and inside knee.

The chair should be low enough or the footrest should be high enough for the hips to be well flexed.

The occupational therapy practitioner measures the distance between the bottom of the child's shoe to the crease behind the child's knee. The proper seat height is 1 to 2 inches less than this distance. The feet should be flat on the floor or footrest, with the child's weight solidly on the heel and the sole, with slightly more weight on the heel.

A common mistake is for a child to use a chair that is too high. If a child's feet dangle or sliding and scooting forward is necessary for the child's feet to be planted firmly on the ground, the seat is too high. If only the sole of the foot is on the ground, stability is insufficient to support upper body control, and increased extensor (straightening) tone can occur in children with high (tight) muscle tone (Figure 13-39).

Determining seat depth

The occupational therapy practitioner measures the distance between the back of child's hip while seated and the crease behind the child's knee. The proper seat depth is 1 to 2 inches less than this distance. The proper seat depth allows the child's hips and back to rest firmly against the back of the chair, promoting hip and trunk stability (see Figure 13-39).

Indicators of positioning problems

Many children with special needs have trouble maintaining the hip and trunk stability required to support hand, head, and eye movements. Signs that the child needs more stability or that the seat may need an adjustment include the following: straddling the seat, wrapping feet around chair legs, sitting using a wide base of support, putting feet up on the seat of the chair, sliding to the side or front edge of the chair, sitting or kneeling on the feet, slouching, banging the chair legs, and rocking. In some schools, many chairs need to be modified but the school has minimal funding to do so. Consider using the following inexpensive methods:

1. Detachable footrests or backrests for small children can be made with cardboard blocks that look like bricks.[33] Attach them to chair legs with sticky Velcro. Cover them with contact paper so that they can be cleaned with a wet sponge. Add weight to the cardboard footrests by filling them with sand.
2. Footrests can be created with sturdy, closed-cell foam for children weighing up to about 100 lb.[33] Cut the foam into blocks with a bread knife. Foam footrests take little time to make and can easily be wiped clean.
3. Covering telephone books with duct tape can make fairly sturdy and cost-effective footrests.
4. Gluing pieces of corrugated cardboard together in the desired width can make firm backrests. Cover them with contact paper so that they look more attractive and can be cleaned.
5. Filling 2- to 3-inch deep rectangular boxes with newspaper can make portable backrests.[58]

Children may need seating alternatives; consider using the following:

1. A child who rocks continuously may pay attention better when sitting in a child-size rocking chair.
2. A child who is fidgety or squirms around a lot in spite of proper positioning can use an air-filled moving seat cushion to increase comfort and ease postural adjustments. A slightly inflated beach ball becomes is an inexpensive seat cushion that can be successfully used by some children.
3. A child who leans heavily on a desk or has trouble staying seated in spite of proper positioning may benefit from sitting on a therapy ball in class. Hold the ball with a stabilizer ring. The bouncy feedback from the ball may facilitate trunk and head control as well as increase alertness. Using the stabilizer ring is important to prevent the child from straining postural muscles. After about 30 minutes the child can be encouraged to use another seating option that provides back support.

4. A child who is unable to stay seated more than a few minutes may be able to stand near the desk and work. Standing next to a desk does not necessarily interfere with learning. Place colored tape on the floor to designate the child's work space.
5. A child who is unable to sit independently because of severe physical limitations may benefit from using a seat belt for hip stability. COTAs may be trained in adaptive seating techniques by an OTR who specializes in the area. Seat belt should not be used on children simply because they frequently get out of their chairs.

CLINICAL *Pearl*

Seat belts are considered restraints and are *not* used on children who are capable of sitting independently.

Typically developing children use a wide variety of positions for learning. Preschoolers use the floor; they crawl with trains and cars, sit sideways to complete a puzzle, or use numerous different sitting postures on the floor with frequent postural transitions to play with dolls or action figures. During all this floor play, the children develop the strength and postural control they will eventually need to sit in chairs. Even children in elementary, junior high, and high schools need to use various positions and participate regularly in strengthening activities to maintain comfortable postures in the classroom, which increases their ability to learn.

CLINICAL *Pearl*

Simply practicing sitting in a chair does not increase postural control. To develop the control needed to sit in a chair for extended periods, children need to perform regular exercises and movements designed to activate and strengthen muscles in the trunk, back, stomach, hips, and neck.

Attending to instruction

Occupational therapy practitioners and educators working in school settings should assess themselves and identify the methods they use to sustain their own attention during class. These individuals often walk around the classroom, sip occasionally from a cup of coffee or glass of water, and talk whenever they want. Teachers and practitioners are allowed to use all these methods to keep them focused on a task, yet children, adolescents, and college students are often expected to pay attention while sitting still for long periods without moving, eating, drinking, or making any noise. It is not surprising that paying attention to class lessons, also known as *attending to instruction,* is a common problem in most schools for all populations.

Children with ADD, hyperactivity, sensory processing problems, anxiety, low tolerance for frustration, impulsivity, or visual- or motor-control problems have even more problems attending to class instruction. They have more difficulty regulating their own levels of arousal (that is, staying alert) than many other children. An optimum level of arousal is required for learning.[54]

The Alert Program for Self-Regulation is a curriculum designed to help elementary school children improve attention to instruction.[56] The program teaches children to become aware of and use the sensory input they need to regulate their own levels of arousal. Sensory input is provided by activities for the mouth, lungs, ears, eyes, muscles, and vestibular (movement-gravity) system.[55,56] The curriculum has been modified for and used successfully with children who have developmental, learning, and emotional limitations.[7,35] The program can also be modified for use with preschool or high school children.

COTAs can play an important role in introducing and reinforcing techniques for regulating children's levels of arousal in the schools. The most skillful teachers already use many of these methods, which include allowing children to keep a water bottle with a straw at their desks, asking fidgety children to run errands or help perform tasks such as sharpening pencils, asking anxious children to pass out heavy books or reposition chairs and tables for class activities, designing group projects in which children are allowed to talk, reducing bright lighting, and incorporating stretching breaks into lessons.

In-class or group treatment sessions provide the best opportunities for occupational therapy practitioners to model techniques for regulation of arousal. Many teachers are eager to integrate the techniques into classes but need demonstrations of how to use them. Team problem solving may be necessary to adapt and implement techniques for special populations. Other strategies such as the following can be incorporated into the classroom schedule:

1. For a child with sensory defensiveness, use the Wilbarger deep pressure and proprioceptive technique every hour or two throughout the day to reduce anxiety and overly negative reactions to harmless events, which allows the child to better pay attention to classroom tasks.[55]
2. A child who is distracted by and unable to screen out background visual input may benefit from using a study carrel (cubicle) that blocks out visual stimulation from the front and sides.
3. A child who is distracted by and unable to screen out background noises may be able to work independently when wearing headphones with (or without) music.
4. A child can be given the option of completing assignments in a quiet area, such as the library, or while sitting just outside the classroom.
5. Discomfort and attempts to maintain an upright position may distract a child with poor postural control. The child may pay so much attention to sitting up that listening to the teacher is secondary. (See the section on Prehandwriting and Handwriting in this chapter for activities to enhance postural control in the classroom.)
6. Using "energizing breaks" may increase self-esteem and attending to instruction.[36] About every 20 minutes, have children participate in positive social interactions and fun movement breaks that last about 2 to 4 minutes. These breaks are designed to increase self-esteem, work muscles, and increase breathing.[36] Oxygen is essential in the brain for carrying out thought processes. The lungs expand and work with the muscles to transport oxygenated blood to the brain. During prolonged periods of sitting, the lungs and muscles have difficulty working properly. One way a teacher could incorporate an energizing break is to have the students act out a silly scene. For example, the teacher could ask each child to get a partner and then tell the children that they are aliens from different planets and need to greet each other. One child could be told communicate only by wriggling on the ground and groaning, whereas the other could be told to communicate only by swaying and singing.

Visual function

Visual function involves visual acuity, oculomotor (eye control) skills, and visual perception. Visual function is required for visual-motor tasks such as handwriting and most work and daily living skills. The occupational therapy practitioner often addresses oculomotor skills, visual perception, and visual-motor skills to improve school participation. Although visual function is needed for most educational activities, some children have severe visual impairments and need specialized intervention.

Visual acuity

Visual acuity is the "capacity to discriminate the fine details of objects in the visual field"[46] or "a descriptive means of expressing the sharpness, clearness, and distinctness of vision."[12] An ophthalmologist or an optometrist assesses acuity. If the COTA notices that a child brings objects very close to the eyes or appears unable to see obstacles or people, the COTA notifies the OTR and team members. Notification of the parents and referral to an outside specialist may be indicated.

Oculomotor skills

Oculomotor skills involve multiple coordinated eye movements produced by eye muscles.[12] These skills are also known as *ocular control* or *ocular-motor skills*. Eyes muscles pull the eyes in horizontal, vertical, and oblique (diagonal) directions. Combinations of eye muscle actions move the eyes in a circle. Children need oculomotor skills for school tasks such as reading as well as communication tasks such as writing and using communication boards.

Oculomotor problems are easily overlooked, but the observant COTA may be able to detect them. When the COTA notices or suspects an oculomotor problem, the COTA notifies the OTR and checks the child's medical record to see whether the child has had a recent eye examination. Parental permission may be obtained to refer a child for evaluation by an ophthalmologist or optometrist.

Some children have so much trouble finding and holding the correct head position that they are unable to maintain a stable **visual field.** The visual field is "the entire area that can be seen while the eye is fixing or gazing steadily at a target in the direct line of vision."[12] Strong neck muscles, which position and steady the head, are needed for a stable visual field. A stable visual field provides a base of support for the eye movements involved in reading, writing, or finding symbols on a communication board.

Some children are unable to maintain visual fixation, or sustain their eye gaze in the direction of a target.[12] Children who have limited **convergence,** or "simultaneous turning of the eyes inward,"[12] are unable to bring their eyes together well enough to see objects close to their faces (that is, within a 12-inch distance). Visual fixation and some convergence are needed to perform many fine motor tasks such as buttoning, stringing small beads, or looking at words or symbols.

Some children have poor **head-eye dissociation,** or ability to move their eyes independently without moving their head. They are unable to separate head and eye movements for reading or finding symbols on a communication board. Instead they move their entire head to look up and down or side to side.

Poor head-eye dissociation makes visual **tracking** (that is, following targets with smooth eye movements) difficult.[12] Children who have poor visual tracking skills often lose focus while trying to follow or find an object. Their eyes may also stop or jump when crossing the midline of the body.

Some children have limited gaze shift skills (that is, the ability smoothly move their eyes from one target to another).[12] These children may be unable to quickly localize (that is, pinpoint with the eyes) items. Limited gaze shift and quick localization skills make tasks such as beginning the next line of text while reading or copying from the blackboard frustrating and time consuming.

Several factors interfering with oculomotor skills include neck or eye muscle weakness, poor discrimination and interpretation of proprioceptive (deep-pressure) feedback in the neck or eyes, or nystagmus (involuntary jerking of the eyes). The OTR may recommend that the COTA carry out specific activities such as the following to help the child improve oculomotor skills:

1. To assist a child with maintaining a stable visual field, use strengthening exercises for neck flexion and extension.
2. To increase convergence, encourage the child to watch an appealing object moving slowly toward the nose. Look at each eye to be sure both are equally directed at the target to within about 4 inches from the face.
3. To help the child coordinate eye, neck, and head control, use specific movement activities such as reaching for toys placed on the floor while riding on a scooterboard in a prone (face-down) position.
4. To improve gaze shift and quick localization, the child can aim at appealing targets while riding on moving equipment. The child can also aim at moving targets, such as a ball or balloon suspended from the ceiling. In a dark room, the practitioner can shine a flashlight on objects, which the child can then point to or identify.
5. To improve head-eye dissociation and tracking skills, move a toy in vertical, horizontal, and circular patterns as the child watches. Touching the chin may gently stabilize the child's head. Playing with toy cars, marbles, balloons, and bubbles can also help.
6. To address quick localization and gaze shift problems and encourage head-eye dissociation and visual tracking, use board games or card or shape-matching activities. Choose activities that require moving the eyes quickly between targets such as the card game Memory and the shape-matching game Perfection.

Visual perception

Visual perception refers to "the ability to interpret and use what is seen"[51] or "the capacity to interpret sensory input, recognize similarities and differences, and assign meaning to what is seen."[12] Visual perception increases with maturity and "occurs through an active process between the child and his environment."[51] It requires cognitive (that is, thinking) analysis as well as perception (that is, receiving information) through sight.

Object perception refers to "visual identification of objects by color, texture, shape and size: what things are."[46] Spatial perception refers to "the visual location of objects in space: where things are."[46]

OBJECT PERCEPTION. Occupational therapy practitioners often work on subskills of the object perception area, including matching and sorting shapes and colors. Teachers also address these skills. An important area of object perception for reading and writing is form constancy, or "the recognition of forms and objects as the same in various environments, positions, and sizes."[46] Form constancy is the skill that allows children to recognize a letter as the same whether it is lowercase, uppercase, or written in cursive. To help improve form constancy, a child can compare details of various pictures or shapes to determine whether forms are the same. The child can use worksheets to find two shapes that are the same, with one being smaller, larger, darker, or lighter, than the other, turned on its side, or inside another shape.

Another area of object perception is visual figure-ground discrimination, which refers to the ability to distinguish important foreground features from background objects. For example, figure-ground discrimination is required to find a pencil in a desk; the child must be able to pick out the pencil (which is in the foreground) while distinguishing it from the desk and other items in the desk. Many activities can be found in bookstores and equipment catalogs that help develop visual figure-ground discrimination. The *Where's Waldo*[25] book series, "Find what's Different" worksheets, "Find the Hidden Figures" pictures, and "What's Wrong with this Picture" worksheets all involve figure-ground discrimination.

SPATIAL PERCEPTION. An area of spatial perception that is commonly addressed by occupational therapy practitioners is "position in space" skills, which "provide the awareness of an object's position in relation to the observer or the perception of the direction in which it is turned."[46] A perception of position in space provides the basis for the development of directional concepts such as in, out, beside, and behind. Position in space perception also allows the child to decipher that one word is separate from another while reading and space letters evenly while writing.[46]

The ability to use the spatial and directional concepts of "in" and "off" usually develops by about 30 months of age. By about 36 months of age the infants usually begin to understand the concepts of "on," "under," "out of," "together," and "away." By about 5½ years of age, children are able to use basic spatial concepts such as "behind," "ahead of," "first," and "last."[51] To improve awareness of position in space and spatial and directionality concepts, use the following activities:

1. Provide obstacle courses or playground activities in which the child must use spatial concepts (for example, going on and over a pillow or a slide).
2. Moving through small spaces may help a child learn about body position in relation to objects in the environment.

3. To teach the child the way to stand next to a person during a conversation, tell the child to extend an arm and use that distance as the correct distance.
4. On an elevator or in other crowded situations, ask the child to look on all sides to ensure that another person is not being touched.
5. During fine motor and self-care activities comment on the child's actions and later ask the child to comment on the activities. For example, as the child places a toy train on the tracks, say, "On," or as the child removes a jacket, say, "Off."
6. To improve spatial and directional concepts, use craft and construction activities that allow the child to imitate or create designs or figures.
7. To teach a child where to start reading or writing, emphasize a starting point. For example, place a sticker at the top left corner of a page.[51]

Visual-motor skills

Visual-motor skills are sometimes referred to as *visual-motor integration skills* or *eye-hand/eye-foot skills*. These skills require coordination of eyes with hands and eyes with feet, such that the eyes guide complex, precise movements. A few examples of visual-motor activities are (1) following dot-to-dot patterns, (2) using mazes, (3) drawing, (4) handwriting, (5) using scissors, (6) playing in obstacles courses, and (7) climbing.

CLINICAL *Pearl*

Use a developmental approach to address visual problems. Higher-level visual-perception and visual-motor skills cannot develop properly unless the lower-level skills of oculomotor control, visual acuity, and maintenance of full visual fields are adequate.[52]

Development of any of the visual skills requires careful grading of activities. The occupational therapy practitioner begins with simple activities and gradually increases their complexity.[51] Because of the intricacy of visual function, the OTR gives precise directions for intervention. The COTA may intervene at different levels during the same session. Teachers and speech therapists also address various visual-perception and visual-motor skills. Coordinate treatment efforts with these professionals whenever possible.

Managing assignments

Knowing how to manage school assignments can help prepare children for future prevocational and vocational responsibilities. The occupational therapy practitioner can provide useful strategies for and assistance to children working on school assignments. The COTA can help children manage schoolwork as part of therapy sessions. Some of the skills needed to manage assignments include organization skills, set-up and clean-up skills, sitting tolerance, eye-hand coordination, sustained focus of attention, sequencing skills, fine motor and graphomotor skills, oculomotor skills, visual-perception skills, self-regulation skills, and head and postural control.

Proper positioning and achieving an optimum level of arousal are essential for managing assignments. The previously listed activities may help children work on their assignments. Several other techniques are as follows:

1. One of the first steps in organizing work involves making a list of assignments. As each assignment is completed, have the child cross it off the list. The child should keep the list in front of a notebook or folder so that it is the first page seen when it is opened.
2. Make sure the child schedules the proper time to work on assignments. To help prepare the child for focusing on schoolwork, allow the child to participate in a physical activity after school and before doing homework. The child may be too tired to concentrate after dinner.
3. Sensory supports play an important role before and during assignments. A routine in which the child has a snack and then prepares needed sensory items before starting work can prevent later disruptions. Sensory supports may include a spout cup filled with water or juice, gum or an edible item for sucking or chewing, an inedible chewing object such as a straw, and a jump rope or swivel chair for short movement breaks.
4. To focus the child on an assignment, only include those items on the table or easel needed for that assignment. Keep other materials in the child's book bag or desk. Once each assignment is finished, the child stores it in the book bag or in the desk again.
5. Children with learning disabilities or oculomotor problems may have trouble completing math problems because the columns of numbers seem to blend together. Simple visual aids for math work include the following: using graph paper, turning an 8½- by 11-inch piece of lined paper horizontally (so that the lines form columns) and writing math problems in the columns, or simply drawing bold vertical lines to separate columns of numbers before starting work.
6. Young children who are unable to read or have limited understanding of writing can use symbols, photographs, or objects attached to a Velcro board for assignments. For example, a pencil could represent a handwriting activity, or a toy bug could represent a science activity. The occupational therapy practitioner attaches the symbols, photos, or objects to the board in the desired order. As each task is accomplished, children pull the related item off the board. Children receive gratification from mastering each task as well as from pulling Velcro items off the board. They also have a visual representation of which tasks were accomplished. The sequence can be varied; children can choose the order of activities and stick symbols, photos, or objects to the board before starting assignments. Using the Velcro board during occupational therapy treatment sessions also helps many children, especially those who learn best through visual means. A Velcro board is relatively inexpensive and easy to make. Cover a piece of cardboard with soft fabric that sticks to hook-style Velcro (The Lockfast Co.; see Chapter 13 Appendix C). Draw symbols on cardboard, cut them out, and cover them with clear contact paper if desired. Attach a piece of sticky hook-style Velcro to the back of the symbols or directly to the back of photographs or objects.

Prevocational Activities

League school prevocational program

The COTA may work directly with children on prevocational skills, depending on their age and the setting. Many prevocational programs are led by special education teachers, such as in a model program at the League School in Brooklyn, NY, designed by Kathryn Norton in 1984. Occupational therapy practitioners consult with vocational teachers about children's work-related talents and limitations as well as useful strategies to use with specific children.

The League School prevocational program promotes movement toward the least restrictive environment, which is the community. All students, who range in age from 5 to 21, attend prevocational classes. They punch in and out on a time card at the beginning and end of each class. They follow either written or picture card directions. They usually fill out a checklist at the end of class, which emphasizes self-awareness of social skills used.

In the prevocational room, students with moderately to severely limited skills may work on sorting, matching, or piecework assembly. Those with higher-level skills may learn to use a cash register, engraver, laminator, computer, copy machine, or vacuum cleaner.

All of the teenagers aged 18 and older are involved in community work. Teenagers with moderate to severe limitations in cognition, language, and environmental awareness receive extra supervision in the community in an enclave. The enclave is a group of students accompanied by a classroom or prevocational teacher. Students go to community sites and work with personnel from other agencies but simultaneously receive behavioral supervision and instruction from school staff.[21]

Students with higher cognitive, language, and social skills are introduced to actual jobs through a gradual process. They first practice interviewing in the school setting. After a successful interview, some get jobs working with school maintenance staff, watering plants after school hours, or setting up and cleaning equipment in the occupational therapy room. Eventually they interview for jobs in the community.

Prevocational staff reach out to community agencies and arrange work positions for students with special needs. Students go on job interviews and if hired receive support from a school job coach during their first months. The job coach works with the student both on and off the job to improve needed skills. Little by little, the coach reduces support until the student works with only periodic school contacts. Many League School graduates have become employed in actual community jobs through this process.

The COTA can assist prevocational specialists in many areas. The COTA can help a child with proper dress, hygiene, and grooming as well as social interactions needed for work. COTAs may also aid in job exploration and development of underlying postural, hand, and visual-motor skills needed for job performance.

Preparing to enter sheltered workshops

Traditionally, many children with disabilities have been trained to enter sheltered workshops at the age of 21 when they graduate from school. Moving toward a sheltered workshop environment may be the right plan for some teenagers with limited cognitive skills and mild to moderate physical limitations. These children need functional sitting tolerance, adequate attention skills, and skills in sorting, counting, matching, and fine manipulation to enter a sheltered workshop. However, little money may be earned for their efforts, and interaction with the community is minimal.

COTAs may help teenagers prepare to enter a sheltered workshop. In a prevocational setting it may be the COTA's responsibility to ensure teenagers are using functional sitting positions, help the adolescent improve sorting, matching, and fine manipulation skills, or to create **templates (jigs)** for specific piecework tasks.

Most sheltered workshops contract with outside agencies for the assembly of small items, such as pens, or to package a specific number and color of items, such as bags of pipe cleaners. Depending on their roles and expertise, either the occupational therapy practitioner or prevocational teacher may create templates, or jigs, to make piecework easier and more accurate. Teenagers with limited coordination or sensory awareness may need specialized templates, which are usually stable holders (such as pieces of wood) with a hole cut that fits the exact size of one or more parts of the item to be assembled. The jig

stabilizes certain parts for the teenager who then attaches other pieces.

Social skills at work

Regardless of whether adolescents have special needs, they need to learn proper social skills for work. Work interactions are different from social interactions in the family, school, or hospital. Poor social skills prevent success at work more often than limited task skills. COTAs work with team members and caregivers to help teenagers learn social skills that will be needed on the job in the future. These skills include respecting personal space; a boss may not be willing to repeat, "You're standing too close to me" as many times as a teacher or parent would.

An adolescent in a prevocational program learns when to ask for help and when to proceed quietly to the next task. Adolescents need to learn the proper way to ask for help. They should address their bosses or supervisors politely and learn to leave to-the-point messages that are neither abrupt nor rude.

Using videotaped role-playing activities can help teenagers, especially when the teenagers themselves review and give feedback on the performances. Topics can include problems on the job, such as a co-worker who calls the teenager names, a boss who does not answer questions, two managers simultaneously requesting help, a co-worker lying about the teenager to the boss, or not knowing what to do on a coffee break. Depending on the COTA's responsibilities and expertise, the COTA may be involved in the videotaped role-playing activities.

Time management

Although managing time at work is extremely important, many teenagers have trouble working at steady pace and planning ways to complete each task within a given time. Using a timer and checklist of tasks that includes an expected time frame for each task helps some adolescents.

During occupational therapy sessions, COTAs may work with adolescents on the timing, rhythm, and timely completion of their work. COTAs may be able to alert vocational specialists to particular problems adolescents may have, such as being excessively distracted by auditory and visual background sensations that disrupt performance. COTAs may also help specialists develop a vocational plan suited to the adolescents' work pace.

Job performance

Vocational teachers usually break job tasks down into small steps and teach each step slowly. COTAs can help considerably by further analyzing sensory, postural, balance, fine motor planning, oculomotor, spatial, and other job demands in relation to a teenager's skills in these areas.

HECTOR'S FILING STORY. *Hector was a 17 year old with learning disabilities, mild mental retardation, and low muscle tone. In his prevocational class, he was asked to find a file at the "back" of a drawer. His teachers patiently explained and demonstrated how to perform the task in numerous ways. Hector still became confused and was unable to find the file in back of the drawer. His COTA was consulted. By observing Hector as he attempted to perform his filing task and from previous information learned about Hector and his learning disabilities, the COTA figured out the problem and a solution.*

The COTA reasoned that when Hector heard the word "back," he could only associate the word with his own physical body part—his own back. He could not figure out what his own back had to do with something in a file drawer. The COTA asked him to turn around and stand next to the open file drawer. His back was then beside the back of the drawer, and the front of his body was beside the front of the drawer. The COTA explained and demonstrated this to him. From then on, when asked to find or put something at the back of the drawer, Hector quietly turned around, stood next to the drawer, and then found the right place.

SUMMARY

Basic treatment planning and intervention methods can be used to help the COTA enhance ADLs and work and productive activities for children with special needs. The role of the COTA involves analyzing, grading, and adapting activities; reading the child in context; consulting and collaborating with the OTR, caregivers, team members, agency administrators, and other professionals; utilizing combined treatment approaches; matching adaptive devices with an individual child's capabilities and caregiver preferences; and utilizing the numerous literature, media, and workshop resources available in occupational therapy and other disciplines. COTAs should consult other resources to learn about areas such as scissor skills, complex visual-perceptual skills (such as seriation and visualization), telling time, and work activities at home.

Numerous treatments and techniques in many areas can be used by occupational therapy practitioners. Other resources contain various additional methods. The COTA may need to work with caregivers and team members to find individualized solutions for children with severe or complex problems.

References

1. American Occupational Therapy Association: Uniform terminology for occupational therapy, *Am J Occup Ther* 48: 1047, 1994.
2. Ball D: *Handwriting issues in school system practice*, Lecture, Charleston, SC, 1998, Trident Technical College.
3. Beauchamp R: *Fine motor activities*, Parent workshop, New York, 1998, Reece School.
4. Benbow M: *Loops and other groups, a kinesthetic writing system*, Tucson, 1988, Therapy Skill Builders.
5. Bergen A, Colangelo C: *Positioning the client with CNS deficit: the wheelchair and other adapted equipment*, Valhalla, NY, 1982, Valhalla Rehabilitation Publication.
6. Boehme R: *Improving upper body control: an approach to assessment and treatment of tonal dysfunction*, Tucson, 1988, Therapy Skill Builders.
7. Bortz S: *Improving classroom behavior with modified use of the Alert Program for Self Regulation*, Masters thesis, Brooklyn, 1997, The League School.
8. Burton GU: Sexuality: an activity of daily living. In Early MB, editor: *Physical dysfunction practice skills for the occupational therapy assistant*, St Louis, 1998, Mosby.
9. Burton L: *Concept and design for weights used during hallway transitions*, Brooklyn, 1996, The League School.
10. Case-Smith J, Humphry R: Feeding and oral motor skills. In Case-Smith, Allen A, Pratt, P, editors: *Occupational therapy for children*, ed 3, St Louis, 1996, Mosby.
11. Early MB: *Mental health concepts and techniques for the occupational therapy assistant*, New York, 1987, Raven Press.
12. Erhardt R: *Developmental visual dysfunction: models for assessment and management*, Tucson, 1993, Therapy Skill Builders.
13. Exner C: In-hand manipulation. In Case-Smith J, Pehoski C, editors: *Development of hand skills in the child*, Bethesda, Md, 1992, American Occupational Therapy Association.
14. Faustin D: *Cardboard brick block footrests*, Brooklyn, 1995, The Joan Fenichel Therapeutic Nursery, League Treatment Center.
15. Feingold B: *Why your child is hyperactive*, New York, 1974, Random House.
16. Feingold B: *The Feingold handbook*, Alexandria, Va, 1982, Feingold Association of the United States.
17. Filemyr J, Spears A: *Techniques for dealing with oppositional behaviors*, Presentation, Brooklyn, 1994, League Treatment Center.
18. Finnie N: *Handling the young cerebral palsy child at home*, ed 3, Boston, 1997, Butterworth-Heinemann.
19. Folio M R, Fewell RR: *Peabody developmental motor scales*, Chicago, 1983, Riverside.
20. Frick S et al: *Out of the mouths of babes: discovering the developmental significance of the mouth*, Hugo, Minn, 1996, PDP Press.
21. Garsia M: *Consultation on prevocational program*, Brooklyn, 1994, The League School.
22. Goldsmith MC: *Expanding children's diets, ketchup isn't the only vegetable*, Presentation, Kennebunkport, Me, 1996, Avanti Summit.
23. Goldstein A et al: *Skillstreaming the adolescent: a structured learning approach to teaching prosocial skills*, Champaign, Ill, 1980, Research Press.

24. Handford M: *Where's Waldo?* Boston, 1987, Little, Brown.
25. Handford M: *Find Waldo now*, Boston, 1988, Little, Brown.
26. Handford M: *The great Waldo search*, Boston, 1989, Little, Brown.
27. Handford M: *Where's Waldo in Hollywood?* 1993, Cambridge, Mass, 1993, Candlewick Press.
28. Heine B: An introduction to hippotherapy, *Strides*, p. 10, 1997.
29. Henderson A: Self-care and hands skill, In Henderson A, Pehoski C, editors: *Hand function in the child, foundations for remediation*, St Louis, 1995, Mosby.
30. Huss AJ: *A neurophysiological approach to central nervous system dysfunction*, Workshop, Ann Arbor, Mich, 1981, Continuing Education Programs of America.
31. Jones L: *Survey of accessibility in group homes for pediatric clients in wheelchairs*, New York, 1982, New York University and United Cerebral Palsy of New York State.
32. Koomar J, Masur S: *Sensory integration treatment*, Workshop, Boston, 1990, Sensory Integration International.
33. Liszkay E: *Closed cell foam foot rests*, Brooklyn, 1998, The Joan Fenichel Therapeutic Nursery, The League Treatment Center.
34. Machover PZ: *Consultation on promoting positive feelings around eating using social-environmental intervention*, New York, 1990.
35. Mandel S: *Classroom structure*, Brooklyn, 1996, The League School.
36. McCarty H: *Energy and stress in the learning process, a neurophysiological approach to learning at any age*, Workshop, Phoenix, 1998, Sensory Integration International.
37. McGinnis E, Goldstein A: *Skillstreaming the elementary school child, a guide for teaching prosocial skills*, Champaign, Ill, 1984, Research Press.
38. McGinnis E, Goldstein A: *Skillstreaming in early childhood: teaching prosocial skills to the preschool and kindergarten child*, Champaign, Ill, 1990, Research Press.
39. Morris S, Klein M: *Prefeeding skills. A comprehensive resource for feeding development*, Tucson, 1987, Therapy Skill Builders.
40. Mosey A C: The concept and use of developmental groups, *Am J Occup Ther* 24(40), 1970.
41. Norton K: *Design of prevocational program*, Brooklyn, 1984, The League School.
42. Oetter P, Richter E, Frick S: MORE. *Integrating the mouth with sensory and postural functions*, Hugo, Minn, 1993, PDP Press.
43. Oetter P, Richter E, Frick S: On MORE. *Integrating the mouth with sensory and postural functions*, Workshop, Greenwich, Conn, 1995, Professional Development Programs.
44. Okoye R, Malden J: Use of neurotransmitter modulation to facilitate sensory integration, *Neurology Report*, 10(4) Fall, 1986, Neurology Section of the American Physical Therapy Association.
45. Olsen J: *Handwriting without tears*, Potomac, Md, 1994, Janice Z Olsen.
46. Schneck C: Visual perception. In Case-Smith J, Allen A, Pratt P, editors: *Occupational therapy for children*, ed 3, St Louis, 1996, Mosby.
47. Stackhouse T, Wilbarger J, Trunnell S: *Treating sensory modulation disorders: the STEPSI: a tool for effective critical reasoning*, Workshop, Boston, 1998, Professional Development Programs.
48. Stoller L: *Low tech assistive devices: a handbook for the school setting*, Framingham, Mass, 1998.
49. Stringer K: *Staff behavior management guidelines*, New York, 1996, The Reece School.
50. Sumar S: *Yoga for the special child*, Buckingham, Va, 1996, Special Yoga Publications.
51. Todd V: Visual perceptual frame of reference: an information processing approach. In Kramer P, Hinojosa J, editors: *Frames of reference for pediatric occupational therapy*, Baltimore, 1993, Williams & Wilkins.
52. Warren M: Evaluation and treatment of visual deficits. In Pedretti LW, editor: *Occupational therapy practice skills for physical dysfunction*, ed 4, St Louis, 1996, Mosby.
53. Wilbarger P, Becker-Lewin M: *Sensory defensiveness & related social/emotional & neurological problems*, Workshop, Long Island, NY, 1998, Professional Development Programs.
54. Wilbarger P, Wilbarger J: *Sensory defensiveness in children aged 2-12: an intervention guide for parents and other caregivers*, Santa Barbara, Calif, 1991, Avanti Educational Programs.
55. Wilbarger P, Wilbarger J: *Intervention for persons with moderate to severe dysfunction*, Workshop, Brooklyn, 1992, Comprehensive Network.
56. Williams M, Shellenberger S: *How does your engine run? A leaders guide to the Alert Program for self-regulation*, Albuquerque, 1994, Therapy Works.
57. Wolf L, Glass R: *Feeding and swallowing disorders in infancy: assessment and management*, Tucson, 1992, Therapy Skill Builders.
58. Zielig S: *Inexpensive backrest*, Brooklyn, 1998, The League School.

Recommended Reading

Amundson S, Weil M: Prewriting and handwriting skills. In Case-Smith J, Allen A, Pratt P, editors: *Occupational therapy for children*, ed 3, St Louis, 1996, Mosby.

Berry J: *Give yourself a hand, an integrated hands skills program*, Framingham, Mass, 1993, Therapro.

Bissell J: *Coping in the classroom: sensory integration special interest section newsletter*, 1991, Bethesda, Md, American Occupational Therapy Association.

Bissell J et al: *Sensory motor handbook: a guide for implementing and modifying activities in the classroom*, ed 2, Tucson, 1998, Therapy Skill Builders.

Bissell J et al: *Trouble-shooting pads: (a) Producing organized written work. (b) Beginning and completing tasks. (c) Sportsmanship & cooperation. (d) Organizing behavior during motor time. (e) Performing tasks while seated. (f) Copying from the blackboard. (g) Cutting with scissors. (h) Writing with pencils. (i) Maintaining order in line. (j) Organizing personal belongings*, Handouts, Tucson, 1998, Therapy Skill Builders.

Bryte K: *Classroom intervention for the school-based therapist*, San Antonio, 1996, Therapy Skill Builders.

Case-Smith J, Allen A, Pratt P, editors: *Occupational therapy for children*, ed 3, St. Louis, 1996, Mosby.

Case-Smith J, Pehoski C: *Development of hand skills in the child*, Bethesda, Md, 1992, American Occupational Therapy Association.

Duran GA, Klenke-Ormiston S: *Multi-play, sensory activities for school readiness*, Tucson, 1994, Therapy Skill Builders.

Early MB, Pedretti L: *Physical dysfunction practice skills for the occupational therapy assistant*, St Louis, 1998, Mosby.

Exner C: Development of hand skills. In Case-Smith J, Allen A, Pratt P, editors: *Occupational therapy for children*, ed 3, St Louis, 1996, Mosby.

Fink B: *Sensory-motor integration activities*, Tucson, 1989, Therapy Skill Builders.

Foti D, Pedretti L, Lillie S: Activities of daily living. In Pedretti L, editor: *Occupational therapy practice skills for physical dysfunction*, ed 4, St Louis, 1998, Mosby.

Ganz J S: *Including SI: a guide to using sensory integration concepts in the school environment*, Bohemia, NY, 1998, Kapable Kids.

Haldy M, Haack L: *Making it easy: sensorimotor activities at home and school*, Tucson, 1995, Therapy Skill Builders.

Henderson A, Pehoski C: *Hand function in the child: foundations for remediation*, St Louis, 1995, Mosby.

Henry D: *Tools for teachers*, Youngtown, Ariz, 1998, Henry Occupational Therapy Services.

Herring KL, Wilkinson S: *Action alphabet, sensorimotor activities for groups*, San Antonio, 1995, Therapy Skill Builders.

Keplinger L: *Movement is fun: a preschool movement program*, Torrance, Calif, 1988, Sensory Integration International.

Levine K: *Fine motor dysfunction: therapeutic strategies in the classroom*, Tucson, 1991, Therapy Skill Builders.

Loiselle L, Shea S: *Curriculum based activities in occupational therapy: an inclusion resource*, Framingham, Mass, 1995, Therapro.

Neistadt ME, Crepeau EB: *Willard & Spackman's occupational therapy*, ed 9, Philadelphia, 1998, Lippincott.

Quirk N, DiMatties M: *The relationship of learning problems & classroom performance to sensory integration*, 1990, Quirk and DiMatties.

Rubell B: *Big strokes for little folks*, San Antonio, 1995, Therapy Skill Builders.

Shepard J, Procter S, Coley I: Self-care & adaptations for independent living. In Case-Smith J, Allen A, Pratt P, editors: *Occupational therapy for children*, ed 3, St Louis, 1996, Mosby.

Sher B: *Different drummers—same song*, San Antonio, 1996, Therapy Skill Builders.

Sher B: *Moving right along*, Hugo, Minn, 1997, PDP Press.

Trombly C, Scott A: *Occupational therapy for physical dysfunction*, Baltimore, 1978, Williams & Wilkins.

Trott M, Laurel M, Windeck S: *Sensibilities: understanding sensory integration*, Tucson, 1993, Therapy Skill Builders.

Tupper LC, Miesner KK: *School hardening: sensory integration strategies for class and home*, San Antonio, 1995, Therapy Skill Builders.

Wilbarger P: The sensory diet: activity programs based on sensory processing theory, *Sensory integration special interest section newsletter*, 18(2), Bethesda, Md, 1995, American Occupational Therapy Association.

Young S, Keplinger L: *Movement is fun: a preschool movement program*, Torrance, Calif, 1988, Sensory Integration International.

REVIEW *Questions*

1. In what ways do activity analysis and reading the child in context help determine intervention strategies for the child with limited independence in ADLs and work and productive activities?
2. In what ways can an occupational therapy practitioner modify the types of limits and verbal cues given to a child to promote positive behaviors and increase self-esteem?
3. Why is s-s-b synchrony important and how would the COTA proceed if the OTR, speech therapist, or parent requested intervention in this area?
4. What are five adapted dressing techniques or devices? What type of child might benefit from using them?
5. Describe some common problems children with disabilities have with hygiene, toileting, and grooming. In what ways can the COTA help address these issues?
6. Describe some activities the COTA might use with a child to promote a functional grasp and controlled handwriting.
7. Describe the three functional pencil grasp patterns. What characteristics are common to all three patterns?
8. What does "separation of the two sides of the hand" mean? How is this related to an early communication skill? Why is separation important for an efficient pencil grasp? What are some activities that help develop separation of the two sides of the hand?
9. In what ways does a COTA work with children in the areas of nutrition, safe mobility, travel in the community, physical fitness, and prevocational skills?
10. Describe the elements that promote functional sitting and support hand, head, and eye function.
11. In what ways can the COTA help children increase their attention span for schoolwork?
12. In what ways can oculomotor problems interfere with communication and school skills?
13. In what ways does the COTA work with the OTR, caregivers, other professionals, and administrators to facilitate children's independence in ADLs and work and productive activities?

SUGGESTED *Activities*

1. Watch a typical child perform an ADL or work or productive activity for 2 minutes. Perform an activity analysis; describe in detail the child's behaviors in response to sensory, motor, cognitive, oculomotor, spatial, social, and environmental demands. How many different behaviors did the child coordinate at one time? Using the same activity analysis, observe a child about the same age who has disabilities. Compare the two children's results.
2. Think of an ADL or work or productive activity for a child. List 8 to 10 directions an adult might give to the child, and incorporate negative words such as "no" or "don't." Change the instructions by using only positive phrases that describe desired behaviors. For example, instead of saying, "Don't yell so much," try "Let's talk in a quiet indoor voice."
3. Using a watch with a second hand, document how often you swallow during a 3-minute period. See how long you can go without swallowing, and describe what happens.
4. Try holding your nose while eating and describe what happens. Try eating without closing your lips and describe what happens.
5. Wearing a thick pair of gloves or mittens, try zipping, buttoning, snapping, buckling, tying a bow, eating with a knife and fork, grooming your hair, and writing a paragraph. In what ways do you compensate for the decreased touch-pressure feedback in your hands? What happens to your motor planning accuracy?
6. Using only one hand, perform your typical bathroom routine, including toileting, showering or bathing, applying deodorant, brushing teeth, and shaving. Which adaptations would make these easier?
7. Imagine you are a child who is able to use only one arm and one leg. Try to dress yourself in clothing with fasteners. Which techniques help you accomplish this? Which are the most difficult parts of the task; why?
8. Grip a pen or pencil tightly against the side of your index finger, keeping your thumb straight and using a lateral grasp (that is, using no thumb opposition). How long are you able to write before this grasp becomes uncomfortable? What does your handwriting look like? If this is your chosen grasp pattern from childhood, what factors influenced this choice and prevented development of a more functional pattern?

9. During a class lecture, look around the room to see in what ways other students are regulating their own levels of arousal. What are they doing with their hands, mouths, eyes, feet, bodies? What do you do to stay focused during a dull presentation? What do you do to calm yourself down before or during a challenging test?

10. Sit on a hard high stool or chair. Do not lean back. Let your arms hang at your sides, and let your feet dangle. Try to stay perfectly still, keeping your head up. Look forward at a visual target. How long are you able to stay comfortable and attentive? List the input or postural changes that might help you. Why do you think these would help?

CHAPTER 13 APPENDIX A

Adapted Clothing Companies

Adrian's Closet
PO Box 9930
Rancho Santa Fe, CA 92067
(800) 831-2577
Fax: (619) 759-0578

Aviano USA
1199-K Avenue
Acaso Camarillo, CA 93012
(805) 484-8138
Fax: (805) 484-9789

eSpecials—Down Syndrome
PO Box 1177
Larkspur, CA 94977
(415) 924-7960
Fax: (415) 927-9043

Kotton Koala
908 West Moffet Creek Road
Fort Jones, CA 96032
(916) 468-5475
Fax: (916) 468-5492

Laurel Designs
5 Laurel Avenue
Belvedere, CA 94920
(415) 435-1891
Fax: (415) 435-1451

Marshons Fashions
PO Box 1848
Calumet City, IL 60409-7848
(708) 849-4610
Fax: (800) 850-4610

MJ Markell Shoe Company
504 Saw Mill River Road
Yonkers, NY 10701
(914) 963-2258
Fax: (914) 963-9293

Plum Enterprises
PO Box 283
Worcester, PA 19490
(800) 321-PLUM
Fax: (610) 584-4151

CHAPTER 13 APPENDIX B

Computer Teaching Resources

AccuCorp, Inc.
PO Box 66
Christiansburg, VA 24073
(703) 961-2001

Aurora Systems
2647 Kingsway
Vancouver, BC V5R 5H4
Canada
(604) 436-2694

Brown Bag Software
2155 South Bascom, Suite 114
Campbell, CA 95008
(408) 559-4545

Bytes of Learning
(800) 465-6428

The Darci Institute of Rehabilitation Engineering
810 West Shepard Lane
Farmington, UT 84025
(801) 451-9191
Fax: (801) 451-9393

Don Johnston Developmental Equipment
PO Box 639
1000 North Rand Road, Building 115
Wauconda, IL 60084
(800) 999-4660

Herzog Keyboarding
1433 East Broadway
Tucson, AZ 85719
(520) 792-2550

Infogrip, Inc.
1141 East Main Street
Ventura, CA 93001
(800) 397-0921

Intelligent Peripheral Devices, Inc.
20380 Town Center Lane, Suite 270
Cupertino, CA 95014
(408) 252-9400

Intellitools, Inc.
55 Leveroni Court, Suite 9
Novato, CA 94949
(800) 899-6687

Interplay/Brainstorm
(800) 428-8200

Keytime
4516 Northeast 54th Street
Seattle, WA 98052
(800) 876-4726

Knowledge Adventure
1311 Grand Central Avenue
Glendale, CA 91201
(800) 542-4240

Macintosh/Apple Computer Systems
(800) SOS-APPL
PO Box 4040
Cupertino, CA 95014-4040
Website: *www.apple.com*

Madenta Communications, Inc.
9411A-20 Avenue
Edmonton, Alberta T6N 1E5
Canada
(800) 661-8406

Microsoft Corporation
One Microsoft Way
Redmond, WA 98052
(800) 876-4726

Microsystems Software
600 Worcester Road
Framingham, MA 01701
(508) 626-8511

NTS Computer Systems, Ltd.
(800) 663-7163

Perfect Solutions
(561) 790-1070

CHAPTER 13 APPENDIX B

Computer Teaching Resources—cont'd

Prentke Romich
1022 Heyl Road
Wooster, OH 44691
(800) 262-1984

Sierra Originals
Sierra On-Line, Inc.
Bellevue, WA 98007

Software Toolworks
(415) 883-3000

Sunburst Communications, Inc
101 Castleton Street
Pleasantville, NY
(800) 786-3155
(800) 321-7511

Thompson Learning Tools
(800) 354-9706

Words+ Inc.
PO Box 1229
Lancaster, CA 93534
(805) 949-8331

CHAPTER 13 APPENDIX C

Adapted Equipment Companies

ABC School Supply, Inc.
3312 North Berkeley Lake Road
Box 100019
Duluth, GA 30096-9419
(800) 669-4222

Achievement Products
PO Box 9033
Canton, OH 44711
(800) 373-4699
Fax: (216) 453-0222

All the Write News
Dixon Ticonderoga Co.
PO Box 67096
Los Angeles, CA 90067
(888) 736-4747
Fax: (888) 329-4747

**Attainment Company for Children
and Adults with Special Needs**
PO Box 930160
Verona, WI 53593-0160
(800) 327-4269

Benik Corporation
9465 Provost Rd NW #204
Silverdale, WA 98383
(800) 442-8910
Fax: (360) 692-5600

Best Priced Products, Inc.
PO Box 1174
White Plains, NY 10602
(800) 824-2939

Callirobics
PO Box 6634
Charlottesville, VA 22906
(800) 769-2891
Fax: (804) 293-9008

Cross Creek
PO Box 289
Millbrook, NY 12545
(800) 645-5816
Fax: (914) 677-9293

Different Roads to Learning, LLC
12 West 18th Street, Suite 3 East
New York, NY 10011

Early Learning Materials
ABC School Supply, Inc.
6500 Peachtree Industrial Blvd.
PO Box 4750
Norcross, GA 30091
(800) 247-6623

Equipment Shop
PO Box 33
Bedford, MA 01730
(800) 525-7681

Flaghouse, Inc.
150 North MacQuesten Parkway
Mount Vernon, NY 10550
(800) 221-5185

Free Spirit Publishing, Inc.
400 First Avenue North, Suite 616
Minneapolis, MN 55401-1724
(800) 735-7323
Fax: (612) 337-5050

Handwriting without Tears
8802 Quiet Stream Court
Potomac, MD 20854
(301) 983-8409
Fax: (301) 983-6821

Imaginart
307 Arizona Street
Bisbee, AZ 85603
(800) 737-1376

Jump-In
1035 Moon Lake Court
Pinckney, MI 48169
(734) 878-0166
Fax: (734) 878-0169

CHAPTER 13 APPENDIX C

Adapted Equipment Companies—cont'd

Kapable Kids
PO Box 250
Bohemia, NY 11716
(800) 356-1564
Fax: (516) 563-7179

The Lockfast Co.
109-04 Deerfield Road
Cincinnati, OH 45242
(800) 543-7157
Fax: (513) 891-5836

MADDAK, Ableware
Pequannock, NJ 07440-1993
(201) 628-7600

Maxanna Learning Systems
9 Greensboro Road
Hanover, NH 03755
(603) 643-9225
Fax: (603) 643-3923

Mealtimes/New Visions
Route 1, Box 175-S
Farber, VA 22938
(804) 361-2285

Milani Foods
2525 West Armitage Avenue
Melrose Park, IL 60160
(708) 450-3354

North Coast Medical
18305 Sutter Boulevard
Morgan Hill, CA 95037-9946
(800) 821-9319
Fax: (877) 213-9300

OT Ideas
124 Morris Turnpike
Randolph, NJ 07869
(973) 895-3622

Oriental Trading Company, Inc.
PO Box 2308
Omaha, NE 68103-2308
(800) 228-2269
Fax: (800) 327-8904

Orvis Fly Fishing Outfitters
PO Box 2861
Vail, CO 81658
(970) 476-3474

PDP Products
14398 North 59th Street
Oak Park Heights, MN 55082
(612) 439-8865

The Pencil Grip
PO Box 67096
Los Angeles, CA 90067
(888) PEN-GRIP
Fax: (310) 315-0607

Pocket Full of Therapy
PO Box 174
Morganville, NJ 07751
(800) PFOT-124

Pro Ed
8700 Shoal Creek Boulevard
Austin, TX 78757-6897
(800) 897-3202
Fax: (800) FXPROED

Rifton
PO Box 901
Rifton, NY 12471-0901
(800) 374-3866

Sammons Preston/Tumble Forms
PO Box 5071
Bolingbrook, IL 60440-5071
(800) 323-5547

Slosson Educational Publications, Inc.
PO Box 280
East Aurora, NY 14052-0280
(888) 756-7766
Fax: (800) 655-3840

Smith & Nephew, Inc.
1 Quality Dr
PO Box 1005
Germantown, WI 53022-8205
(800) 558-7681

CHAPTER 13 APPENDIX C

Adapted Equipment Companies—cont'd

Southpaw Enterprises
PO Box 1047
Dayton, OH 45401-1047
(800) 228-1698
Fax: (937) 252-8502

Sportime Abilitations
1 Sportime Way
Atlanta, GA 30340
(800) 850-8602
Fax: (800) 845-1535

Stanfield Publishing Co.
PO Box 41058
Santa Barbara, CA 93140
(800) 421-6534

TFH (USA) Ltd.
4537 Gibsonia Road
Gibsonia, RI 15044
(412) 444-6400

TherAdapt Products, Inc.
17 West 163 Oak Lane
Bensenville, IL 60106
(800)261-4919
Fax: (630) 834-2478

Therapro
225 Arlington Street
Framingham, MA 01702-8723
(800) 257-5376
Fax: (888) 860-6254

Therapy Skill Builders
(Division of the Psychological Corporation)
355 Academic Court
San Antonio, TX 78204-2498
(800) 211-8378
Fax: (800) 232-1223

Therapy Shoppe
4445-B Breton Rd, Southeast, Suite 226
Grand Rapids, MI 49508
(800) 261-5590

Toys to Grow On
Lakeshore Curriculum Materials
2695 East Dominique Street
PO Box 17
Long Beach, CA 90801
(800) 542-8338

Velvasoft
MW Sales and Service, Inc.
7730 Marigold Trace
San Antonio, TX 78233
(210) 656-5228
Fax: (210) 656-1150

CHAPTER 13 APPENDIX D

Workshop Sponsors for Continuing Education

AOTA
4720 Montgomery Lane
PO Box 31220
Bethesda, MD 20824-1220
(800) 729-2682

Boehme Workshops
8642 North 66th Street
Milwaukee, WI 53223
(414) 355-8744
Fax: (414) 355-6837

Clinical Developmental Seminars
6407 Overbrook Avenue
Philadelphia, PA 19151
(215) 879-2929
Fax: (215) 879-9979

Continuing Education Programs of America
PO Box 52
Peoria, IL 61650
(309) 263-0310

Dove Rehabilitation Services
3305 Jerusalem Avenue
Wantaugh, NY 11793
(516) 679-3683

Education Resources
266 Main Street, Suite 12
Medfield, MA 02052
(800) 487-6530

North American Riders for the Handicapped Association
PO Box 33150
Denver, CO 80234
(303) 452-1212

Occupational Therapy Associates
124 Watertown Street
Watertown, MA 02472
(617) 923-4410

OT Kids, Inc
PO Box 1118
Homer, AK 99603
(907) 235-0688
Fax: (907) 235-0688

Professional Development Programs
14398 North 59th Street
Oak Park Heights, MN 55082
(612) 439-8865
Fax: (612) 439-0421

Sensory Integration International
1514 Cabrillo Avenue
Torrance, CA 90501
(310) 320-9986
Fax: (310) 320-9982

Vital Sounds
PO Box 46344
Madison, WI 53744
(608) 278-9330
Fax: (608) 278-9363

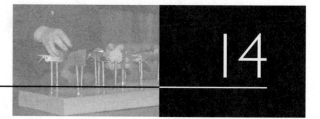

Play

JANE CLIFFORD O'BRIEN

After studying this chapter, the reader will be able to accomplish the following:

- Describe the characteristics of play and playfulness and differentiate between the two
- Describe ways to facilitate play and playfulness in children with special needs
- Describe the way play is used as a tool in therapy sessions to increase skills
- Describe how play is used as a goal of occupational therapy
- Identify occupational therapy assessments used to evaluate play and playfulness
- Describe techniques that promote play and playfulness

KEY TERMS

CHAPTER OUTLINE

Think about a time in your childhood when you were playing.

What were you doing?
Who was with you?
Where were you?
How did you feel?
What was the expression on your face?
What did you learn?
Was playing an important aspect of your day?

Perhaps you are thinking about a time you and your friends sat on your grandmother's porch and played house. Maybe you were playing school. Recalling these moments brings many happy memories to mind. People remember laughing, making friends, learning and testing skills (such as who could jump the highest), problem solving, and negotiating. These skills are critical to a child's development and provide a foundation for the future.

Children learn motor, social-emotional, language, and cognitive skills through play.* To illustrate this fact, consider a 12-month-old girl playing in the water sprinkler. The child bends down to feel the cool water in her hand. She is practicing motor planning, squatting, and balancing while receiving a tactile sensation of the water on her hands. As she cups her hands on the sprinkler, she must coordinate her tiny fingers to grasp the nozzle. Cognitively, she pays attention to the water and tries to figure out what happens when she changes her hand position. She is learning the ways liquid differs from the solid ground on which she stands. She problem solves to keep the water in her hands and tries to understand the reason it leaks through. Orally, she feels the water on her tongue and swallows the droplets. She sticks her tongue out and gathers the liquid in her throat to swallow it. Her 4-year-old brother joins the play activity, and now she must share the sprinkler. He laughs and jumps. She watches and smiles and tries to imitate his skills. She is developing social skills. The children repeat the play activities. By watching them it becomes clear that play requires many skills.

Children learn and refine skills during play.† This is demonstrated as children show off feats of strength and agility, problem solve to play a game or perform a motor skill, and work out problems that arise. They communicate to satisfy their needs and decide on rules for the activities by negotiating with group members. Often children spend the entire playtime deciding on the rules of the game or the way the story will unfold. They use their

---

*References 1, 5, 21, 24, 33, 34.
†References 1, 4, 5, 10, 13, 19.

language skills and must become keen observers of nonverbal communication.[5,8]

Maximizing a child's ability to play interests occupational therapy practitioners because play is the primary occupation of childhood and critical to the development of skills.[8,20,27] To appreciate its importance, imagine life without play. Life would certainly be lacking without play. Parham and Primeau underscored the importance of play by stating that play may reveal what makes life worth living.[31]

With this appreciation of the importance of play, imagine making a difference in a child's ability to play. Developing a child's play skills comprehensively affects both the child and the child's family. The child is better able to interact with friends, family, and the environment.

Occupational therapy practitioners work with children to enhance their ability to play and therefore make a difference in children's lives.

PLAY

Most adults smile when asked to remember a time they were playing. They reminisce about childhood memories of favorite toys and activities. They laugh and relate humorous stories such as the time they attempted to jump over a ditch and failed and fell into the mud. They remember being lost in the woods, falling into the water, having mud fights, and conducting elaborate neighborhood play events. Adults recall historic events such as pretending they were astronauts landing on the moon. They are able to describe the activities, feelings, and skills they gained during play. Most agree that play was and still is fun!

Play is generally defined as a pleasurable, self-initiated activity of which the child is in control. **Intrinsic motivation** is the self-initiation or drive to action that is rewarded by the activity itself, rather than some external reward.[8] Intrinsic motivation is demonstrated when children repeat activities over and over.[8] **Internal control** is the extent to which a child is in control of the actions and to some degree the outcome of an activity.[8] Internal control is observed when children spontaneously change the play (for example, when a 6-year-old boy declares in the middle of a pretend game, "Now I am going to be the good guy.") Intrinsic motivation and internal control are important for the development of problem solving, learning, and socialization skills.

Another element of play is the **freedom to suspend reality,** which is sometimes seen as the ability to participate in make-believe activities, or **pretend play**[8] (Figure 14-1). Pretend play develops as children are able to engage in higher cognitive functioning.[33] Children begin by role playing simple everyday actions such as feeding a doll. They are able to engage in elaborate, make believe scenarios as their language and cognitive skills develop.

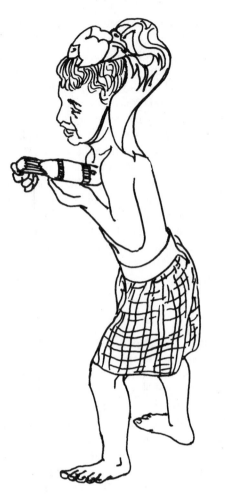

FIGURE 14-1   Pretend play allows children to break free from rules.

Freedom to suspend reality also includes teasing, joking, mischief, and bending the rules.[8] Children turn old games into new ones by changing the rules, creating new situations, and using objects imaginatively during play.

CLINICAL *Pearl*

Occupational therapy practitioners can evaluate the characteristics of play to design intervention. Emphasis is placed on using the child's strengths to improve weak areas. For example, a child who is highly motivated to play but lacks the needed physical skills may be encouraged to perform activities in an alternative way. A child who focuses on the end product versus the process of play (winning the game, for example) may benefit from participating in play activities that have no end product such as imaginative play.

Play is the primary occupation of children and a medium for intervention.* Play affords skillful occupational therapy practitioners unlimited opportunities to teach, refine, or enable more successful functioning and play.

PLAYFULNESS

Playfulness is the disposition to play.[4,9] It is a style individuals use to flexibly approach problems and can be regarded as an aspect of a child's personality.[9] Playfulness, like play, encompasses intrinsic motivation, internal control, and freedom to suspend reality, all of which occur on a continuum.[8,15,24,27]

Children who are engaged in the play process are intrinsically motivated. They show signs of enjoyment and seem to be having fun.[8] Internal control is evidenced in sharing, playing with others, entering new play situations, initiating play, deciding, modifying activities, and challenging themselves.[8] Children who use objects creatively or in unconventional ways, tease, and pretend show the element of freedom to suspend reality.[8]

Children lacking playfulness exhibit problems fulfilling their roles as players. For example, Sam is a 6-year-old boy with sensory integrative dysfunction. He has difficulty with motor tasks and does not play well with friends. Sam is not spontaneous in activities. He requires time to plan the way he will accomplish motor tasks. Sam becomes very upset when he does not get his way. Sam does not like the rules to change and has trouble changing pace once involved in an activity. Moreover, he does not read the other children's cues and frequently plays roughly. He shows poor body awareness by getting too close to the other children. Sam does not initiate play with his peers. His slow and awkward movements cause him to lag behind. Sam states during the occupational therapy evaluation that he has no friends and no one likes him. His parents are worried that Sam does not have any friends. The goal of his occupational therapy sessions is to improve Sam's playfulness so that he can interact with friends at home, at school, and in the community.

The occupational therapy practitioner works to develop a rapport with Sam and plans fun and playful activities. Sam does not initiate play activities but is cooperative and attempts all activities. The occupational therapy practitioner strives to see the child have fun and be spontaneous during the therapy sessions hoping that this behavior extends to home and school.

*References 9, 16, 20, 27, 32, 33.

During one session the occupational therapy practitioner and Sam engage in a game of Star Wars. *Sam is Darth Vader and runs after the practitioner saying, "I will get you, Luke." The occupational therapy practitioner is thrilled that Sam is initiating play. However, shortly thereafter Sam stops playing, looks at the practitioner, and says, "Is it time to go yet?"*

Sam exhibits a low level of playfulness. He is not engaged in sustained intense enjoyment. He focuses on the end product (completing therapy) rather than being intrinsically motivated to play. Poor internal control is characterized by an inability to enter new play situations, initiate play with peers, share, decide what to do, or challenge himself. Sam is able to engage in pretend play when acting out Star Wars *with the occupational therapy practitioner, but has difficulty reading others' cues, which is evident when he plays too roughly and gets too close to his peers during interactions.*

Considering Sam's limitations and the long-term goal that he be able to play with peers, Sam's therapy objectives include the following:

1. *Spontaneously initiate a change in activity at least 3 times during a 45-minute, supervised play situation.*
2. *Respond positively (smile, cooperate with the occupational therapy practitioner) when he does not get his way at least 3 times during a supervised play situation.*
3. *Enter a group of peers already playing on the playground and participate in the activity without interrupting the play at least 3 times a week.*
4. *Engage in a motor challenge during play at least 3 times during a supervised play situation.*

Framing situations as play allows children to know what play is so that they may interact accordingly. They are free to pretend, challenge each other, and tease without malice. All of these actions require that children read nonverbal and verbal cues. Reading nonverbal cues allows children to realize when they have pushed a boundary too far during play.

Scott and Alison are playing in a sandbox pouring sand on each other. They laugh and watch for cues from each other that say, "This is okay. We are still playing." The game continues, and Alison begins to pour sand on Scott's head. She receives a serious look from Scott. The nonverbal cue says, "Hey, that is a little too close to my eyes. I do not like that." Alison responds with a smile that says, "Oops! I'm sorry," and pours sand on Scott's arm instead. Her nonverbal response says, "Okay, I'll be more careful." This exchange of cues allows the play to continue while they learn to be attentive to each other. They are learning the rules and boundaries of play.

Assessment of a child's playfulness provides information about the way the child processes, problem solves, and manages emotional stress. These skills are important to the child's development and social well being.

NATURE OF PLAY AND PLAYFULNESS

Occupational therapy practitioners must understand the nature of play and playfulness to use play effectively as an intervention technique. When children play and are playful they may laugh, smile, and be active. They may also be serious, quiet, and totally absorbed in play depending on the activity. Play can be frustrating and it can involve failures. The flexible and spontaneous nature of play and playfulness is demonstrated when children change themes or use toys in unpredictable ways.

The process (doing) rather than the product (outcome) provides the primary source of the reward in play activities.[8] Children engage in play for the sake of play itself.[9] Playful children discover, create, and explore. Thus no way of playing is right or wrong. Playing is a safe outlet for children to challenge themselves and helps them develop skills.

Occupational therapy practitioners must remember to maintain the nature of play and playfulness during therapy. Children with special needs may require additional assistance to play.[23] Occupational therapy practitioners are knowledgeable about the abilities of children with special needs and are therefore in an ideal position to promote play and playfulness.

CONSIDERATIONS FOR PLAY

The normal sequence of the development of play is often delayed in children with special needs.* (See Chapter 7 for a discussion of this sequence.) This may be a result of limited physical, cognitive, or social-emotional skills.[19,21,25] For example, a young girl unable to bring her hands to her mouth has trouble exploring her environment. Children who are unable to experience sensations in a normal manner often require intervention to engage in normal play opportunities, which stimulate their growth and development. If children are not afforded these opportunities they may exhibit poor play skills.[25,29] Children with special needs may require environmental

---

*References 17, 19, 21, 23, 25, 28.

and play adaptations and intervention to provide them with these experiences.[25,28,29] For example, children who are unable to sit independently may benefit from sitting in an adapted chair. This way they can interact and play at the same level as their peers without fear of falling over.[29]

CLINICAL *Pearl*

Children play in various positions. Occupational therapy practitioners make sure that children with special needs spend time in many positions such as supine, quadruped, sitting, and standing. Playtime is not the time to work on positioning. Children should be free to use their arms and hands and feel safe.

Children with special needs require time to develop their abilities. They may take longer to respond, make less obvious responses, initiate activities less frequently, and be less interactive than other children.[23,28] Researchers and theorists report that children with special needs are often passive in their play.[21,23,25] In cases involving children with mental retardation, children have been described as exhibiting a restricted repertoire of play and language, decreased attention span, and less social interaction during play.[21,23,25] In cases involving children with autism, children are described as demonstrating more stereotypical movements and less diversity in play.[21] Children with visual impairments are less interested in reaching out to explore and in engage in social exchanges during play.[21] Children with hearing impairments show less symbolic and less organized play.[21]

Children with special needs require assistance to meet developmental challenges and learn ways to play.[21,23,25,28] Occupational therapy practitioners must understand typical play patterns and support children when teaching skills and facilitating play. For example, occupational therapy practitioners can increase **spontaneity** in children by allowing them to discover play materials that have been hidden or placed within reach.[11,25,28]

Occupational therapy practitioners must identify the child's strengths and weaknesses, as well as the family's, to design effective intervention. Capitalizing on strengths can increase the success of therapy and facilitate advanced play skills.

RELEVANCE OF PLAY

Twelve-month-old Frankie cannot sit up because of hydrocephalus and poor trunk tone. He is nonverbal. He can move his arms, but he is unable to reach and grasp objects. He occasionally smiles and laughs. His vision is poor. The occupational therapy practitioner places a mercury switch attached to a flashlight on his arm after positioning him. If he raises his arm the flashlight lights up in his face. Frankie raises his arm soon after the switch is placed on his arm and smiles when the flashlight lights up in his face. He puts his arm down and the light turns off. Frankie laughs and laughs. He repeats this activity numerous times. It is evident that he realizes he is in control of the light. His mother has tears in her eyes. She turns to the practitioner and says, "Frankie is playing."

Occupational therapy changed this family's perception of Frankie by showing them his ability to play. Play is both a powerful tool and an important outcome in occupational therapy.

CLINICAL *Pearl*

Observe the child's movements when deciding where to position a switch. Place the switch where the child can activate it by using movement patterns he uses automatically. This promotes play and provides the child with control and immediate success.

Occupational therapy practitioners work with family, educators, and other professionals to improve the quality of life for children and their families. Play is vital to a child's development and an important outcome of intervention. Occupational therapy practitioners who use play may be faced with parents and professionals who do not take them seriously.[7,9,16] Engaging the parents in discussions from the beginning educates them about the importance of play during therapy sessions. Practitioners should discuss with parents how the session went and the progress made toward the goals. Occupational therapy practitioners who recognize that the parents do not value play as a goal may decide to emphasize the use of play as a tool to increase the child's skills in other areas. Professionals may take occupational therapy practitioners more seriously once they see the progress a child makes in therapy. Practitioners may frequently need to educate parents and professionals as to the purpose of the use of play.

Activities recommended for home should be limited to those that are fun and nonthreatening for the child to promote play and playfulness. The child can engage in activities where he can show off his abilities to his parents. This is motivating for both the child and the parents. Occupational therapy practitioners investigate the role of play in the child's life and focus on providing the child with a means to play.

Play as a Tool

Play is often used as a tool to increase skill development. Therapy is designed around play activities that will increase skills such as strength, motor planning, problem solving, grasping, and handwriting necessary for the child to function. Using play as a tool to improve a child's ability to function has many advantages. Children typically cooperate and readily engage in play. Most goals can be addressed during a play session because play encompasses a variety of activities.

The characteristics of play (that is, intrinsic motivation, internal control, and suspension of reality) need to be present when using play as a tool to improve a child's skills. These characteristics occur within the framework of a play setting. The occupational therapy practitioner arranges the environment so that children choose activities that help them meet their goals while having fun. The practitioner allows the child to tease, engage in mischief, and face challenges.

CLINICAL *Pearl*

Many household items make novel toys for the clinic and can also be used at home. Pots and pans can be musical instruments, containers, or even hats. They promote pretend play. Use cardboard boxes, grocery bags, and laundry baskets for a variety of play activities. Bring them into the clinic to allow children to explore and create (Figure 14-2).

Making therapy sessions fun through play is not always easy. Occupational therapy practitioners must set up an environment to encourage the child to choose activities that foster therapy goals. This is considered the *art* of therapy.[2,9] The occupational therapy practitioner sets up the just *right* challenge, which is one that is neither too hard nor too easy.[2,9] The occupational therapy practitioner must know the child's strengths and weaknesses to do this effectively. Some children are competitive and enjoy such games. Other children fear failure and may be easily intimidated by competitive games. Some children enjoy roughhousing and others do not. Making a therapy session fun means observing a child's subtle cues and spontaneously adapting the session to maintain a level of excitement and motivation.

A physically and emotionally safe environment allows the child to feel in control. The occupational therapy practitioner designs activities to target specific skills. The child is only aware that the activity is fun. Often the practitioner may need to discreetly change the way the task is performed to get the maximum benefit from the activity. This must be done playfully to keep the flow of the play session going.[15] Sometimes practice of a skill takes priority over playing.

A critical element of play is that activities are free from rules. This does not mean that rules are not present in play activities but that they are negotiable. Children may make up new rules and change them during play. Occupational therapy practitioners should provide enough rules for children to feel secure and safe without imposing so many rules that the children do not feel free to play. Both the child and practitioner must have the freedom to change the activity. Thus if a child is performing an activity that does not promote the therapy goals, the practitioner can modify the challenge. This is illustrated in a therapy session challenging David's balance.

David is kneeling on a platform swing and propelling it forward and back. The practitioner increases the skill level required by saying, "Oh, here come the asteroids," and throwing large balls under the swing. David looks at the occupational therapy practitioner, smiles, and says, "Hey, no fair, I didn't know that was coming." The practitioner responds, "The asteroids came out of nowhere! Luckily you are Superman and were able to stay on the space ship!" The changes are skillfully made so that the session remains playful.

CLINICAL *Pearl*

Children love to swing. Remember that swings are not just for children with sensory integrative dysfunction. Many children benefit from the sensations and movement patterns that accompany swinging.

Children can imagine a therapy session to be a space ship ride, an Olympic quest, a deep-sea diving expedition, a skiing event, or a leisurely stroll down the alley. Through pretend play the child gains skills in imagination, verbalization, and communication. Pretend play allows the practitioner to use the same equipment in countless ways that tap into the child's imagination. Teasing, joking, and mischief are parts of play. The child may teasingly throw a softball to hit the practitioner's head. They may joke that the occupational therapy practitioner can not perform a skill. Children develop their sense of humor during play.

Play provides an excellent tool for intervention when used correctly because children are highly motivated to participate.*

---

*References 9, 10, 11, 16, 21, 26, 28.

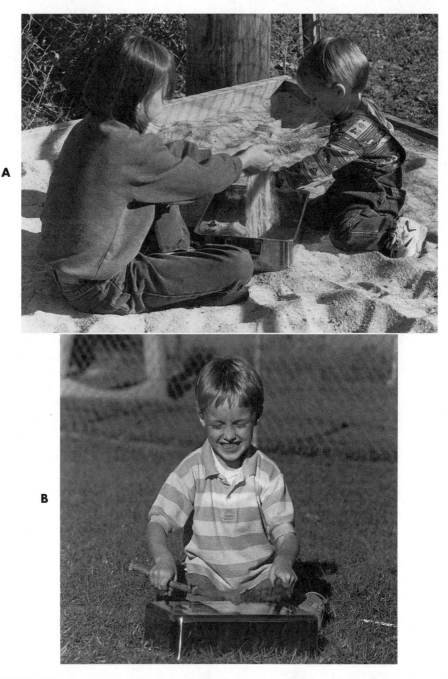

FIGURE 14-2   Everyday household objects allow for pretend play and creativity. **A,** A brother and sister are using a stainless-steel cake pan to build sandcastles. **B,** The same cake pan has now been turned upside down and, with some sticks from the yard, is being used as a drum.

Angie is a 2-year-old girl with hemiplegia on the right side of her body. She lives with her two brothers, ages 8 and 9, and her parents. Angie attends day-care daily. She receives occupational therapy services for 1 hour weekly. Her parents report she does not play well with other children. She grabs their toys, pushes them, and screams to have her needs met. She does not like to be touched on her right side and does little weightbearing on this side. Angie has a difficult time engaging in play activities. She screams and cries when the practitioner touches her on the right arm. She does not initiate play. Angie exhibits decreased active range of motion (AROM) in her right arm.

The occupational therapy practitioner designs treatment that involves play to increase Angie's use of her right side. (See Chapter 7 for a description of the sequence and development of typical play and useful information for designing this type of intervention.) The occupational therapy practitioner considers Angie's age when choosing the play activities. Based on knowledge of 2-year-old children, the practitioner chooses active and messy play activities. According to Parten, 2 year olds usually participate in solitary play but do make some effort to interact with other children.[33] The practitioner notes that 2-year-old children enjoy sensory activities such as playing in sandboxes, water play, and working with Play Doh. They also enjoy manipulative toys such as Legos, pop-up toys, and blocks, and gross motor toys such as balls, riding toys, and swings. Table 7-1 includes a list of suitable toys and activities for various ages.

The child's age and gender, the setting, and the concerns of the parents must be considered when writing goals and objectives of therapy. The occupational therapy practitioner considers the child's physical capabilities and the factors interfering with her ability to play. Angie has right-sided hypersensitivity. She is not weight bearing on the right side. Considering Angie's limitations and the long-term goal that she will use her right hand spontaneously for bimanual activities, Angie's therapy objectives include the following:

1. She will spontaneously reach for objects placed above her head with her right hand at least five times during a 45-minute therapy session.
2. Using two hands, she will catch a 20-inch ball tossed underhand from two feet away at least three times in a 45-minute session.
3. She will walk at least ten feet while holding on with both hands to a push toy such as a shopping cart.
4. She will use both hands to take apart small objects such as pop-beads.

BOX 14-1

Sample Objectives When Play is the Tool for Occupational Therapy Intervention

- Child will catch a large object such as a beach ball, with both hands at least five times when it is thrown directly from three feet away.
- Child will utilize a neat pincer grip to pick up ten small objects for use in daily activity.
- Child will ride a bike at least 20 yards in a straight line without falling.
- Child will make at least three out of ten baskets from the free-throw line.
- Child will put on and button a shirt independently.

Box 14-1 contains sample objectives involving play as a tool for occupational therapy intervention.

CLINICAL *Pearl*

Children love little packages. Wrap little items in small boxes and allow the children to unwrap them to work on fine motor skills through play. Have them wrap up surprises for other children as a fun way to work on hand skills.

The practitioner designs play activities that incorporate the use of Angie's right side. She plays games rolling a large ball, wheelbarrow racing, and climbing a ladder. She pulls pop beads apart, dresses baby dolls, pours sand and water into containers, and makes confetti out of newspaper. The activities all require Angie to use both arms. The practitioner stages the activities so that Angie is successful. The occupational therapy practitioner frequently provides Angie with hand-over-hand assistance. The occupational therapy practitioner watches for cues from Angie when placing a hand on Angie's arms. The practitioner uses humor and laughter to keep the session playful. Treatment focuses on keeping the atmosphere fun and playful while increasing the functional use of Angie's right arm. The emphasis of the treatment session is to promote bilateral hand skill development. The occupational therapy practitioner assists Angie in using her right hand during play.

Table 14-1 lists toys associated with the development of specific performance components. Angie's case demonstrates the use of play as a tool to improve a child's physical skills. The practitioner uses play activities to increase the ability of the child to use her right side.

TABLE 14-1

Toys and Play Activities Designed to Target Selected Performance Components

PERFORMANCE COMPONENT	TOYS AND ACTIVITIES
SENSORIMOTOR	
Sensory	
Sensory awareness and sensory processing	
Tactile	Water play, massage, Play Doh, koosh balls, glue, beans, sand play, tactile boards, brushing, lotion games, stickers
Proprioceptive	Trampolines, jumping, pulling on ropes, climbing ladders, tug-of-war, pulling a wagon, wheel-barrow walking, pushing
Vestibular	Riding a bike, skateboarding, see-saw, sliding, swinging, Sit and Spin, rocking horse
Visual	Mobiles, toys that move, bright colored rattles and toys, mirrors
Auditory	Musical toys, bells, rattles, tape recorders, songs
Gustatory	Foods, gums, candy
Olfactory	Smelly markers, Play Doh, smelly stickers, food
Perceptual processing	Puzzles, building blocks, doll houses, farms, building logs, model cars and airplanes, paper dolls, coloring books, mazes, computer games, dress-up, obstacle courses, Simon Says, Follow-the-Leader
Neuromusculoskeletal	
Strength	Ball games, bike riding, manipulative games, jump-rope, Red-Rover, London Bridge, swimming, sports
Endurance	Repetitive games, walking, sports, hiking, swimming, bike riding climbing
Postural control	Trampolines, bike riding, sports, swimming, climbing, walking an uneven trail
Motor	
Gross coordination	Outdoor playground equipment, bikes, sports, water, outdoor play
Fine motor	Manipulative, arts and crafts, small toys, figurines, dolls, dress up, sewing, coloring, cutting
Oral motor	Musical instruments, whistles, bubble blowers, pinwheels
COGNITIVE	
Memory, sequencing	Board games (for example, Memory, Clue, Monopoly, Candy Land)
Categorization	Card games (for example, Hearts, Go Fish), sorting, matching games
Spacial operations	Puzzles, models, arts and crafts, Legos, Lincoln Logs
Problem solving	Board games, card games, arts and crafts, puzzles
PSYCHOLOGICAL	
Psychological	Self-esteem board games, art projects, motor challenges
Social	
Interpersonal	Pictionary, team games, Twister, new games
Self-expression	Arts and crafts, pottery, clay, dance
Self-management	
Coping skills	Monopoly, life skills game, role playing

Modified from American Occupational Therapy Association: Uniform terminology for occupational therapy, *Am J Occup Ther* 48(11):1047, 1994.

BOX 14-2

Sample Objectives When Play or Playfulness Is the Intended Outcome of Occupational Therapy Intervention

- Child will initiate one new activity during an adult-supervised play session.
- Child will enter into a play activity (already in progress) without disrupting the group during an adult supervised play session.
- Child will stay with the same basic play theme for at least fifteen minutes during an adult supervised play session.
- Child will use an object in an unconventional manner spontaneously at least once during an adult supervised play session.
- Child will share toys with another child (trading toys at least three times) during a fifteen-minute play session.

Play as a Goal

Occupational therapy practitioners must be careful to avoid "teaching" play. Practitioners model play, cultivate skills needed for play, and set up the environment to facilitate play. Occupational therapy practitioners must ensure that play is enjoyable. Increasing the skills required to play is important and beneficial to the child.

Occupational therapy practitioners must maintain the quality of play.[9,20,32] A child who has the skills needed for play but does not engage in spontaneous and intrinsically motivated activity is at risk. That child may show deficits in play that will carry over to school, home, and the community. Play deficits in childhood may inhibit a child's ability to gain needed skills for adulthood.* Therefore it is important for occupational therapy practitioners to target play as a goal of therapy.

The occupational therapy practitioner emphasizes the child's approach to activities and the manner in which the child plays when play is the goal of therapy. If play is viewed as a goal of therapy, rather than merely a tool of intervention, the practitioner notices the way Angie engages in play, not only whether she uses her right hand to manipulate a toy. A short-term objective to increase Angie's play might be for her to spontaneously initiate play with a peer at least three times during an adult supervised play session. Box 14-2 contains sample objectives when play is the goal of occupational therapy intervention.

Angie's occupational therapy sessions include playmates because she needs assistance playing with others. The practitioner designs the environment to encourage Angie to respond to changes and be spontaneous. Angie participates in bilateral activities such as playing with balls, wheelbarrow racing, and ladder climbing. The practitioner provides a playful attitude while allowing Angie to pick the activities and choose the way she will perform them.

The practitioner facilitates sharing, negotiating, and taking turns. The occupational therapy practitioner encourages the child's parents and teachers to facilitate the skills of sharing, negotiating, and taking turns at home and school, providing Angie with many opportunities to improve her play skills.

CLINICAL *Pearl*

Invite another child or practitioner to keep the play sessions exciting. This is a great way to learn new activities and methods for playing.

*Angie's second session differs from the first session, which targeted the use of Angie's right hand, in that the emphasis is now on both interaction and motor skills, as opposed to motor skills alone. The occupational therapy practitioner pays close attention to Angie's ability to engage in spontaneous activity, choose a variety of tasks, initiate changes, and read the cues of her peers. The Test of Playfulness (ToP) is used as a framework for the observation, evaluation, and documentation of playfulness.[8] (O'Brien and others were able to design **play goals** after a parental interview and a 30-minute observation of free play using the ToP as a guide.[30])*

It is possible to use play as both a tool for therapy and as a goal of therapy sessions. In Angie's case, it would be appropriate to work on increasing the use of her right side as well as on improving play. This takes skill on the part of the occupational therapy practitioner. The practitioner must have the trust of the child and read the child's cues very carefully to maintain the child's engagement in play.

*References 10, 12-14, 19, 22, 32.

ROLE OF OTR AND COTA DURING PLAY ASSESSMENT

Observation of children during play provides occupational therapy practitioners with important information. **Play assessment,** in combination with a parent, child, and teacher interview, provides the practitioner with necessary information. Bryze supported the contributions of narratives in collecting information on play.[6] These narratives focus on the interviewing of parents, caregivers, and children.

Occupational therapy practitioners use a variety of play assessments when working with children with special needs. (See Chapter 14 Appendix A for descriptions of several play assessments.) The OTR is responsible for the evaluation and analysis of information when evaluating play but can delegate portions of the assessment to the COTA. COTAs can assist in interviewing the teachers and caregivers and observing the children during play. The occupational therapy practitioner uses the results of the play assessments to design therapy goals and provide effective intervention. Play assessments provide a foundation for organizing information.

TECHNIQUES TO PROMOTE PLAY AND PLAYFULNESS

There is an art and science to fully utilizing play in occupational therapy practice. Just as with any treatment, occupational therapy practitioners must practice the techniques. The science of using play involves understanding the characteristics, components, and settings that facilitate play. Occupational therapy practitioners must identify the desired outcome of therapy and evaluate the motor, psychological, or social factors interfering with the child's ability to play.

Creating a therapeutic environment involves analyzing a child's skills and determining the way to adapt activities. Knowledge of the development of motor, cognitive, language, social-emotional, and play skills of children is essential to designing effective treatment. Examination of the environment and knowledge of the child's culture helps occupational therapy practitioners determine appropriate play activities.

Therapy using play requires occupational therapy practitioners to find the child within themselves. Playful practitioners practice play and are able to support the child's playful nature. Clinical expertise in the therapeutic use of self is important for understanding the way to evoke play in children and is considered part of the art of therapy. Occupational therapy practitioners engage in the art of therapy when they connect with the child. Skillful practitioners play effortlessly with children while challenging them to acquire and master new skills. The art of therapy involves weaving clinical judgment, skill, and individual style into successful therapy sessions.

CLINICAL *Pearl*

Get in touch with your playful side. Spend the day with a child to remember the way it feels to play. Let the child lead you and show you the way to play.

Characteristics of Playful Occupational Therapy Practitioners

Occupational therapy practitioners may cultivate specific characteristics in themselves that promote play (Box 14-3). Occupational therapy practitioners must be playful themselves if they wish to treat children effectively and facilitate play and playfulness. Children view a happy, smiling practitioner, who is able to interact joyfully with a child, as playful.

It is important for the practitioner to establish goals and structure the treatment setting. However, the occu-

---

BOX 14-3

Characteristics of Occupational Therapy Practitioners that Promote Play and Playfulness in Children

- *Playfulness.* Has warm, inviting, sincere personality
- *Flexibility, creativity, and spontaneity.* Changes activities and pace based on the needs of the child. Able to stop activities and create new ones if needed
- *Child friendliness.* Interacts at the child's level and is familiar with child's terms and current trends such as *Dalmatians, Power Rangers, Barney, Teletubbies*
- *Sense of humor.* Tries out silly things and laughs at self
- *Intuition.* Is able to read child's cues (nonverbal and verbal) and is aware of signs of boredom, fatigue, or frustration
- *Positive reinforcement.* Offers sincere praise when child has performed well, has tried very hard, or is in need of support
- *Patience.* Allows child to experience some frustration. Helps the child work on frustration tolerance through play
- *Observational skills.* Able to watch and not intervene at every turn. Allows the child to be in control
- *Openness.* Learns new games and play activities from children. Watches children in many settings to keep activities novel
- *Fun.* Smiles, laughs, and plays with the child

pational therapy practitioner must be flexible enough to change the activity based on the child's responses. The occupational therapy practitioner needs to be skillful in planning and setting up a playful environment so that the child will choose activities that further the therapeutic goals. This ensures that therapy is fun for the child. Facilitating play requires that the practitioner keep goals clearly in mind while structuring the environment and adjusting the mode of interaction.[16,21]

Occupational therapy practitioners acting as play facilitators attend to the child's interests, elaborate on the child's verbalizations, and model play behaviors.[21] If an activity is not challenging to a child but the child is enjoying it, the practitioner may decide to continue the activity before increasing the skill required. The child may need to practice the task to gain mastery.[32] Children need to be challenged in all areas of development. Occupational therapy practitioners need to provide social, cognitive, and motor challenges.

Practitioners need to be creative to spark children's imagination during a play session. (See Chapter 14 Appendix B for a resource list of play ideas.) A sense of humor is vital; practitioners may have to act silly, make mistakes, and even act as a peer to encourage the child to play. From children's point of view, practitioners may seem to demand that they perform tasks that seem much harder to them than to the adult. When a child asks to play the role of the practitioner and then says, "Okay, now stand on your head and clap your hands together behind your back three times. I will time you," this suggests that the degree of challenge the child has experienced during treatment sessions is too difficult.

CLINICAL *Pearl*

Provide children with a theme for play activities. Ask them to bring in something from home and use that during therapy.

Reading a child's verbal and nonverbal cues provides occupational therapy practitioners with information that may change the play activities. This is important in gaining the trust of the child. Children need to feel that someone is listening to them. Skillful occupational therapy practitioners use the child's cues as indicators of stress and emotions. Practitioners can assist children in learning to listen to and give cues by noting and listening to the child's nonverbal and verbal feedback.

Praising children is highly effective if done properly. Children appreciate honest and specific praise. Children realize that play can be frustrating and not always successful. Occupational therapy practitioners need to allow children with special needs to feel frustration and experience failure sometimes.

Playful practitioners allow children to make mistakes occasionally. Some of the most playful sessions are those in which the children make mistakes along the way. It is the process that is important.

An obstacle course in the clinic is difficult for Jon to climb on without falling. He tries numerous times and each time falls into the pillows laughing. He is determined to succeed. He works on this activity until he succeeds in doing it properly. Once he masters the task he moves on to something new. For Jon, falling into the pillows is almost as fun as staying on the course.

Practitioners must have a sense of humor. They must take into consideration the setting and the play frame. Therefore if the child says, "I have a laser gun," during a pretend game, the practitioner does not become alarmed. However, a child may be crying out for help during play. Occupational therapy practitioners should take these opportunities to reach out to the child. Perhaps the most important characteristic of playful practitioners is that they have fun. Children learn the way to play from practitioners who get involved in play. They smile, laugh, and enjoy playing.

Characteristics of Optimum Play Environment

The optimal **play environment** has specific characteristics (Box 14-4); first and foremost is a safe environment.[3,33]

Children must be and feel physically and emotionally safe. The environment should have a variety of age-appropriate toys from which the child can choose.* These toys need not be expensive; children enjoy playing with household items such as pots and pans.

The occupational therapy practitioner should design an environment that promotes novelty, opportunity for exploration, repetition, and imitation of competent role models.[16] Novelty makes the session fun and enjoyable, fosters creativity, and creates arousal. Providing an environment that allows for exploration requires arranging toys so children can look for them, reach them, and investigate the surroundings. Children learn from repetition and should be allowed to do this during play. Repetition is encouraged by initiation of the same activity with a different theme, goal, or object. For example, the practitioner may ask a child to throw a ball at a new target to continue the activity. Being a competent role

---

*References 3, 11, 16, 21, 28.

Characteristics of Optimum Play Environment

- *Playful.* Provides cheerful, warm, and safe feeling
- *Fun and inviting.* Is child friendly; is decorated in such a way that children enjoy being there
- *Safe.* Keeps children physically and emotionally safe, so they feel free to explore and play; has mats available
- *Novel.* Provides various new toys and challenges
- *Flexible and creative.* Allows children to play in different ways with the toys; is arranged to promote a variety of play activities
- *Encouraging.* Includes adults who facilitate play, are not directive, ensure that the children are safe, assist when needed, and disappear when appropriate
- *Creative.* Materials and supplies are available to promote creativity and do not necessarily have an end product. Children enjoy sand, water, clay, and Play Doh
- *Quiet.* Allows children some space to be alone if they desire

Safety in the Play Environment

THE BEST SAFETY PRECAUTION IS TO WATCH ALL CHILDREN CAREFULLY AT ALL TIMES.
- Plug all electrical outlets with safety caps.
- Ensure that bookshelves are sturdy and will not topple. Anchor to the wall at top.
- Do not place toys so that they will fall on toddlers' heads when they pull them down.
- Cut all cords so that children cannot get caught in them.
- Have plenty of mats under equipment.
- Pad corners of walls and furniture.
- Know infant CPR.
- Be sure cleaning supplies and medications are out of reach.
- Be sure water tables are closed when not in use.
- Watch and mop up slippery surfaces.
- Have a first-aid kit available and review emergency procedures.
- Check out all equipment periodically to ensure it is in good working order.
- Clean and disinfect toys and surfaces after each use.
- Follow universal precautions for cleaning spills.

model requires the practitioner to demonstrate playful behavior. Parents and professionals need to give children space to work out play scenarios and this space must be safe (Box 14-5).

The play space should be arranged to promote a variety of types of play[1,3] (see Chapter 7). Ways to promote different types of play include the following:

1. *Pretend play.* This type of play promotes make-believe and may include kitchen table, play food, puppets, and dress-up clothes.
2. *Constructive play.* This type of play is designed to allow children to build and create things and includes blocks, Legos, Lincoln Logs, various other building toys, arts and crafts, paper; crayons, clay, markers, and paint, chalk, scissors, wind-up toys, beads, and small manipulative toys.
3. *Reflective or reading area.* This is a quiet area where children can go to read or write. Items included in this area may include books, audiotapes, videotapes, paper, and pencils.
4. *Sensorimotor area.* This area is for large motor movements. Toys and equipment present in this area include mats, balls, bikes, swings, balance beams, and trampolines.
5. *Exploratory play.* This type of play includes water, sand, and other tactile play activities.
6. *Computer play.* This play area includes a computer with a variety of games.

7. *Musical play.* This type of play promotes music and includes whistles, rattles, drums, pianos, rhythm games, singing, and tapes.

The occupational therapy practitioner should allow children to express creativity and spontaneity. Toys have many uses in addition to those suggested by the manufacturer. Unless the children are being harmful to others or themselves, allow them to use toys in different ways. Some children are not aware of the way the toy is typically used. After they have taken some time to explore it, the practitioner may demonstrate the expected way without imposing one method of playing with the toy.

CLINICAL *Pearl*

Musical games are fun and playful ways to help a child become more attentive to verbal directions. The child must pay attention to the words of the song or beat of the music to follow along.

Many children enjoy roughhousing. Children with special needs may also enjoy this. Gentle roughhousing can provide sensory input to children and is often therapeutic and fun. Children of all ages learn through physical contact and therapy sessions can provide a safe environment for this type of contact. Children may push each other playfully. Adults do not always need to intervene.

Playful environments take advantage of themes and are decorated for the occasion. Make sure that the play environment is not too stimulating. Use warm colors such as pinks, melons, and yellows.[2] The temperature of the room should be warm, not too hot or cold. Children enjoy being outdoors, so they should be able to play in outdoor settings as well. They should have places for quiet time and concentration.

The best way to promote play and playfulness in children is to be a playful adult in a playful environment. Arranging the play environment helps occupational therapy practitioners become skillful at utilizing the environment therapeutically.

SUMMARY

Occupational therapy practitioners view play as the major occupation of childhood and believe it is crucial to a child's development. They facilitate the development of play in children with special needs. Thus practitioners must understand the characteristics of play if they wish to make significant changes in the play of the children they treat. Practitioners play an important role in helping parents, teachers, and peers play with children with special needs. They may be able to make simple **play adaptations** that allow children with special needs to be included in play with their peers.

Play is a fun, spontaneous, internally motivated, and self-directed activity that is free from rigid rules. *Playfulness* is defined as an individual's disposition to play. Occupational therapy practitioners typically use play as a tool to improve a child's skills and as a goal for therapy.

Occupational therapy practitioners should expand their use of play by exploring the characteristics of play and practicing these techniques in the treatment of children. Occupational therapy practitioners can have a tremendous impact on the lives of children and their families through fun, creative, enjoyable, and spontaneous activities, allowing children to develop play skills that will carry over to home, school, and the community and help prepare them for adult roles.

References

1. Axline VM: Play therapy procedures and results. In Schaefer C, editor: *The therapeutic use of play*, New York, 1976, Jason Aronson.
2. Ayres AJ: *Sensory integration and learning disorders*, Los Angeles, 1972, Western Psychological Services.
3. Bantz DL, Siktberg L: Teaching families to evaluate age-appropriate toys, *J Pediatr Health Care* 7(3):111, 1993.
4. Barnett LA: The adaptive powers of being playful. In Duncan MC, Chick G, Aycock A, editors: *Play & culture studies*, vol 1, Greenwich, Conn, 1998, Ablex Publishing.
5. Berger KS: *The developing person through the lifespan*, ed 3, New York, 1994, Worth Publishers.
6. Bryze KC: Narrative contributions to the play history. In Parham LD, Fazio LS, editors: *Play in occupational therapy for children*, St Louis, 1997, Mosby.
7. Bundy AC: Assessment of play and leisure: delineation of the problem, *Am Occup Ther* 47: 217, 1993.
8. Bundy AC: Play and playfulness: What to look for. In Parham LD, Fazio LS, editors: *Play in occupational therapy for children*, St Louis, 1997, Mosby.
9. Bundy AC: Play theory and sensory integration. In Fisher AG, Murray EA, Bundy AC, editors: *Sensory integration: theory and practice*, Philadelphia, 1991, FA Davis.
10. Carlson BW, Ginglend DR: *Play activities for the retarded child: how to help him grow and learn through music, games, handicraft, and other play activities*, New York, 1961, Abingdon Press.
11. Cass JE: *The significance of children's play*, London, 1971, Batsford.
12. Clifford JM, Bundy AC: Play preference and play performance in normal boys and boys with sensory integrative dysfunction, *Amer J Occup Ther* 9:202, 1989.
13. Cohen D: *The development of play*, New York, 1987, New York University Press.
14. Coster W: Occupation-centered assessment of children, *Am J Occup Ther* 52(5):337, 1998.
15. Csikszentmihalyi M: *Beyond boredom and anxiety*, ed 1, San Francisco, 1975, Jossey-Bass.
16. Florey L: Development through play. In Schaefer C, editor: *The therapeutic use of play*, New York, 1976, Jason Aronson.
17. Greenstein DB: It's child's play. In Galvin J, editor: *Evaluating, selecting, and using appropriate assistive technology*, Gaithersburg, Md, 1996, Aspen.
18. Hart R: *Therapeutic play activities for hospitalized children*, St Louis, 1992, Mosby.
19. Jernberg AM: *Theraplay: a new treatment using structured play for problem children and their families*, ed 1, San Francisco, 1979, Jossey-Bass.
20. Kielhofner G, editor: *A model of human occupation*, Baltimore, 1985, Williams & Wilkins.
21. Linder TW, editor: *Transdiscipinary play based assessment*, Baltimore, 1990, Paul H Brookes.
22. Llorens LA: *Application of a developmental theory for health and rehabilitation*, Bethesda, Md, 1976, American Occupational Therapy Association.
23. Marfo K, editor: *Parent-child interaction and developmental disabilities*, New York, 1988, Praeger.
24. Millar S: *The psychology of play*, New York, 1974, Aronson.
25. Moran JM, Kalakian LH: *Movement experiences for the mentally retarded or emotionally disturbed child*, Minneapolis, 1974, Burgess.
26. Morrison CD, Bundy AC, Fisher AG: The contribution of motor skills and playfulness to the play performance of preschoolers, *Am J Occup Ther* 45:687, 1991.

27. Morrison CD, Metzger P, Pratt P: Play. In Case-Smith J, Allen A, Pratt PN, editors: *Occupational therapy for children*, ed 3, St Louis, 1996, Mosby.

28. Musselwhite CR: *Adaptive play for special needs children*, San Diego, 1986, College-Hill Press.

29. O'Brien JC et al: The impact of positioning equipment on play skills of physically impaired children. In Duncan MC, Chick G, Aycock A, editors: *Play & culture studies*, vol 1, Greenwich, Conn, 1998, Ablex Publishing Corporation.

30. O'Brien JC et al: The impact of occupational therapy on a child's playfulness, *Occup Ther Healthcare* 12(2), 1999.

31. Parham LD, Primeau L: Play and occupational therapy. In Parham LD, Fazio LS, editors: *Play in occupational therapy for children*, St Louis, 1997, Mosby.

32. Reilly M, editor: *Play as exploratory learning: studies in curiosity behavior*, Beverly Hills, 1974, Sage.

33. Rubin K, Fein GG, Vandenberg B: Play. In Mussen PH, editor: *Handbook of child psychology*, ed 4, New York, 1983, Wiley.

34. Sutton-Smith B: Play in cognitive development. In Schaefer C, editor: *The therapeutic use of play*, New York, 1976, Jason Aronson.

Recommended Reading

Britton L, Turner S: *Montessori play and learn: a parent's guide to purposeful play from two to six*, New York, 1993, Crown Publishers.

Featherstone H: *A difference in the family: life with a disabled child*, New York, 1980, Basic Books.

Florey L: Studies of play: implications for growth, development and clinical practice, *Amer J Occup Ther* 35(8):519.

Greenstein D et al: *Backyards and butterflies—ways to include children with disabilities in outdoor activities*, Ithaca, NY, 1993, New York State Rural Health and Safety Council.

Linder T: *Transdisciplinary play based intervention*, Baltimore, 1993, Paul H Brookes.

Singer D, Singer J: *Partners in play—a step by step guide to imaginative play in children*, New York, 1977, Harper & Row.

Sutton-Smith B: *The ambiguity of play*, Boston, 1998, Harvard University Press.

Young S: *Movement is fun*, Torrance, Calif, 1988, Sensory Integration International.

REVIEW *Questions*

1. Describe the characteristics of play and playfulness.
2. What is the difference between play and playfulness?
3. How would you facilitate play and playfulness in children with special needs?
4. What characteristics do you possess that would promote play and playfulness in children with special needs?
5. How is play used as a tool in the treatment of children?
6. Describe the ways play can be the goal of therapy.
7. List three play assessments used by occupational therapy practitioners. Describe the ways they are administered and the information you gain from them.
8. How can the environment stimulate play and playfulness?

SUGGESTED *Activities*

1. Volunteer to baby-sit for a child with special needs. Play with the child. Reflect on the experience by writing a one-page paper describing the way you felt about the time you spent with the child.
2. Plan and participate in an activity you enjoy with others. Describe the activity, materials needed, and the environment. How did you feel during this activity?
3. In a small group, discuss your favorite childhood games and playmates. What types of skills did you learn as a child during play? What feelings do these memories bring to mind?
4. In a small group, role-play the characteristics of occupational therapy practitioners that promote playfulness in children.

CHAPTER 14 APPENDIX A

Play Assessments

KNOX PRESCHOOL PLAY SCALE[2,5,7]

The Knox Preschool Play Scale (PPS) provides a developmental description of play behavior in four domains: space management, materials management, imitation, and participation. The Knox PPS is designed for children 0-6 years old. It is easy to administer and score. The Knox PPS requires two 30-minute observations of free play (indoors and outdoors). The revised scale provides age equivalencies to six months for children 0 to 3 years of age and yearly for children 3 to 5 years of age.[7]

TEST OF PLAYFULNESS[3]

The Test of Playfulness (ToP) provides objective measurement of playfulness. Children are observed playing in familiar play environments with peers for 15 minutes inside and 15 minutes outside. Administration of the scale requires training by viewing of videotapes of children playing and scoring them according to ToP guidelines. Occupational therapy practitioners can use the information to systematically examine playfulness in children.[3]

TRANSDISCIPLINARY PLAY-BASED ASSESSMENT[6]

The Transdisciplinary Play-Based Assessment (TPBA) is a procedure for administering a comprehensive transdisciplinary assessment for children 0 to 3 years of age. The TPBA provides structured guidelines for performing this assessment. Clinicians can use this procedure to design intervention. The TPBA is an observational assessment that may take as long as 1½ hours to administer. Team members participate in the assessment. Information is gained in cognitive, social-emotional, communication and language, and motor skills.[6]

PLAY HISTORY[8,9]

A play history is a semistructured interview designed to obtain information about the child's behavior. The play history is based on the developmental progression of play and examines behaviors in five developmental phases: (1) sensorimotor, (2) symbolic and simple constructive, (3) dramatic and complex constructive, (4) games, and (5) recreational. Practitioners using this scale must have a firm knowledge of the normal progression of play. The scale provides a framework for gathering information on play.[8]

CHILDREN'S PLAYFULNESS SCALE[1]

The Children's Playfulness Scale* scale consists of 23 Likert-type format items using a five-point response scale: "sounds exactly like the child," "sounds a lot like the child," "sounds somewhat like the child," "sounds a little like the child," and "does not sound at all like the child." Children receive a playfulness score. This scale is efficient and inexpensive and requires no direct observation of the child. Bundy and Clifton questioned the use of this scale for children with disabilities.[4]

Appendix References

1. Barnett LA: Playfulness: definition, design, and measurement. *Play and culture*, 3: 319, 1990.
2. Bledsoe N, Shephard J: A study of the reliability and validity of a preschool play scale. *Am J Occup Ther*, 36(12):783, 1982.
3. Bundy AC: Play and playfulness: What to look for. In Parham LD, Fazio LS, editors: *Play in occupational therapy for children*, St Louis, 1997, Mosby.
4. Bundy AC, Clifton JL: Construct validity of the children's playfulness scale. In Duncan MC, Chick G, Aycock A, editors: *Play and culture studies*, vol 1, Greenwich, Conn, 1998, Ablex.
5. Knox S: A play scale. In Reilly M, editor: *Play as exploratory learning*, Beverly Hills, 1974, Sage.
6. Linder TW, editor: *Transdisciplinary play based assessment*, Baltimore, 1990, Paul H Brookes.
7. Parham LD, Primeau L: Play and occupational therapy. In Parham LD, Fazio LS, editors: *Play in occupational therapy for children*, St Louis, 1997, Mosby.
8. Reilly M, editor: *Play as exploratory learning*, Beverly Hills, 1974, Sage.
9. Takata N: Play as a prescription. In Reilly M, editor: *Play as exploratory learning*, Beverly Hills, 1974, Sage.

---

*Scales that may be administered by COTAs on establishing service competency with supervising OTR.

CHAPTER 14 APPENDIX B

Resources for Play Activity Ideas

PUBLICATIONS

Burkhart LJ: More homemade battery devices for severely handicapped children with suggested activities, College Park, Md, 1982, Linda J Burkhart.

Cole J, Tiergreen A, Calmenson S: *Eentsy, weentsy spider: fingerplays and action rhymes*, New York, 1991, Mulberry Books.

Coleman K, McNairn P, Shioleno C: *Quick tech music*, Solana, Calif, Mayer-Johnson Company.

Dexter S: *Joyful play with toddlers: recipes for fun with odds and ends (tool for everyday parenting series)*, 1996, Seattle, Parenting Press.

Hamilton L: *Child's play around the world: 170 crafts, games and projects for 2-6 year olds*, 1996, New York, Beverly.

Judith G, Ellison S: *365 days of creative play for children 2-years and up*, 1995, Trabuco Canyon, Calif, Sourcebooks.

Kranowitz CS: *101 activities for kids in tight spaces: at the doctor's office, on car, train and plane trips, home sick in bed*, New York, 1995, St Martin's Press.

Miller K: *Things to do with toddlers and twos*, West Palm Beach, Fla, 1984, Telshare.

Morris LR, Schultz L: *Creative play activities for children with disabilities*, Sportime Abilitations

Munger EM, Bowden SJ: *Beyond peek-a-boo and pat-a-cake: Activities for baby's first twenty-four months*, ed 3, Clinton, NJ, New Win Pub.

Nipp S, Beall PC: *Wee sing childrens songs and fingerplays*, audiocassette, New York, 1994, Price Stern Sloan Audio.

Nolan A: *Great explorations: 100 creative play ideas for parents and preschoolers from playspace at the children's museum*, Boston, 1997, Pocket Books.

Silberg J: *300 3-minute games: Quick and easy activities for 2-5 year olds*, Beltsville, Md, 1997, Gryphon House.

Totline Staff: *1001 rhymes and fingerplays*, Pomona, Calif, 1994, Warren Publishing House.

Ulene A, Shelov S: *Discovery play: loving and learning with your baby*, Berkeley, Calf, 1994, Ulyss Press.

Wright C, Nomura M: *From toys to computers: access for the physically disabled child*, Wauconda, Ill, Don Johnston.

COMPANIES AND PUBLICATIONS HELPFUL IN ADAPTING PLAY FOR CHILDREN WITH SPECIAL NEEDS

Ablenet
1091 Tenth Avenue, Southeast
Minneapolis, MN 55414-1312
(800) 322-0956

Linda Burkhart
8503 Rhode Island Avenue
College Park, MD 20740
(301) 345-9152

Crestwood Company
6625 North Sidney Place
Milwaukee, WI 53209-3259
(414) 352-5678

Exceptional Parent Magazine
PO Box 5446
Pittsfield, MA 01203-9321
(800) 247-8080

Don Johnston
PO Box 639
Wauconda, IL 60084-0639
(800) 999-4660

National Therapeutic Recreation Society
2775 South Quincy Street, Suite 300
Arlington, VA 22206
(703) 820-4940

Toys for Special Children
385 Warburton Avenue
Hastings-on-Hudson, NY 10706

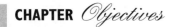

Sensorimotor
Treatment
Approaches

GLORIA GRAHAM
PAULA McCREEDY
JEAN W. SOLOMON

CHAPTER *Objectives*

After studying this chapter, the reader will be able to accomplish the following:

- Describe the current movement concepts influencing occupational therapy treatment
- Broadly explain sensorimotor approaches to treatment
- Discuss the major goals and principles of three sensorimotor treatment approaches
- Apply treatment strategies from the described sensorimotor treatment approaches to clinical case example

Sensorimotor treatment approaches have traditionally been defined as those treatment approaches concerned with the impact of sensory input on a person's motor responses and motor recovery. These approaches assume that abnormal motor responses can be altered through specific sensory input and that the central nervous system (CNS) can learn more normal motor control. Sensorimotor treatment approaches are used with children and adults suffering from CNS dysfunction. This chapter presents three sensorimotor treatment approaches and discusses key principles, concepts, and clinical applications to pediatric practice for each. The three approaches are the neurophysiological treatment approach, the neurodevelopmental treatment (NDT) approach, and the sensory regulatory approach. These approaches are rarely used in isolation. Rather, the occupational therapy practitioner combines treatment techniques from one or more of the approaches according to the child's motor responses and sensory needs.

All three approaches are based on reflex-hierarchical theories of motor control. **Motor control** is concerned with what processes control movement. In **reflex-hierarchical models** of motor control, movement is viewed as being controlled by a central process (the CNS) in a top-down format. Higher levels of the CNS are thought to control the lower levels; the cerebellum and cerebrum controlling voluntary movements and the spinal cord controlling reflexes.[20] Contemporary theories of motor control question this linear, top-down view. New research shows that motor control occurs independently of sensory input and that although important the CNS is not the primary determinant of motor output.[1,20,24] The system model of motor control views movement as the result of the interaction of multiple systems, including various body systems, the environment, the task, and the child's motivation and interest (Table 15-1) (see Chapter 8).

NEUROPHYSIOLOGICAL TREATMENT APPROACH

Margaret Rood was a physical and occupational therapist who developed treatment techniques in the 1940s based on clinical observations, developmental literature, and reflex-hierarchical models of motor control.[12,21,27,32] She originally developed the **neurophysiological treatment approach** for individuals with cerebral palsy but believed the techniques were applicable to any individual with motor

Acknowledgement: A special thank you to Gretchen Parker for her detailed review of this chapter.

TABLE 15-1

Current Movement Concepts

CONCEPT	DEFINITION	CLINICAL IMPLICATIONS
Motor control	The motor control concept focuses on the set of processes that organize, control, and coordinate posture and movement.	Two major perspectives exist: a hierarchical view and a systems model of motor control. Current practice has shifted to systems perspective.
Motor learning	The motor learning concept focuses on the process of the ways motor skills are acquired and permanent changes occur.	Intervention should provide instruction, feedback, and opportunities to practice in multiple contexts.
Hierarchical model of motor control	Motor control is centrally controlled by the CNS. Information flows in top-down format.	Treatment intervention emphasizes the use of reflexes and sensory input to change motor performance.
System model of motor control	Motor control is a result of cooperative and interactive processes, including the CNS and other biological systems, as well as physical, psychological, and social environments.	Treatment intervention is multifaceted and incorporates the environment, adaptation of the environment, the child's interest, and biological, cultural, and social systems with the purposefulness and relevance of the activity to function.

Modified from Cech D, Martin S: *Functional movement across the lifespan,* Philadelphia, 1995, WB Saunders, 1995; Kaplan M, Bedell G: *A motor skill acquisition frame of reference* (in press).

control problems. Her basic premise was that the motor responses of clients with neurological dysfunction could be altered by the application of specific sensory stimulation. She believed motor skills are developed from reflexes that are used and gradually modified by sensory stimuli until the highest motor control is gained on a conscious level.[27]

General Considerations

The goals and principles Rood emphasized to guide treatment intervention include the following [21,27,32]:

1. Normal muscle tone precedes desired motor responses and depends on specific and appropriately applied sensory stimuli. Motor responses should be elicited on a reflexive level initially and modified as control is achieved at higher levels. For example, swinging a child through space may facilitate righting reactions and normal muscle tone.

2. Sensorimotor control follows a developmental progression with treatment aimed at repeating the normal sequence of motor development until a higher level of control is attained. Rood used the cephalocaudal (head-to-tail) and proximal-to-distal (closer to the trunk, farther away from the trunk) rules to guide the sequence of treatment. For example, a child develops head control before trunk control (cephalocaudal rule). A child develops shoulder stability before wrist stability (proximal-to-distal rule).

3. Purposeful movement and activities are necessary to elicit the desired motor response. The repetition or practicing of movement patterns is needed to ensure motor learning and effective intervention. Activities should motivate the child to practice movement skills and patterns (for example, encouraging a child to play repetitively in the all fours (quadruped) position while reaching for and playing with a favorite toy.

TABLE 15-2

Selected Neurophysiological Intervention Techniques and Applications

TECHNIQUES	SENSORY METHOD	CLINICAL APPLICATION
FACILITATION TECHNIQUES		
Light moving touch	Apply tactile input using fingertip or soft object, such as a cotton swab.	Activates superficial muscles
Stretch-muscle tapping	Apply proprioceptive input with three to five taps over muscle belly using fingertips.	Facilitates a stronger motor response in a contracting muscle. Tapping is critical. Tapping should be done just before an active muscle contraction
Heavy joint compression	Apply proprioceptive input manually or with weights through the long axis of bone.	Promotes holding and maintaining of postures
Battery-activated vibration	Apply tactile and propioceptive input using battery operated vibrator over muscle belly.	Increases muscle tone and contractions. Lasts only while input is being provided
Fast vestibular input	Apply vestibular input by spinning, rocking, or other movements in a quick and irregular way.	Increases muscle tone and general arousal state
INHIBITION TECHNIQUES		
Wrapping	Apply tactile and proprioceptive input as child is wrapped in a blanket.	Decreases muscle tone and general arousal state (calms)
Slow stroking of spine while child is in prone position	Apply tactile and proprioceptive input using fingertip pressure.	Decreases muscle tone and general arousal state
Slow rocking or rolling	Apply vestibular input slowly and rhythmically.	Decreases muscle tone and general arousal state
Applying sustained pressure to tendon	Apply tactile and proprioceptive input.	Decreases tone in specific muscle

Specific Intervention Techniques and Applications

Rood integrated the use of controlled sensory stimulation during treatment with a sequence of developmental postures and activities to facilitate specific motor responses.[21,27] She described several key developmental postures used to achieve mobility and stability.[10,12,21,22] These postures include prone-on-elbows, prone-on-extended arms, quadruped, semisquat, and standing and walking postures. For a complete review of Rood's developmental postures, see McCormack's work.[21]

Rood also devised several methods and tools to administer controlled sensory input. She used tactile (touch), thermal (hot and cold), olfactory (smell), gustatory (taste), visual (seeing), and proprioceptive (input to the muscles and joints allowing for sense of position in space) sensory stimuli to facilitate or inhibit motor responses.[27] **Facilitation techniques** increase the contraction of a muscle or a reflex response. Facilitation techniques make movement easier and promote normal motor responses. **Inhibition techniques** decrease muscle contractions or reflex responses and are used to decrease spasticity and stop abnormal motor responses. (See Chapter 17 for additional discussion and clinical application of inhibition and facilitation techniques.) Table 15-2 summarizes selected Rood's sensory techniques and their clinical applications. COTAs should be properly trained in these and other sensory stimulation techniques by an OTR because these techniques though valuable are unpredictable.

The Rood approach guides the child through the developmental progression until skilled movement control is obtained.[21] Controlled movement develops as the child learns to shift weight in stable positions.[10] Sensory techniques of inhibition and facilitation reinforce the child's developmental postures and prepare the child for engagement in functional activities. The practitioner should use positioning techniques based on normal development when using the Rood approach.[13] For example, a child in the prone-on-elbows posture is encouraged to weightshift when reaching for toys with one hand. This posture allows the child to maintain or develop stability while moving (reaching) with an extended arm. In this position, if shoulder muscles are active about a joint while supporting the joint, the use of compression (aligning and pushing the articulating surfaces of a joint together) can be applied to facilitate holding of the posture. Mobility and stability in the squatting posture is reinforced by having the infant retrieve objects from the floor. As the child progresses along the developmental continuum, activities that require standing and reaching, weightshifting, and balance reactions are incorporated. Developmental postures integrate easily into a child's play routine and activities. Practitioners should encourage and provide ample opportunity for repetitive play in developmental postures to promote controlled and skilled movement.

NEURODEVELOPMENTAL TREATMENT APPROACH

A physical therapist named Berta Bobath and her husband, neurologist Dr. Karel Bobath, developed the **neurodevelopmental treatment (NDT) approach** in the 1940s based on their work with children neurologically impairments and adults who exhibited abnormal movement patterns. The goal of NDT is to promote the development of functional skills by improving the control and quality of movement.[6] The NDT approach continues to evolve as new research information on motor development, motor learning, and motor control is integrated into the theoretical base and clinical practice of NDT.

General Considerations

The focus of contemporary NDT intervention is to enhance the child's performance of functional activities by increasing the quality of the child's postural control and movement. Children with movement disorders or CNS disorders typically have resulting impairments that affect their ability to perform skilled movements and functional activities. Often these children have symptoms such as abnormal postural control and muscle tone that affect their ability to perform voluntary movements (see Chapters 8 and 11). Postural control is viewed as the basis for functional movement and is essential for smooth, efficient, and coordinated movements.[10] **Postural control** is defined as the ability to maintain a certain posture against the forces of gravity while simultaneously stabilizing or controlling forces that result from movement.[29]

Various postural control strategies can be used initiate and maintain movement and postures in response to environmental demands.[29] Postural reactions (that is, righting, equilibrium, and protective reactions) occur in response to sensory stimuli and are automatic responses to disturbances in the center of gravity. A child makes anticipatory postural adjustments before, during, and after movement. These postural adjustments allow the child to prepare the body for movement, maintain proper body alignment, sustain controlled movement, and shift the base of support as needed.[1]

The human postural control system develops from birth and continues to change throughout the life span as individuals acquire new motor skills. The developing infant uses certain postures that provide stability when postural control is immature. For example, W-sitting helps position the child's legs in a wide base of support. Children with abnormal movement seek postural stability by fixing at proximal joints so that body parts do not move.[22] For example, shoulder elevation is used to stabilize and support head control. The focus of treatment in the contemporary NDT approach is to activate the child's postural system to support functional movement. This is achieved by providing the child with various sensory inputs to normalize movements and muscle tone. Sensory input, sensory feedback, and sensory experiences are crucial to the development of postural control and movement. A child's sensory system helps to organize and guide functional movements.

Specific Intervention Techniques and Applications

The NDT approach uses specific handling techniques to enhance the child's performance of functional activities. Handling is defined as the use of the practitioner's hands to provide graded sensory input to a child's body to influence the child's muscle tone and movement patterns.[7,26] The goal of handling is to provide the child with feedback about what normal sensation and movement feel like within the context of a task. Current NDT practice advocates that practitioners decrease direct handling as soon as possible to allow the child more active participation and opportunity to control the speed and flow of movement during functional activities.[15]

CLINICAL *Pearl*

Skilled observation is essential during the intervention process. This includes constant monitoring of the child's observable emotional, sensory, and motor reactions. Skilled observation assists the practitioner in knowing when to change gears and allow the child to engage in a different activity or simply rest and regroup.

Children who have abnormal muscle tone and movements are restricted in their abilities to explore the environment. Specific sensorimotor techniques are used during handling to assist the child in developing and expanding a sensory and motor repertoire.[8] Box 15-1 provides a brief summary of inhibition and facilitation techniques used in NDT.

Weightbearing and weightshifting techniques are used in NDT to promote normal muscle tone and postural alignment and to facilitate the child's ability to move through space. All functional movements require weightshifts.[10] A child with movement problems often has difficulty controlling the amount of weightshift required to initiate or engage in an activity. Children with high tone tend to move in a blocklike fashion and show limited ability to

---

BOX 15-1

Selected NDT Intervention Techniques

FACILITATION TECHNIQUES
Weightbearing and Weightshifting
Active movement against gravity promotes increased muscle tone and postural control.

Joint Compression
Gentle compressing of well-aligned joints promotes muscle activation.

Sweeping or Alternate Tapping Over Muscles
Using cupped hands, the practitioner lightly sweeps or taps the muscle belly to promote activation.

INHIBITION TECHNIQUES
Weightbearing and Weightshifting
Active movement can have an inhibitory effect on spastic muscles.

Rotation
Rotating upper body on lower body can help to break up total patterns of movement and decrease the influence of abnormal tone.

Oscillations or Hand Vibration
Briskly shaking an extremity in small increments or shaking the practitioner's hand over a muscle belly can promote decreased abnormal muscle tone.

---

weightshift. Activities that vary the speed and amount of weightshift are used with these children. Children with low tone lack the muscle tone needed to maintain stability and tend to collapse into lower-level developmental postures using excessive weightshifts. Weightshifting activities that require midrange control are encouraged when working with children with low tone. An occupational therapy practitioner may engage a child in weightbearing activities to prepare the limbs for active and skilled movements before participation in functional activities. For example, a child performs weightbearing tasks before reaching and writing tasks.

Another important NDT technique used by occupational therapy practitioners is positioning. Proper positioning of the child during movement and non-movement activities is crucial. It promotes the child's experience of normal tone and sensory input while maintaining optimal postural alignment.[13,26] Positioning is a technique that incorporates easily into the child's daily routine and if carried out by parents, teachers, and other caregivers continually supports the child's experience of normal sensation and movement (see Chapter 17).

Functional activities that provide cognitive and perceptual stimulation are incorporated into the treatment process when working with children with movement disorders.[26] Play activities offer the practitioner a natural and powerful intervention tool because they focus the child's attention and may provide the motivation for the child to "move and interact with the environment."[8,26] The facilitation of normal movement responses is easier when the child's attention is focused on the activity instead of the movement.[26] During the treatment session the practitioner continually monitors and adapts environmental variables, such as extraneous noises, play surfaces, and bright lights, which may affect the child's performance. Creating safe spaces and conditions in which a child can explore and experiment with various movement patterns helps a child gain confidence, overcome fears, increase movement exploration, and enhance sensory motor skills (see Chapter 15).

Opportunities to practice skills are built into the treatment session. The practitioner monitors the child's emotional and sensory responses to determine when a break in the action is needed. According to Kaplan, children need opportunities to process information and self-direct their activities and movements.[15] This is especially true of children with low tone who tend to process information slowly and "needs ample time to receive, interpret, and respond to input."[8]

CLINICAL *Pearl*

The intervention process can be likened to a dance in which the practitioner and child are equal partners and take turns following and leading. Opportunities for the child to both lead (initiate) and follow should be created and integrated into every clinical treatment session. Leading and following activities promote independent and self-directed functioning and are based on the child's abilities.

Assessment and intervention intertwine in the NDT process. Information collected through the clinical observation process is used to identify problem areas and make adjustments in treatment as needed. Strong observation skills are a must for the NDT practitioner because the assessment process consists of observation of the child's normal and abnormal movement patterns in relation to the task and environment. The assessment provides a map that is used to plan intervention strategies. The child's quality of movement (presence of symmetry and body alignment in relation to tasks) is continually assessed during the intervention process. Inhibition and facilitation techniques are used throughout the NDT treatment process.

Treatment is focused on preparing the child to experience normal sensation and movement in the initial stage. Sensory techniques such as tapping or joint compression normalize the child's tone before engagement in functional activities. For the child with low tone, facilitation techniques increase muscle activity. Inhibition techniques decrease hypertonicity in the child with high tone. Engaging the child in functional activities that incorporate the improved tone and normal movement patterns immediately follows these techniques in this stage of treatment. The practitioner follows the child's lead and slowly guides the child's movements as the child engages in selected activities.

A child with abnormal tone may need assistance getting into the quadruped position or making the transition to a sitting position. The practitioner's hands placed at key points of control (hips, shoulders, wrists) initiate the weightshift and gently guide the child into the desired position. The practitioner usually begins at more proximal key points and gradually moves distally (guiding the movements from the shoulder to the elbow). The practitioner experiments with varying speed and amount of sensory input. This promotes the child's ability to respond to increased environmental demands. The practitioner uses less handling as the child gains more active control of movement patterns, until no physical handling is required.[12] Handling requires skill and practice to learn to feel the subtle changes that occur in a child's body and movements as sensory input is provided. Handling techniques are best learned under the guidance and supervision of an experienced OTR.

Experienced OTRs closely supervise COTAs who desire to incorporate the NDT approach into their clinical work with children. Supervision should also be supplemented by attending a certified NDT course to gain hands-on experience and knowledge of specific techniques. Strong observational skills are a key component of both the assessment and treatment process. The COTA should have basic knowledge and the ability to identify normal and abnormal movements to effectively engage the child in treatment activities that reinforce normal motor patterns.

SENSORY REGULATORY TREATMENT APPROACH

Treating children who have been diagnosed with sensory integration dysfunction or sensory regulatory disorder is extremely complex. Children who have sensory integration dysfunction often exhibit defensiveness or hypersensitivity in one or more sensory systems. Most often a child demonstrates tactile defensiveness. These children may withdraw from touch or become aggressive in situations in which touching occurs naturally. Disorders may be observed in other sensory systems that are too responsive or not responsive enough as a result of inadequate processing of sensory information. The sensory systems affected may be vestibular, proprioceptive, tactile, gustatory, olfactory, auditory, or visual (see Chapter 11). This area of practice involves advanced training for the occupational therapy practitioner. A close, collaborative, and working relationship is required between the OTR and the COTA when the COTA is involved in the delivery of care to this population and the application of this treatment approach. Both practitioners are responsible for the continuous and close monitoring of the child's sensory life and the child's response to intervention.

The **sensory regulatory treatment approach** is a collaborative process among therapists, parents, caregivers, teachers, and others. Some children have an expanded team of physicians, nutritionists, speech therapists, audiologists, physical therapists, psychologists, social workers, after school instructors, coaches, and counselors. Teams may vary depending on the child's age, specific goals for the child, cultural standards, and expected behaviors within the child's social context.[9] Treatment options have grown as our profession has moved from a reflex-hierarchical model for evaluating problems and strengths to a broader, multiple-systems approach to the child's disorder. This expanded professional thinking allows the occupational therapist to consider a child's situation and reality more specifically. Approaches to treatment can be combined to find solutions to a child's problems.

General Considerations

The field of sensory integration has received a great deal of attention in recent literature.[31] The original work by Dr. A. Jean Ayres[4] defining sensory integration and its effects on the child's functional behavior has been expanded. Dr. Ayres defined sensory integration as the child's ability to organize sensations for use.[3] Ayres' original sensory-processing theory provides a broad understanding of the way that all the sensory systems interact.

New theories help explain the ways sensory regulation and sensory modulation effect behavior. Individuals receive information about their environment through their senses. The senses also provide awareness and increase understanding of the inner workings of the body. This information is received, transmitted, integrated, and interpreted for use. Information can be stored for future use. If a child's sensory perception is inaccurate or the response to sensory input is extreme, the child may function poorly. The child's ability to respond effectively to the demands of the body, mind, and environment depend on two important processes known as *sensory regulation* and *sensory modulation*.[31] Sensory regulation is the child's ability to accurately respond to sensory input from many sensory experiences. For example, a child is able to si-

multaneously respond to the taste of food, the touch of a spoon, and the temperature of ice cream while eating it. Sensory modulation is the child's ability to accurately perceive sensory input and adjust responses accordingly. For example, an irritable child will calm when rocked and cuddled. Internal processing of stimuli strongly affects a child's social and emotional success as well as the way child functions in the occupational performance areas.[3,18]

The therapist must understand the way sensory-processing problems may affect the child's ability to perform activities, tolerate input from the environment, and respond to that input. Sensory input is necessary for typical growth and development. The processing of sensory input is used to live fully and to adapt to the demands of life. When a person has atypical sensory experiences, either through regulatory or modulation disorder, behavior is disrupted and performance is affected.[31] Dunn and Westman, Reismont and Hanschu, and Wilbarger have created scales for rating sensory dysfunction.[11,25,30] These scales are useful in determining whether a child's sensory processing difficulties are mild, moderate, or severe.

Occupational therapists describe classic, sensory integration therapy as those interventions used to observe, explain, and change a child's behavior in terms of brain-behavior theory. Lorna Jean King's description of three goals of practitioners using this therapy follows:

1. Assist the child in reaching a state of calm alertness.
2. Enhance the organization of sensation into information.
3. Acquire concepts that underlie learning.[16]

Sensory regulatory therapy begins by evaluating the sensory systems' ability to modulate sensory information. Sensory-system modulation is the effective increase or decrease in neural activity in synchronicity with all the functions of the nervous system.[17] A part of this process is the child's ability to regulate the amount of sensory information received so that attention to relevant details occurs and responses are accurate and adaptive. The occupational therapy practitioner observes and treats the child in structured and unstructured situations that require familiar as well as new responses. The practitioner designs experiences and opportunities that require the child to use organizational skills. The design must include experiences that require both initiative and the ability to follow directions, such as an obstacle course that challenges a child's sequencing and motor skills. As the practitioner becomes more experienced in working with the child, it becomes easier to use the child's own initiative to guide the therapeutic activities. This is unlike other intervention plans, in which skill-building approaches are used to compensate for disability. The child with sensory regulatory disorders needs first to develop a sensory-processing foundation from which skills will emerge. A balance between structure and freedom is the ideal approach.

Traditional sensory integrative treatment is child guided and addresses the following three sensory systems: tactile, proprioceptive, and vestibular. Treatment is usually individual and long-term, lasting from 6 months to 3 years.[19] Traditional sensory integration therapy uses special equipment in a room designed for the safe use of suspended climbing equipment that can provide a great deal of proprioceptive, tactile, vestibular, and other sensory input. Some practitioners who treat children with sensory regulatory issues incorporate passive techniques such as massage or brushing stimulation into the treatment session.

The child's state of alertness and temperament must be considered if the practitioner is to understand and normalize sensory processing, sensory regulation, and sensory modulation problems. A child must manage varied arousal states in many contexts over a long period and at many times throughout the day.[33] The practitioner should observe the way a child does this so as to design an intervention plan to improve the child's ability to function.[33]

The child feels understood when parents and peers accept the child's needs; this may lead to more effective therapy.[3] Therapy with children ideally proceeds in a planned sequence. The occupational therapy practitioner addresses sensory system modulation before functional support capabilities (that is, physical abilities such as contraction of muscles and coordination of sucking, swallowing, and breathing). Once the child develops behaviors indicative of proper functioning, the therapist provides opportunity for the child to work on functional support capabilities, followed by end-product abilities (such as eye-hand coordination and praxis or motor planning).[3,17]

The occupational therapy practitioner can use sensory regulatory treatment approaches within a classroom setting rather than exclusively in a traditional sensory integration clinic using the one-to-one therapy matrix and suspension equipment (Figure 15-1). A child who needs increased tactile, proprioceptive, and vestibular stimuli to improve attention to a school task may be successful with small adaptations in a classroom setting. A child and practitioner can work on fine motor skills while using a therapy ball to enhance proprioceptive arousal (Figure 15-2). The same child may then be able to concentrate while seated in a regular classroom chair with the practitioner providing increased shoulder stabilization through firm touch (Figure 15-3).

Another important thing to consider when using a sensory regulatory approach in therapy is the affective or emotional component of behavior.[2,14] Children with sensory defensiveness and regulatory problems often have difficulty handling the emotions and effects that accompany

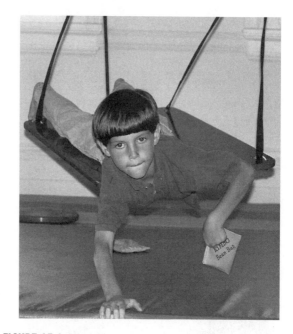

FIGURE 15-1 A child uses suspension equipment in a traditional sensory integration clinic.

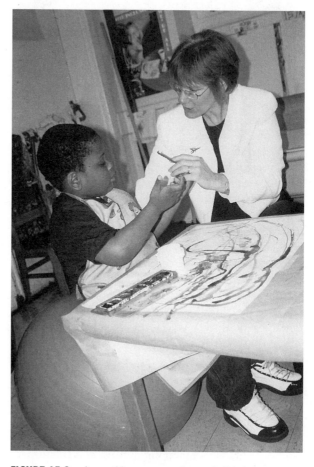

FIGURE 15-2 A practitioner uses a therapy ball to increase proprioceptive input as the child engages in a fine motor activity.

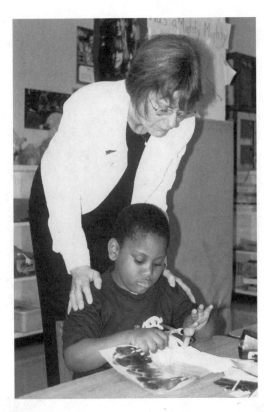

FIGURE 15-3 A practitioner uses firm touch to increase shoulder stability during a classroom activity.

responses to sensory reactions. The feelings associated with the disorganizing effects of sensory defensiveness can be traumatic. If the child's ability to self-regulate or the child's specific sensory needs are not accommodated by adaptation of the environment, the child can find the demands overwhelming. If the child is consistently overwhelmed, the child perceives the experiences as negative. If this continues without intervention and understanding from significant adults and peers, a child's self-confidence and self-concept may be harmed. Occupational therapy practitioners, primary caregivers, and teachers can help a great deal by assisting the child and being aware of the child's needs. Treatment staff and others can help by teaching the child coping strategies that improve emotional reactions and change emotional responses.

Specific Intervention Techniques and Applications

The occupational therapy practitioner helps each child use activity purposefully to gain skills, practice skills, improve the quality of skills, and generalize skills learned in one way to broader functioning. Sensory regulatory interventions focus on the integration of sensory systems and their optimal functioning. The concept of arousal

and the *just right* challenge are essential to designing effective treatment activities.[3] For example, encouraging a child with poor sitting balance to swing in the prone or supine position may improve the child's balance. As the child's sitting balance improves, swinging seated on the platform swing is encouraged. An **adaptive response** is achieved when a child is able to make appropriate responses to environmental demands.

Some children cannot appropriately perceive the sense of touch and may accidentally injure themselves while seeking stimuli. Other children are overly sensitive to touch and need control over the tactile experience to prevent them from becoming overwhelmed or overly aggressive. This imbalance of insufficient and overwhelming arousal can happen with any one sensory system or within multiple systems. Levels of arousal and defensiveness can vary with the time of day and environmental stimuli. Certain activities have a calming effect and others have an exciting effect. A calming activity can simply be a tight hug or slow, rhythmic rocking in a rocking chair (Figure 15-4).

A calming activity for one child may be a stimulating activity for another. The use of therapeutic brushing and adaptive strategies, such as telling the child before touching and using firm rather than light touch, are important intervention techniques when working with a child with tactile defensiveness. A child whose tactile system is excessively alert cannot successfully use activities until arousal has been decreased. A child whose tactile system is not sufficiently aroused must be stimulated to use activities to learn and make adaptive responses. The occupational therapy practitioner must use a child's response to determine the manner in which an intervention is used and when to intervene. Some children may resist brushing initially but quickly accommodate and use the technique to their advantage. Other children may need to brush themselves with a rag, a favorite toy, and then a therapeutic surgical brush, slowly adjusting to the process over time. The practitioner must be careful not to intrude on or overwhelm a child with a powerful sensory technique, such as brushing or joint compression. Adaptive techniques such as asking the child to take the practitioner's hand rather than the practitioner taking the child's hand gives the child control over physical contact.

Vestibular receptors within the inner ear provide a sense of movement and position of the child's head in space. For children experiencing vestibular defensiveness, such as gravitational insecurity (that is, an inability to know where they are in space when their feet are not touching the ground or another supporting surface), rocking slowly on an air pillow with their feet off of the ground may be overwhelming. Allowing children to keep their feet on the floor can help the practitioner achieve the right arousal level.

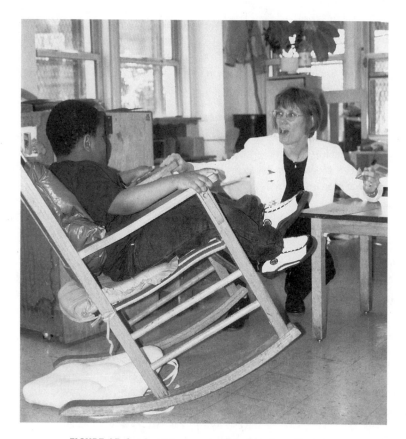

FIGURE 15-4   A child uses a rocking chair for self-calming.

The proprioceptive system registers the child's body position from information in muscles, joints, and tissue surrounding the joints. Proprioceptive discrimination difficulties are often linked with vestibular deficits. Some children seek an excessive amount of proprioceptive input by falling on purpose, bumping deliberately into objects, or constantly jumping and climbing. The child's response may be giggling instead of expressing discomfort or repetition of the painful experience rather than withdrawing from the pain or stopping before contact. This behavior indicates to the practitioner that the child's proprioceptive system needs excessive stimulation and is not easily aroused. A child with this problem often responds by paying more attention to a task and increasing adaptive responses when provided with extra therapeutic input.

Praxis is the functional end result of the following processes: (1) thinking of an action, (2) planning the motor action, and (3) executing the motor action.[19] Multiple types of sensory input can be effectively combined with cognitive strategies when planning activities for children with praxic disorders. The child must be given opportunities to repeat learning experiences. Practice is critical for helping the child develop organization and adaptive skills. A child may have difficulty in one or more of the processes involved in praxis. If the child

has difficulty thinking of or developing a mental image of an action, the intervention techniques include teaching strategies to compensate for ideational deficits to improve sensory processing. For example, a child with a praxic disorder can learn to catch a ball. However, if the ball is not thrown directly to the child, the child may not make the correct body position adaptations needed to catch the ball. This child can be taught strategies to anticipate changes in ball movement and can be emotionally supported while attempting to perform activities that the child has failed in the past. However, practitioners must understand that a child needs to learn specific skills through experiences designed to challenge the child while avoiding failure (the *just right* challenge). Skill building must occur with sensitivity to the emotional issues that a child might experience as a result of poor performance, previous failures, and fear of new tasks. Activities designed to address underlying sensory deficits should be combined with a skill building opportunity.

The treatment of sensory regulatory disorders is a complex area of practice, an area of specialization within the occupational therapy profession in which each practitioner is encouraged to pursue advanced training before using it or any of its techniques.

CASE *Study*

Hannah is a bright and friendly 2-year-old girl. She is one of a set of triplets, with one brother and one sister. Hannah was the first of the three neonates to come home from the hospital following a brief stay in neonatal intensive care unit (NICU). All three children relied on breathing monitors for several months after their discharge from a hospital in a neighboring city. The triplets live with their mother and father, Linda and Larry, and an older sister, Marie, in a small town. Hannah has a medical diagnosis of spastic quadriplegia cerebral palsy.

Jeannie is an occupational therapist who lives in the same small town, several minutes from Hannah's home. Jeannie has been providing Hannah with direct occupational therapy services since she was 8 months old. Jeannie visits Hannah at home twice a week. Jeannie sees Hannah on Monday mornings and Thursday afternoons.

Morning Session

Jeannie arrives on Monday while Linda is fixing breakfast for the triplets. Hannah is propped up in the corner of the couch in the living room and greets Jeannie on her arrival. All of the children are in their pajamas. Jeannie sits down beside Hannah and tells her that this morning they will work on self-feeding skills using an modified spoon and scoop dish. Linda calls the children to the kitchen for breakfast. After telling her what she is going to do, Jeannie gently lifts Hannah onto her lap. Stabilizing Hannah's pelvis with one hand, Jeannie rotates Hannah's upper body to the left and then to the right until she feels Hannah's overall tone in her arms and legs decrease. Jeannie carries Hannah into the kitchen, continuing the rotational activities before placing her into her modified high chair.

As Hannah begins to feed herself, Jeannie notices that Hannah is having difficulty straightening her left arm while scooping her food. After repositioning the scoop dish, Jeannie applies deep pressure to the tendon of the biceps muscle until she feels the muscle relax and sees that Hannah is no longer struggling to scoop her food. When Hannah has finished half of her meal, she asks Linda to feed her the rest of her food because she is tired. Because the other children have finished their breakfast and are anxious to leave the table, Linda and Jeannie agree that Hannah has worked hard, and Linda can feed Hannah the rest of her breakfast.

Afternoon Session

Jeannie arrives on Thursday while Linda is playing with the children in the sunroom. Hannah is seated in a corner chair made of triwall (thick and durable cardboard), which gives her trunk adequate support so that she can use her hands to play. The children greet Jeannie and Hannah asks Jeannie to help get her favorite baby doll out of the toy box. Jeannie removes the tray from the corner chair. With one hand on Hannah's pelvis and the other hand under her arms and around her chest, Jeannie assists Hannah in rotating from a modified long-sitting position to a prone-on-the-floor posture. Using both hands on Hannah's shoulders, Jeannie helps to guide Hannah's weightshift gently into the prone-on-elbows position. Hannah's extensor tone in her legs increases, so Jeannie places one hand on Hannah's buttocks and shakes her hand back and forth until she feels the abnormal tone decrease. To prepare Hannah for bearing weight on her open palms, Jeannie spends time providing deep tactile input to both hands. When Hannah is ready, Jeannie places both hands on Hannah's pelvis to guide her weightshift backward so that Hannah's hips and knees are flexed (bent). Jeannie then cups Hannah's elbows and guides her weightshifts side to side and backward until Hannah is in the quadruped position on extended arms. Jeannie cups her hands and alternately taps the fleshy parts of Hannah's hips as if to say, "Hold it here." Jeannie assists Hannah in creeping to the toy box using Hannah's shoulders, hips, and elbows to guide her movements. Jeannie helps Hannah transition from the quadruped position to standing so that she can reach into the toy box. Hannah becomes very excited at the sight of her favorite doll. The excitement causes her arms to become stiff, making it difficult for her to straighten her arms enough to grab the doll. Jeannie takes one arm and then the other, rotating them until she feels Hannah's tone decrease. Hannah is now able to get her doll out of the toy box.

SUMMARY

The neurophysiological treatment approach, the NDT approach, and the sensory regulatory treatment approach can each contribute, individually or combined, to the treatment of children with CNS dysfunction, movement disorders, and sensory processing deficits. All of these approaches emphasize the use of sensory techniques. Current research on motor control, motor learning, and motor development contributes to occupational therapy practitioners' knowledge of functional movement. Practitioners know that movement is dynamic and the result of multiple forces interacting to produce function. Motor-learning theory contributes to practitioners' knowledge base by providing information on how learning skills are acquired. Occupational therapy practitioners now understand that a reflex-hierarchical model is insufficient to explain the development of functional movement and adaptive responses.

A COTA must gain a thorough knowledge base and collaborate with a trained OTR before using any sensorimotor treatment approach. The occupational therapy practitioner must be sensitive to the family and the child's goals to promote independent functioning. The child, family, OTR, and COTA must work as a team to achieve the best results from these advanced approaches in occupational therapy treatment.

References

1. Alexander R, Boehme R, Cupps B: *Normal development of functional motor skills*, Tucson, 1993, Therapy Skill Builders.

2. Anzalone ME: Sensory contributions to action: a sensory integrative approach, *Zero to Three*, 14:17, 1993.

3. Ayres AJ: *Sensory integration and the child*, Los Angeles, 1979, Western Psychological Services.

4. Ayres AJ: *Sensory integration and learning disorders*, Los Angeles, 1972, Western Psychological Services.

5. Deleted in proofs.

6. Bobath B: Sensorimotor development, *NDT Newsletters* 7:1, 1975.

7. Boehme R: *Improving upper body control: an approach to assessment and treatment of tonal dysfunction*, Tucson, 1995, Therapy Skill Builders.

8. Boehme R: *The hypotonic child: treatment for postural control, endurance, strength and sensory organization*, Tucson, 1990, Therapy Skill Builders.

9. Bundy AC, Fisher AG, Murray EA: *Sensory integration: theory and practice*, Philadelphia, 1991, FA Davis.

10. Cech D, Martin S: *Functional movement development across the life span*, Philadelphia, 1995, WB Saunders.

11. Dunn W, Westman K: The sensory profile: the performance of a national sample of children without disabilities, *Am J Occup Ther* 51:25, 1997.

12. Dutton R: Neuromuscular treatment: sensorimotor techniques. In Neistadt ME, Creapeau EB, editors: *Willard and Spackman's occupational therapy*, ed 9, Philadelphia, 1998, Lippincott-Raven.

13. Gentile PA et al: Sensorimotor approaches to treatment. In Early MB, Pedretti LW, editors: *Physical dysfunction practice skills for the occupational therapy assistant*, St Louis, 1998, Mosby.

14. Greenspan SI, Wieder S: An integrated developmental approach to intervention for young children with severe difficulties in relating and communication. In *Diagnostic classification: 0-3*, Washington, DC, 1994, Zero to Three.

15. Kaplan M, Bedell G: *A motor skill acquisition frame of reference* (in press).

16. Kientz MA, Dunn W: A comparison of the performance of children with and without autism on the sensory profile, Bethesda, Md, 1997, American Occupational Therapy Association.

17. Kimball JG: Sensory integrative frames of reference. In Kramer P, Hinojosa J, editors: *Frames of reference for pediatric occupational therapy*, Baltimore, 1993, Williams & Wilkins.

18. King LJ: Sensory integration: an effective approach to therapy and education, *Autism Res Rev* 5:3, 1991.

19. Koomer JA, Bundy AC: The art and science of creating direct intervention from theory. In Fisher AG, Murray EA, Bundy AC, editors: *Sensory integration: theory and practice*, Philadelphia, 1991, FA Davis.

20. Mathiowetz V, Haugen JB: Motor behavior research: implications for therapeutic approaches to control nervous system dysfunction, *Am J Occup Ther* 48:733, 1994.

21. McCormack GL: The Rood approach to treatment of neuromuscular dysfunction. In Pedretti LW, editor: *Occupational therapy: practice skills for physical dysfunction*, ed 4, St Louis, 1996, Mosby.

22. Nichols DS: The development of postural control. In Case-Smith J, Allen AS, Pratt PN, editors: *Occupational therapy for children*, St Louis, 1996, Mosby.

23. Pedretti LW et al: Treatment of disturbance in tactile sensation, perception, cognition, and vision. In Early MB, Pedretti LW, editors: *Physical dysfunction practice skills for the occupational therapy assistant*, St Louis, 1998, Mosby.

24. Deleted in proofs.

25. Reismont J, Hanschu B: *Sensory integration inventory revised for individuals with developmental disabilities*, Hugo, Minn, 1992, PDP Press.

26. Scheon S, Anderson J: Neurodevelopmental treatment frame of reference. In Kramer P, Hinojosa J: *Frames of reference for pediatric occupational therapy*, Baltimore, 1993, Williams & Wilkins.

27. Trombly CA: Rood approach. In Trombly C, editor: *Occupational therapy for physical dysfunction*, ed 4, Baltimore, 1994, Williams & Wilkins.

28. Trott MC, Laurel MK, Windeck SL: *Sensibilities: understanding sensory integration*, San Antonio, 1993, Therapy Skill Builders.

29. Deleted in proofs.

30. Wilbarger JL, Wilbarger P: *Sensory defensiveness in children aged 2-12*, Santa Barbara, Calif, 1991, Avante Educational Programs.

31. Wilbarger P: The sensory diet: activity programs based on sensory processing theory, *Sensory Integration Special Interest Section Newsletter* 18:1 1995.

32. Williams G: The Rood approach to treatment of neuromuscular dysfunction. In Pedretti LW, editor: *Occupational therapy: practice skills for physical dysfunction*, ed 4, St Louis, 1996.

33. Williams MS, Shellenberger S: *How does your engine run? A leader's guide to the alert program for self-regulation*, Albuquerque, 1992, TherapyWorks.

34. Williamson CG, Anzalone M: Sensory integration: a key component of the evaluation and treatment of young children with severe difficulty in relating and communicating. In *Diagnostic classification: 0-3*, Washington, DC, 1994, Zero to Three.

Recommended Reading

Byarm LE: Neurodevelopmental therapy. In Kurtz L, editor: *Handbook of developmental disabilities: resources for interdisciplinary care*, Gaithersburg, Md, 1997, Aspen.

Coling MC: *Developing integrated programs: a transdisciplinary approach for early intervention*, Tucson, 1991, Therapy Skills Builders.

Dunn W, Westman K: The sensory profile: the performance of a national sample of children without disabilities, *Am J Occup Ther* 51:25, 1997.

Giuffrida CG, Hallway M: *Contemporary neurodevelopmental therapy and motor control and learning*, Paper presented at American Occupational Therapy Association Conference, Baltimore, April 1998.

Kaplan M: Motor learning: implications for occupational therapy and neurodevelopmental treatment, *Developmental Disabilities Special Interest Newsletter* 17:1, 1994.

Kinnealey M, Oliver B, Wilbarger P: A phenomenological study of sensory defensiveness in adults, *Am J Occup Ther* 49:444, 1995.

Kurtz LA: Sensory integration therapy. In Kurtz LA, Childrens' Seashore House, editors: *Handbook of developmental disability*, Gaithersburg, Md, 1996, Aspen.

Vansant AF: Development of posture: motor control and motor learning. In Cech D, Martin S, editors: *Functional movement development across the life span*, Philadelphia, 1995, WB Saunders.

REVIEW *Questions*

1. What is the difference between the reflex-hierarchical model and system model of motor control?
2. List two treatment principles of the neurophysiological approach.
3. List two treatment principles of the NDT approach.

4. What is the significance of postural control to functional movement development?
5. List two treatment principles of the sensory regulatory approach.

SUGGESTED *Activities*

1. Practice handling techniques with classmates. Have them place their hands on your hip joints and experiment with giving you both firm and light tactile input as you attempt to walk. Note how the techniques impact your movements and performances. Exchange places; discuss and share your observations.
2. Carefully analyze changes in your body posture (noting any postural adjustments you make) as you move from a sitting to standing position. Reverse the process and move from a standing position to a sitting position. Compare and discuss your observations with a classmate.
3. While performing a functional activity, such as washing dishes or writing a paper, note and write down all environmental elements that affect your performance. Consider ways you can change elements of environment to improve your performance.

4. Keep a record of your state of alertness and arousal for an entire day. Record your responses and the actions you take to alter your states of arousal and alertness.
5. Be a child for a day. Visit a well equipped playground or park. Climb, swing, and explore all the play equipment. Note your responses. Identify the sensory systems used during your play activities. Write a brief summary of your experience.
6. Identify whether the techniques used are neurophysiological, neurodevelopmental or sensory regulatory techniques during Hannah's treatment sessions. Discuss and practice techniques in small groups.
7. Practice the facilitation and inhibition techniques described in Box 15-1 and Table 15-2 on a classmate.

Assistive Technology

KAREN S. CLAYTON

CINDY TIMMS MATHENA

CHAPTER *Objectives*

After studying this chapter, the reader will be able to accomplish the following:

- Define the concepts of assistive technology devices and services
- Understand the role of federal legislation as it relates to assistive technology and people with disabilities
- Discuss the role of the certified occupational therapy assistant as part of the assistive technology team
- Provide examples of light technology and the ways they might be used to assist a child to achieve a goal
- Discuss the use of a switch in relation to adapting a child's environment
- Describe the importance of independent access to a computer system for children with disabilities
- Provide examples of accommodation using universal design and accommodation that can be added to a computer
- Define two types of augmentative communication and provide examples of each
- Discuss the importance of a team approach when using augmentative communication for a child with a disability
- Provide examples of who might benefit from an environmental control unit and how it might be used
- Describe how an environmental control unit operates and the components necessary to use it
- Discuss various types of mobility devices and provide examples of each
- Define features of a wheelchair and discuss the ways they might be used for different needs

KEY TERMS	CHAPTER OUTLINE

Assistive technology (AT) is a two-word concept that redefines independence for people with disabilities. Occupational therapy practitioners have always been the primary providers of **adaptive equipment** and were recommending and creating this type of equipment long before the information age and the rapid advances in technology. The birth of this age of technology necessitates mastering new skills to advance the realm of adaptive equipment to include AT.

The computer, computer-related technology, and AT are no longer areas in which skills are optional for the occupational therapy practitioner; they have become a part of daily living. Practitioners must be prepared to be on the forefront of the continuing growth and development in the field of AT.

DEFINITION

Although AT involves many types of equipment and services, one universally accepted definition has been established by federal legislation.[3] This legislation states that an **AT device** is ". . . any item, piece of equipment, or product system, whether acquired commercially off-the-shelf, modified, or customized, that is used to increase, maintain, or improve the functional capabilities of individuals with disabilities."[3]

The same report defines an **AT service** as ". . . any service that directly assists an individual with a disability in the selection, acquisition, or use of an assistive technology device."[3] AT services might include assistance with design, fit, adaptation, customization, maintenance, repair, training, or coordination of AT devices.

RELATED LEGISLATION

Understanding the evolution of AT requires a review of the legislation pertaining to this subject. The first law to mandate provisions of reasonable accommodations, including technologies, was Public Law 100-407, the Technology-Related Assistance for Individuals with Disabilities Act (also known as the *Tech Act*). This law, which was passed in 1988, provides funding to states that are able to implement a system for the provision of AT services to its residents with disabilities. This law was the first attempt at defining AT devices and services.

In 1990, Public Law 101-336, the Americans with Disabilities Act (ADA), was enacted. The purpose of the bill is to eliminate discrimination against people with disabilities in all realms of society, including in schools, jobs, public services, accommodations, and transportation. To meet the requirements of this law, many schools, employers, and city officials turned to AT (as described within the law) as a medium of adaptation and accommodation.

In the same year, Public Law 101-476, the Individuals with Disabilities Education Act (IDEA), called for the reauthorization and amendment of an earlier educational law entitled Public Law 94-142, the Education of the Handicapped Act (EHA). IDEA specifically addresses the educational needs of children with disabilities and refers to the use of AT devices and services as part of a free and appropriate education. In 1998, this legislation was amended to include specific terminology that addressed the use of AT for inclusion and transitional services.

Although these laws made AT more readily available to people with disabilities, occupational therapy played a significant role in the establishment of AT. Some occupational therapists involved in the early development of AT include Dennis Anson, Beverly Bain, Jennifer Angelo, Miriam Struck, and Judy Timms. Occupational therapy practitioners are the primary providers of AT.

ROLE OF THE COTA

The role of the certified occupational therapy assistant (COTA) in AT varies depending on the setting, team, and COTA's level of experience. The COTA and registered occupational therapist (OTR) are important members of a team comprising family members and professionals who attempt to evaluate, provide services and equipment, secure funding, develop a plan for the purposeful use of AT, and supervise the use of equipment or related activities.

More specifically, the COTA may be involved in collecting observation and interview data, implementing the use of equipment, or providing client and family education. Examples of a COTA's role might include the instruction of an early childhood educator in the use of an adaptive toy for a child with cerebral palsy or trial of various placements for an environmental control system being used with a child who is paralyzed.

TEAM APPROACH

Regardless of the roles COTAs may assume, they are never alone; the team approach is the key to all AT programs. No one person can possibly make all AT recommendations or carry out all services because AT encompasses numerous aspects of a person's life. For example, a psychologist may assess a child's emotional issues whereas a speech therapist assesses the child's language skills. A physical therapist may comment on the child's physical abilities whereas an occupational therapy practitioner, the child, and the child's family members examine the child's needs for proper positioning and use of AT equipment. Other specialists may be consulted regarding funding (such as a social worker) or training (such as a teacher). The **AT team** works together to decide not only which equipment to use but also the ways in which it will be used, maintained, and reevaluated (Box 16-1).

CLINICAL *Pearl*

One of the most important aspects of any AT program is the use of a team approach.

LIGHT TECHNOLOGY

Light technology (also known as *low technology*) involves devices that are inexpensive, easy to obtain, and simple to make.[4] A principle of AT is to use the simplest method or least complicated device that can be used to meet the needs of the child and the child's family members. Light technology is often preferred to **high technology** and may present a means by which a child can practice important prerequisite skills with little or no cost involved.

Computers, environmental control units, and powered wheelchairs are examples of high technology. Examples of light technology include typing sticks, modified

---

BOX 16-1

Potential Members of the Pediatric AT Team

Child
Family
Caregivers
Teachers (regular education and special education)
Occupational therapy practitioner
Physical therapist
Speech therapist
Physician
Case worker or social worker
Funding specialist
Rehabilitation engineer
Rehabilitation technology supplier (vendor)
Other specialists (such as vision and hearing
  specialists)

---

eating utensils, and pencil holders. In its broadest context, light technology includes adaptation or alteration of the placement of such items. Thus turning the angle on the handle of a spoon to adapt it for easier use by a child with limited range of motion or mobility is an example of light technology.

CLINICAL *Pearl*

Light technology is preferred to high technology if it is the best way to achieve the goal.

Categories

Light-technology devices can promote successful functioning in children with limited ROM, strength, or dexterity; the use of only one limb; impaired cognition; limited communication skills; or impaired or absent sensory functions such as vision or hearing (Table 16-1). Every occupational therapy practitioner should become familiar with commercially available AT products by reviewing catalogs, attending exhibits at conferences, getting to know local vendors, and subscribing to on-line product services (see Chapter 16 Appendix). Devices that are not commercially available can be designed, fabricated, and individually tailored to meet the requirements of a child.

Occupational therapy practitioners have unique skills in understanding the full scope of varying disabilities, including motor, sensory, cognitive, psychosocial, and environmental domains. A holistic frame of reference promotes the occupational therapy practitioner's role on AT teams as the interface specialist. Smith describes the human environment interface model (HETI) as a conceptual theory used to examine the interface assessment between a human and technology[9] (Figure 16-1). Smith's model indicates that human performance (sensation, cognition, motor control) must be interfaced with the environment (method of input, way to process the task, method of output). Each of these six areas of human and technological function can be evaluated for AT solutions

---

TABLE 16-1

Examples of Light Technology

DIAGNOSIS	IMPAIRMENT	LIGHT-TECHNOLOGY SOLUTION
Muscular dystrophy	Limited endurance	Pegs on wheelchair
Retinopathy	Vision impairment	Cane
Developmental dyspraxia	Language delay	Picture board
Spastic cerebral palsy	Limited mobility	Head pointer
Athetoid cerebral palsy	Limited coordination	Computer keyboard

if a deficit is keeping the child from accomplishing goals that should be within reach.

Light-technology devices are frequently used in conjunction with high technology. For example, a child with a motor impairment is not able to access the computer (high technology), so the therapist uses positioning of the child and a universal cuff to hold a dowel, which is used as a pointer (light technology).

Jason has a learning disability, which affects his visual motor skills, fine motor skills, and ability to read and write. His COTA works with his classroom teacher to provide light-technology adaptations, such as adapted books with small tabs to assist him in turning the pages. A special pencil grip assists him with handwriting, and paper with raised lines allows him to learn where and how to write on the lines. Sometimes he utilizes highly technical adaptations, such as a talking word processor, to assist him with language arts activities.

Switch Technology

A **switch** is a simple electrical unit that involves a phone jack, two wires, and two plates (Figure 16-2). The plates are the movable parts of the switch; when pressed together, they bring the two wires into contact. When the wires come into contact, electricity flows into the device and provides power for operation.

A simple, commercially available or easily assembled, inexpensive switch can help children to control items in their environment; this type of simple switch corresponds

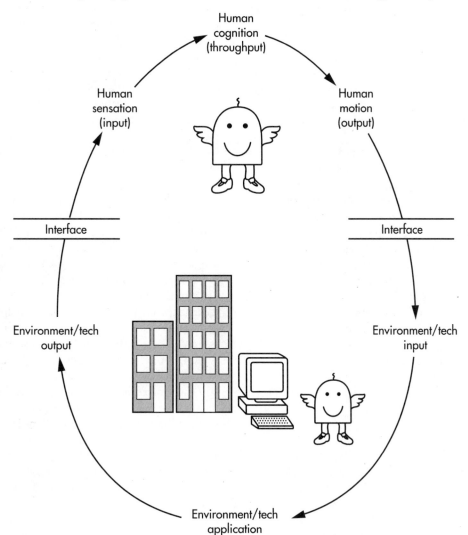

FIGURE 16-1 Human environment and technology interface model (HETI). (From Smith RO: Technology part II: adaptive equipment and technology. In Royeen CB, editor: *AOTA self-study series: classroom applications for school-based practice,* Bethesda, Md, 1992, American Occupational Therapy Association.)

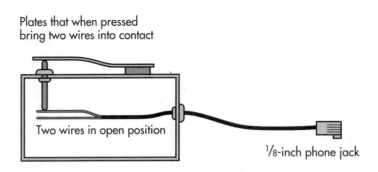

FIGURE 16-2 Anatomy of a switch.

to Cook and Hussey's definition of a light-technology device—one that is inexpensive, easy to make, and readily available.[4] However, the selection and use of the switch for a specific problem requires the skills of an occupational therapy practitioner to successfully interpret the child's needs.

Children with physical, sensory, or cognitive impairments often have difficulty interacting with and learning from the environment. Young children use play as their primary occupation and as a vehicle of learning. A carefully selected and placed switch may help children develop their play and cognitive skills through interactions with the environment.

Using switches to operate age-appropriate toys fosters a sense of control over the environment and facilitates cause-and-effect learning. Operating a simple switch-activated jumping dog or battery-operated train as part of a play activity can lead to mastery of more complex tools in the environment, such as appliances and computers.

Occupational therapy practitioners should consider the many features of, types of, and ways to adapt switches before determining which switch is best for the child who is being evaluated and trained to use the device. Switches can be designed to provide momentary or latching connections. *Momentary* refers to a switch that requires constant pressure to keep the device it controls operating. An example is a doorbell. *Latching* involves pressing the switch once to activate the device and then pressing the switch again to deactivate the device. An example of this type of switch is a radio.

Switch Features

Numerous **switch features** exist to accommodate all types of children. Children can operate switches using various methods, including by limb, eye, head, or tongue movements; airflow; sound; or voice. Carefully assessing children's needs determines the most effective type of switch for each child. A switch may be chosen based on the force needed for activation. Children with severe hypotonia may need a switch that is activated with minimal force,

whereas children with athetosis may need a switch that can be activated by (and endure) forceful movements. Children who do not have sufficient control of a limb can use head and neck movements or a mouth stick to operate a switch. Using a high-technology method such as pneumatic control, sound or voice activation, or a light pointer system may help when simpler switch operation methods are unsuccessful.

The occupational therapy practitioner determines the shape and size of the switches and the spacing between them. Although a single switch can initially be the size of a notebook, as the child develops the switch can be made smaller and less conspicuous. The smaller the switch's contact area and the more closely together it is to other switches, the better motor control the child must have to successfully use it.

Switches should provide the child with some sort of feedback so that the child knows when the switch is activated. This knowledge is usually gained from visual, auditory, or tactile feedback. An example of visual feedback is a light that turns on when the switch is active, which can be particularly helpful in a classroom because it does not disturb others (as auditory feedback would). Auditory feedback, such as a click, particularly helps children who cannot see the switch because of impairments or the switch is out of the visual field (for example, a head switch). Some switches vibrate, and some are covered with special textured materials.

The practitioner must carefully evaluate the placement of the switch. Switches are often mounted to something in the environment, such as a bed frame, wheelchair laptray, or tabletop. Occupational therapy practitioners should have several equipment-mounting options available so that they can assess which type and position provides optimal switch control. Switch-mounting kits containing clamps, tubes, rods, and gooseneck arms are commercially available. A careful assessment and an initial home trial of the mounting system can promote successful use of the switch. Permanent mounting systems are commercially available, and customized mounting systems may be used when nothing else works. The mounting system should not interfere with daily activities and should be as visually appealing as possible. Family members, teachers, and other caregivers must be able to assemble and position the mounting system if necessary.

Sarah is in a first-grade class with her peers. She has delayed cognitive skills because of a chromosomal disorder that has affected her development. Although she is unable to speak, an AT team has designed a switch that allows her to operate many devices. She can use it to activate a tape recorder with a prerecorded tape that allows her to sing along with her class during music time, or she can use it to turn on a fan when the class discusses wind during science. Her AT team thought of numerous creative ways in which Sarah can use her switch to participate with her class. The other children in her class enjoy helping her use the switch, and she has made many friends this year.

COMPUTER-RELATED ASSISTIVE TECHNOLOGY

The ability to use a computer has become an important and necessary life skill and an integral part of numerous individuals' lives, from the preschooler who is learning preliteracy skills by interacting with an animated CD-ROM to the business person who is researching products on the Internet. **Computer access** can provide independence and learning experiences not available through any other type of technology or media for individuals with disabilities. Any child with a disability can benefit from using a computer for communication, leisure, learning, and socialization.

Computer-related AT involves adapting the computer or its devices and usually involves specialized hardware or software or both. AT related to hardware is known as *input* or *output AT*. Examples of adapted input are an enlarged keyboard, a touch window, or a switch and switch interface box. Examples of adapted output include a Braille printer and a speech synthesizer to read words on the computer screen. Examples of software adaptations, which are becoming more universal, include software with enlarged text and graphics, speech output, and accessible websites.

Mobility and Sensory Impairments

A child with a mobility impairment may have difficulty using a computer keyboard and mouse. The occupational therapy practitioner plays an important role in determining the most appropriate method of adapted input and needs to be familiar with the child's movement quality and available adaptive input. Input adaptations should be

TABLE 16-2

Universal Design Computer Features

MOBILITY IMPAIRMENT	UNIVERSAL DESIGN FEATURE
Difficulty using two hands to hit a modifier key at the same time as another key	Sticky keys
Difficulty releasing a key before it starts to repeat	No-repeat key setting
Difficulty hitting correct keys because of lack of coordination or ataxia	Slow keys
Difficulty using a mouse	Mouse keys

TABLE 16-3

Adaptive Equipment for Computer Use

MOBILITY IMPAIRMENT	ADAPTIVE EQUIPMENT
Cannot accurately target keys on keyboard	Keyguard, enlarged or mini keyboard
Cannot interact with keyboard	Touch sensitive monitor screen, alternative keyboard
Cannot interact with mouse	Joystick track ball or on-screen software

simple and involve direct selection when possible. Direct selection includes typing with a mouth stick or pointer or using a keyboard or touch window to activate an alternate keyboard or input device. Indirect selection includes scanning letters or pictures and selecting choices with a switch.

CLINICAL *Pearl*

Direct selection is almost always more accurate and simpler to use than an indirect method.

Many standard features of computer systems and operating software are appealing and useful not only to individuals with disabilities, but for anyone using a computer. Engineering technology that has equal appeal to numerous individuals is called technology that has a **universal design** (Table 16-2). Other features may not be inherent in the software or computer's design. Table 16-3 provides several examples of adaptive equipment for computer use. Commercially available software allows a switch user to access the games and activities by simply plugging in a switch through a switch interface box.

Computer adaptations for individuals with sensory impairments are becoming increasingly affordable and easy to use. For example, with the advent of multimedia computers, speech synthesis became a standard feature and the purchase of a separate speech synthesizer was no longer necessary. Software, such as the popular talking word processors Intellitalk (Intellitools, Inc., Novato, Calif.) and Write:OutLoud (Don Johnston Developmental Equipment, Inc., Wauconda, Ill.) take advantage of the speech output features of multimedia and provide enlarged text for a reasonable cost.

Many of the most popular children's games and CD-ROMs feature large graphics and sounds. Adaptive keyboards and customized overlays provide endless possibilities for adapting school curricula and leisure activities for children with sensory impairments. Hardware adaptations include Braille printers, scanners, and software that include American sign language (ASL) translations for children who use sign language.

Learning Disabilities

Children with any type of learning disability can benefit from the computer, particularly in schools. Special software can read text, help with spelling, or assist with grammar. Typing on a keyboard is sometimes easier and neater for children who have difficulty with handwriting and allows them to keep up with their schoolwork. The occupational therapy practitioner works with the AT team to identify which types adaptive software would be beneficial and to set up a keyboarding curriculum.

Autism

Computers can help children with autism participate with their peers. The computer is a valuable means of learning, writing, and interacting for many children who are otherwise unable to communicate. In many cases the structured content of the software, graphics, sound, or nonhuman contact provides a type of interaction that brings out the highest potential in children who are unable to communicate. Computers are and must remain an important aspect of education and communication for children with autism.

Amy is blind. She attends high school and would like to pursue a career in music. She has been accepted at a prestigious music college but is worried that her disability will make it difficult for her to fully participate. An AT team has been training Amy to use a portable Braille note taker, a

Braille music translator, and adaptations that allow her to hear the computer. Amy currently uses these adaptations to perform research for school projects, translate her music assignments to Braille, and take notes in class. Highly technical adaptations have made it possible for her to fully and independently participate in high school activities. However, the AT team recognizes that Amy's needs will change when she reaches college. Additional adaptations will be provided for Amy as needed.

AUGMENTATIVE COMMUNICATION

Lewis has defined **augmentative communication** (AC) as ". . . a set of approaches used to improve the communication skills of persons who do not speak or whose speech is not intelligible."[6] Although the terms *augmentative* and *alternative* are often linked, their meanings are slightly different. AC approaches supplement, enhance, or support the communication process for persons who have difficulty with expressive communication. Mathena and Snyders further defined AC as a total communication approach involving the use of multiple systems, or modes, that are unaided (such as gestures, signs, word approximations) and aided (such as pictures or symbol boards with light- or high-technology devices).[7]

Team Approach

The roles of occupational therapy practitioners vary depending on their experience level, the setting, the AT team members, and the model of service delivery being used. Particularly in the field of AC, the team needs to adhere to a transdisciplinary model in which all members are familiar with all aspects of the child's abilities and development and use their expertise to develop recommendations and implement programs. The team members may find that their roles tend to overlap more than usual, but this can help them focus on all aspects of a child. Occupational therapy practitioners should keep in mind that even a simple switch or a picture on the wall can be considered a form of augmentative or alternative communication. The way the system is incorporated in the child's life is a responsibility of the occupational therapy practitioner.

Light-Technology Augmentative Communication Systems

Simple communication systems are a great way to introduce, evaluate, or practice AC, especially for children. Hastily purchasing expensive equipment can be costly and impractical, especially because many children readily

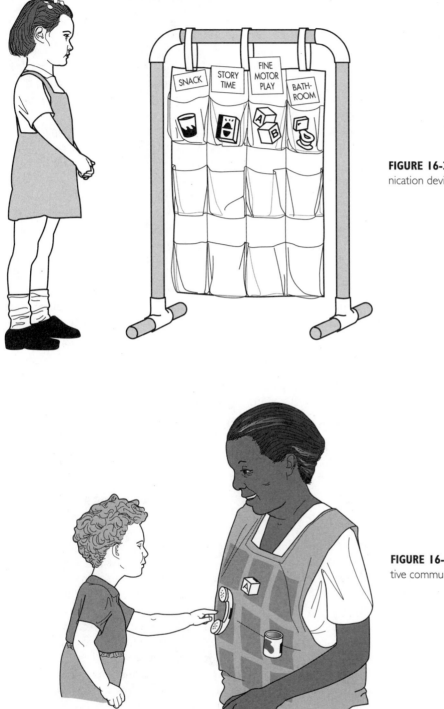

FIGURE 16-3 Shoe bag used as a simple communication device.

FIGURE 16-4 Adapted vest used as an augmentative communication device.

use and enjoy simpler systems. Examples of simple systems include objects or realistic pictures, pictures in books, or portable systems. Occupational therapy practitioners can put their creative skills to good use while designing these systems. For example, a hanging shoe bag can be used to hold objects from which a child can choose activities (Figure 16-3). Placing pictures on a schedule board or near activity centers also provides a simple and effective means of communication for some children. Other examples of light-technology communication include a communication vest (Figure 16-4), an eyegaze chart, and talking switches and toys.

High-Technology Augmentative Communication Systems

High-technology methods of communication are probably what most people envision when they think of AC. Unfortunately, some studies show that as many as 80% of individuals stop using these devices after 6 months. In most cases, the lack of use can be attributed to poor planning, education, and implementation, not poor selection of appropriate devices. Developing a plan for a device's use is as important as the actual selection of the device.

Features of high-technology devices include digitized speech (recorded human speech), synthesized speech (computer-generated speech); direct selection, switch input; scanning, portability; size, selection, and number of sites, and additional features. Special software is integrated into a computer and thus provides a greater variety of features and uses. These are called dynamic display devices.

Regardless which type of device a child needs, successful use of a communication system depends on several factors. A supportive and knowledgeable team, appropriate programming, meaningful language and activities, maintenance planning, and creativity all affect the success of a high-technology device. A positive attitude should be used when introducing the child to and training the child in use of the system.

Jacob is a young man with autism. His parents and teachers have always suspected that he is a bright young man but is frustrated because he is unable to communicate his needs and wants. Jacob becomes angry and aggressive when others do not understand him. A team consisting of an occupational therapist, a speech therapist, a teacher, a parent, and an administrator have worked for 3 months to determine the best methods and equipment to use to allow Jacob to become more independent in communication. They began with simple, structured activities that Jacob enjoyed; he was given a simple picture book to use to initiate an activity. Once he mastered using the book, his team added voice output to his activity. Soon he was using a digitized voice feedback device with eight choices. His AT team instructed others on the ways to program it for different activities throughout the day. Now eight choices are not enough. Jacob is ready for a device with more choices and different levels of information. The device should be portable and easy to program. The team is confident that he will be able to use the device successfully based on his previous practice and mastery of other devices.

ENVIRONMENTAL CONTROL UNITS

Children with severe musculoskeletal limitations such as high quadriplegia or progressive muscular disorders can learn methods to control various items in their environment. An **environmental control unit** (ECU) increases independence by providing a method for the child to operate electrical devices such as telephones, room lights, bed controls, call buttons, and televisions.

The major parts of the ECU include the input device, control unit, and output devices (the appliances that are to be controlled by the ECU) (Figure 16-5). The child's ROM and ability to consistently operate the unit are factors in the selection of the input device. Angelo describes the control of the input device as being accomplished by either direct selection, a set of switches, or voice control.[1] An example of direct selection is the positioning of a keyboard (especially if the ECU is used in conjunction with a computer) and a joystick or control panel so that the child can operate the input device. The child can control the switch mechanisms by using a single switch for each device being controlled or using one switch that operates the device as well as the features of the device (for example, being able to control the volume of a television after turning it on).

The occupational therapy practitioner may need to explore using voice control for children who do not have the motor capabilities to operate an ECU. An ECU can be designed to recognize key sounds from the user's voice, which activate the devices controlled by the ECU.

Types of Transmission

The signal from the input device is sent to the control unit. The control unit contains the circuits that interpret the signal and send it to the devices the ECU controls. Most ECUs use some form of remote control to activate their devices. Cook and Hussey describe four ways that this can be accomplished: (1) house wiring, (2) ultrasound, (3) infrared transmission, and (4) radio frequency transmission.[4] Using the existing wiring in the child's house makes installation easier. (However, if several devices are to be activated by the ECU, too many electrical outlets may be required.) Ultrasound is sound waves whose frequency are beyond human hearing ranges. The control unit picks up the sound waves and activates the devices attached to the ECU. Although the ultrasound setup is wireless, the child is confined to controlling the devices from within one room.

Infrared transmission requires the user to point the input device directly at the control box. An infrared input device would be appropriate for a child with enough motor control to line up the infrared input device with the control unit. Remote controls of most television sets use infrared transmission. Just as a television set remote does

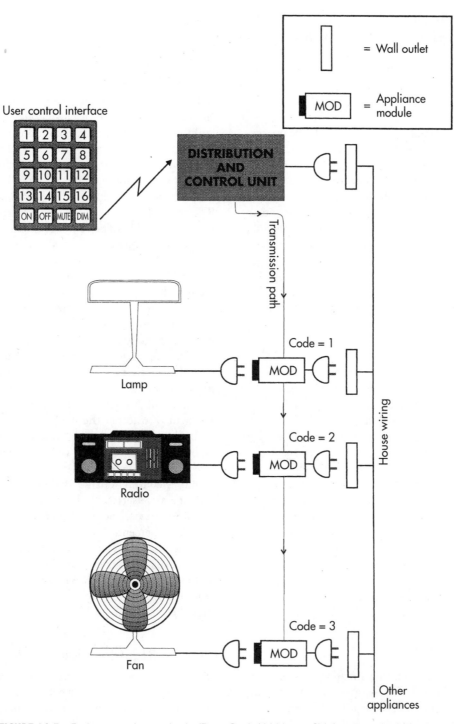

FIGURE 16-5 Environmental control unit. (From Cook AM, Hussey SM: *Assistive technologies: principles and practice,* St Louis, 1995, Mosby.)

not work when blocked by someone or something, infrared transmission does not activate an ECU if something or someone is blocking the transmission.

Radio frequencies are not blocked when someone or something is between the control unit and the devices being activated. However, the ECU can be activated unintentionally by someone using another radio frequency device such as a garage door opener nearby.

The output devices or appliances to be controlled by the ECU should be selected with input from the child, family members, and the AT team. Depending on the child's situation, addressing safety issues (such as the ability to place an emergency call or activate a call button) may be a higher priority than television or radio access.

Assessment

Angelo provides a list of questions to answer before recommending an ECU,[1] several of which involve the assessment of the child and the child's family. The occupational therapy practitioner must determine exactly what the child and the child's family want the ECU to do, the child's functional capabilities (including cognitive status), where the ECU will be used, and the position the child will be in when using the ECU. Issues to consider about the equipment include the space that the ECU will require, the portability of the ECU, the type of feedback (that is, visual or auditory) the unit provides, funding constraints, installation, and maintenance responsibilities.

Chris is a young man who has been introduced to ECUs through his occupational therapy practitioner. He has muscular dystrophy and in recent years has become increasingly dependent on his parents and siblings for assistance at home. Being so dependent bothers him because he is a teenager and thinks he needs more privacy and independence. He tells his practitioner that he wants to be able to use a remote control to operate the television, play CDs on the stereo, and operate the lights and fan in his room. His practitioner recommends an ECU that would allow him to do this through use of a switch. The unit also has the capability to control up to 30 other devices so as his needs change, he can control additional devices. A local service organization donates a portion of the ECU cost so that Chris's parents can afford it.

MOBILITY DEVICES

Mobility is essential for learning and quality of life. Improving mobility through the use of AT supports the additional goals of greater independent functioning, better social interactions, and improved self-esteem. **Mobility devices** can be introduced successfully at any age; however, in normal developing infants, the mastery of motor skills in the first 3 years of life are extremely closely linked with cognitive and social development. Therefore children should be introduced to mobility at as young of an age as possible—the younger the better.

A pediatric mobility system is not only smaller than an adult mobility system but also must accommodate growth changes over several years. A pediatric mobility

system is also used in environments such as schools or playgrounds.

Selection Process

Selecting the best mobility device for a child requires the AT team to work in close collaboration with the child, parent or caregiver, prescribing physician, school personnel, and the rehabilitation technology supplier (RTS). A COTA cannot evaluate a child or prescribe wheelchairs without input from others but is usually part of the team that is making the recommendations. The RTS should be knowledgeable about current mobility devices and be able to present choices in accordance with the desired features.

The occupational therapy practitioner must identify the child's mobility needs and recommend features that promote function and successful use. Once the mobility device has arrived, the practitioner needs to reassess the fit and train the child, family members, and caregivers in its use and maintenance.

The occupational therapy practitioner should ask the RTS whether the device being considered could be loaned to the family or at least brought to an evaluation session. A trial period allows a more realistic assessment of whether the device will meet the goals of optimal mobility. Many funding agencies do not replace mobility devices for 3 to 5 years after purchase. Therefore all parameters of the device must be carefully evaluated. A comprehensive evaluation includes current age, age at onset of disability, type of disability, and prognosis. Assessments of motor, sensory, cognitive, and visual-perceptual abilities include evaluation of endurance, tone, reflexes, musculoskeletal abnormalities, and functional transfer skills. Environmental demands, including any additional AT items that may need to be mounted to the wheelchair (such as an AC device), should be assessed.

Children Requiring Mobility Aids

Hays has categorized children without locomotion (that is, the ability to move their body from one place to another) into the following four functional groups[5]:

1. Children who will never ambulate and need a power wheelchair, such as children who have severe cerebral palsy or spinal muscle atrophy
2. Children who have inefficient mobility because of limitations in speed, rate, or endurance and need a power wheelchair, such as children with moderate cerebral palsy or spinal deformities (such as myelomeningocele spina bifida with upper extremity involvement)

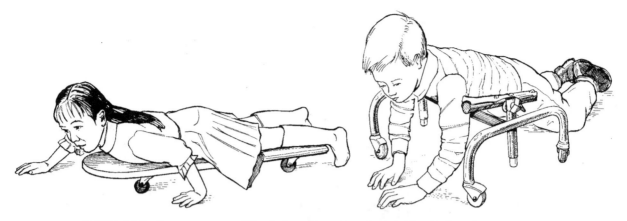

FIGURE 16-6   Prone scooter mobility devices. (From Case-Smith J, Allen AS, Pratt PN: *Occupational therapy for children,* ed 3, St Louis, 1996, Mosby.)

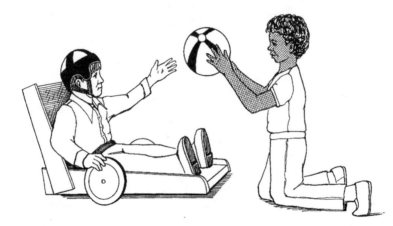

FIGURE 16-7   Caster cart mobility device. (From Case-Smith J, Allen AS, Pratt PN: *Occupational therapy for children,* ed 3, St Louis, 1996, Mosby.)

3. Children who have lost their mobility through head injuries or progressive neuromuscular conditions and often have many psychosocial issues associated with adapting to an assisted mobility device when one was previously not needed
4. Children who may eventually become independently mobile and temporarily need a mobility device, such as children with arthrogryposis or juvenile rheumatoid arthritis

The previous four categories describe children who are not mobile. They do not include children with impaired mobility skills who would benefit from an assistive light-technology device to enhance their existing skills.

Light-Technology Mobility Aids

Of the many appropriate and useful **mobility devices** in the category of light-technology aids, examples include crutches, canes, walkers, and scooters. A prone scooter may be helpful for a young child while engaging in play on the floor (Figure 16-6). The child needs head and neck control and upper extremity function to propel the scooter. Although the scooter allows access to playing on the floor, maintaining head and neck extension is fatiguing. Therefore this device may only be useful for limited amounts of time in an indoor environment. A caster cart is another means of mobility for a young child and can be used indoors and outdoors for limited distances over smooth terrain (Figure 16-7). The child must be able to tolerate a long leg sitting position.

Wheelchairs

The most important considerations in selecting a wheelchair are the mobility base and the postural support system. According to Sylvester, three kinds of mobility bases exist: (1) independently user propelled by hand or foot,

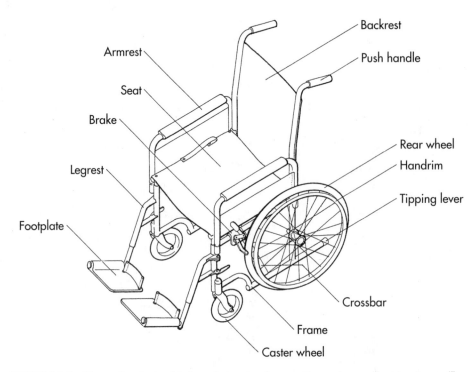

FIGURE 16-8 Conventional wheelchair: major parts of supporting and propelling structures. (From Ragnarsson KT: Prescription considerations and a comparison of conventional and lightweight wheelchairs, *J Rehab Res Devel* 2(suppl):8, 1990.)

(2) electronically user propelled, and (3) propelled by someone other than the user, such as a parent or caregiver.[10] A classification system has been developed to help therapists understand the hundreds of different types of wheelchairs available.

Wheelchair features

The most recognizable features of the standard wheelchair are the frame, push handles, rear wheels, front casters, armrests, legrests, and wheel locks (Figure 16-8). A wheelchair prescription form outlines chair specifications (Figure 16-9). The weight of the materials used in the construction of the chair frame often serves as a classification for the chair (that is, heavy duty, lightweight, ultralight). The appearance of the chair is important, so the child should be encouraged to participate in selecting the style, fabric, and color if possible.

The seat surface may be firm or a sling type made of vinyl fabric. The sling feature allows a chair to fold. However, solid seats can be designed for foldable wheelchairs. Many pediatric chairs and strollers are built to increase in width as the child grows. A reclining backrest may be a necessary feature for a child with contractures or spinal deformities.

The rear tires may be solid or air-filled (pneumatic). The air-filled tires may be easier to push or manipulate over sandy or rough terrain such as a playground surface.

However, they are not as durable as solid tires. Adaptations such as plastic coatings or knobs on the handrims can improve the child's traction and make manual propulsion easier. Some children may need a one-arm drive system that allows both wheels to be operated from one side.

Armrests can be fixed or removable, full length, desk length, or elevating. Removable and desk-length armrests allow a child to roll up under a table. Removable armrests make transferring easier. Full-length armrests provide a more stable surface for mounting trays or other AT devices as the child grows.

Powered wheelchairs

Powered wheelchair bases are either belt driven or direct drive. Traditional powered wheelchairs are usually belt driven; a motor turns pulleys on each side of the wheelchair, which turn the wheels. Direct drive is a system in which the motor is connected directly to the wheels, making the wheelchair more maneuverable outdoors than the belt-driven models. Powered bases have direct drive systems, with the powered unit being a separate section from the seating section. Although they are not technically wheelchairs, scooters are in same category as direct-drive wheelchairs, even though some have the drive system applied to the front wheel. Three-wheeled scooters are more suitable for indoor use and older children with

Name:_____   Diagnosis (1): _____
Date of evaluation: _____   (2):_____
Date of birth: _____   _____
Ht (Lt): _____   Wt: _____   Sex: _____   Prognosis:_____
Patient residence: Home _____   Institution _____
Mode of transportation: Car _____   Van _____   Van with lift _____
Functional level:
    Head control: Absent _____   Poor _____   Fair _____   Good _____
    Sitting balance, unsupported: Absent _____   Poor _____   Fair _____   Good _____
    Transfers: Independent _____   Assisted _____   Dependent _____
    Hand function: Requires support of distal arm?   Yes _____   No _____
    Propulsion (current or future):   Self _____   Motorized self _____   Dependent _____
    Can patient communicate comfort?   Yes _____   No _____
    Can patient relieve pressure?   Yes _____   No _____
Anticipated use of seating device:
    Hours of expected daily use: _____hours
    Classroom use: Yes _____   No _____
    Feeding positioning: Yes _____   No _____   (Oral _____   Gastrostomy _____)
    Support communication device: Yes _____   No _____

Predominant Reflex Activity, Seated Position

	Present*	Absent	Predominant Tone Pattern (Seated)	Upper extremity	Lower extremity	Trunk
Asymmetrical tonic neck to right	_____	_____				
Asymmetrical tonic neck to left	_____	_____	Normal	_____	_____	_____
Symmetrical tonic neck	_____	_____	Hypotonic	_____	_____	_____
Tonic labyrinthine	_____	_____	Hypotonic, flexor	_____	_____	_____
Extensor thrust	_____	_____	Hypertonic, extensor	_____	_____	_____
Marie Foix	_____	_____	Fluctuating	_____	_____	_____

*Record as 1 to 4+

Skeletal Review

1. Pelvis: Fixed tilt   Yes _____   No _____
    If yes: Anterior _____   Posterior _____
        Obliquity   Yes _____   No _____
        Rotation   Yes _____   No _____
2. Hips: Normal   Right _____   Left _____
        Subluxed/dislocated   Right _____   Left _____
        Contracted*   Right _____   Left _____
        Abduction   _____   _____
        Adduction   _____   _____
        Flexion   _____   _____
        Extension   _____   _____
*Record in degrees
3. Knees: Contracture   Right _____   Left _____
4. Ankle/foot: Contracture   Right _____   Left _____
        Deformity: Right _____   Left _____
        Describe: _____
        _____

5. Leg length discrepent: Yes _____   No _____
6. Trunk: Kyphosis: Yes _____   No _____
        Scoliosis: Yes _____   No _____
        Flexible: Yes _____   No _____
        Degrees: _____
        Convex to: Right _____   Left _____
7. Shoulders: Protracted: Yes _____   No _____
        Retracted: Yes _____   No _____
        Asymmetrical: Yes _____   No _____
8. Neck: Torticollis   Yes _____   No _____
        Chin to: Right _____   Left _____

Sensation: Normal _____   Impaired _____   Skin intact: Yes _____   No _____
Recommendations:_____

FIGURE 16-9   Sample wheelchair prescription form. (Courtesy Children's Hospital of the King's Daughters, Norfolk, Va.)

good trunk control and balance. Some children using manual wheelchairs may benefit from using an add-on power pack, a feature that allows a manual wheelchair to be turned into a powered chair.

Some children may use all three mobility bases. Parents of a young child may use a stroller for quick trips because it is easier to handle and not as heavy as the standard or powered wheelchair. Some environments are not accessible to powered chairs, and powered chairs periodically have to be repaired. Although powered chairs have the advantages of increased speed, less energy expenditure, and independent maneuvering, they have the disadvantages of increased weight, decreased portability, and more maintenance and repair issues.

Input devices

The method a child uses to operate a powered wheelchair must be determined according to safety and efficacy. Based on the child's abilities, the practitioner assists in selecting the control device and the positioning of this device. Angelo divides **input devices** into the two categories: (1) proportional and (2) digital (or microswitch).[1] Proportional controls allow for gradation of the chair's speed and angle of movement. The proportional joystick is the method most frequently used to operate a powered chair. The size, style, and positioning of the joystick are critical factors. Many children use an upper extremity to operate the joystick; however, the optimal joystick placement for children who are unable to use their upper extremities is under their chin or behind or beside their head. Customizations of joysticks include tremor-damping mechanisms and short-throw features that allow joysticks to be maneuvered with less movement.

The digital joystick operates by an on or off directional mechanism. Control efficiency can be more difficult to achieve with the digital control. A pneumatic, sip-and-puff type of control exemplifies the on or off directional method because the child uses a hard puff of breath to go forward and a hard sip to reverse. To go left, the child uses a soft sip, and to go right, a soft puff. Switch boxes, or switch-scanning, systems are another method of digital control. The child must be able to respond quickly enough to avoid objects and people in the environment. Although not a substitute for actual practice, computer-training programs help a child learn the sequence of steps necessary to operate the digital joysticks.[7]

A COTA named Jane is working in a school system in which she addresses the needs of children with physical disabilities as part of her job duties. The majority of the children are in wheelchairs. She is committed to ensuring that the medical team and school AT team work closely together to evaluate and determine mobility aids a child might use. After making recommendations and purchasing the wheelchair, she began working with her school AT team to monitor positioning, use of adaptive equipment, and any modifications the system might require. She often assists with training children who have received powered mobility aids. She adapts lap trays for computers, modifies wheelchairs to hold books, and attaches switches to chairs for use with computers. She knows that a child who spends a great deal of time in a wheelchair needs to be monitored constantly and that the wheelchair needs frequent modifications.

DOCUMENTATION AND FUNDING

Documentation and funding are inextricably related; securing funding is difficult without proper AT documentation. Documentation exists in several formats that may entail questionnaires, checklists, narrative reports, and formal evaluation tools. Regardless of the report format used, the documentation should be a team effort. Many AT teams have found alternative reporting formats, such as videotapes or portfolios of a student's work, to be extremely successful for securing funding or services. Another important aspect of documentation includes the goals and objectives. Goals should be functional and achievable. Objectives should focus on performance of specific, activity-related tasks that are performed within the child's natural setting.

With proper documentation, a child's services or device might be funded through a school system, insurance company, vocational rehabilitation system, or charitable organization. For a school system to fund a device, its use must be educationally necessary. Likewise, for a third-party reimburser to purchase equipment, it must be considered **durable medical equipment** (DME), which means that the company recognizes it as being medically necessary for the child to function. Schmeler offers tips for successful documentation of the need for AT.[8] Though he stresses that no particular statement or style ensures funding, he does provide advice for describing the child's currently used technology, describing the technology with pictures, and providing alternatives.

CASE *Study*

Mariah is a 10-year-old girl who has cerebral palsy and athetoid movements (Figure 16-10). She does not vocalize and uses a wheelchair as her primary means of mobility. She is the only child of divorced parents, both of whom are very supportive and involved in her life. Mariah is a bright student who attends a school that allows her to receive

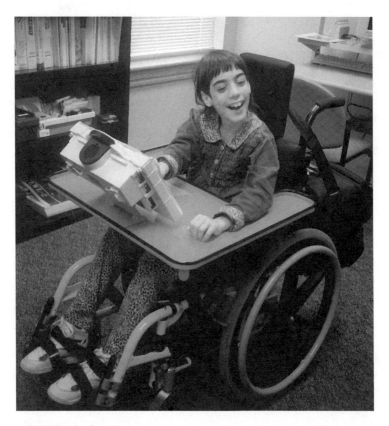

FIGURE 16-10   Mariah in powered wheelchair with mounted AC device.

special instruction and therapy as well as participate in integrated regular education classes. She has a personal assistant who accompanies her to class and helps her with note taking and written work.

It became evident that Mariah was a good candidate for AT when she entered an early childhood special education program at the age of 2. Her occupational therapy practitioner noted her need for adapted toys and alternative communication and began to assemble a team of people to address these needs. Initially the two greatest concerns were the adaptation of toys and learning materials and the provision of light-technology communication aids. With Mariah and her mother, the teacher, OTR, COTA, physical therapist (PT), and speech and language patholo-gist (SLP) designed switches for Mariah's favorite battery-operated toys. The switches also allowed her to communicate simple messages for social greetings or to make simple requests, such as requesting a certain item at snacktime. Mariah easily mastered the concept of switch use and was soon using more complex communicators and beginning to enjoy switch-operated games on the computer.

Although this was a good start, it has become apparent that as Mariah has grown older, her needs have changed. Not only would AT be helpful in other areas of her life, but she is now accomplishing more academically in school, and the simple communication devices and switches are not sufficient for the level of work she is capable of performing. A new AT team has been formed, and this time many more people are involved.

Because Mariah needs a stand-alone communication device for all aspects of her life and not just school, the AT team decides to refer her for a medical evaluation of her AC needs. The AT clinic at a local hospital recommends a device that is deemed to be a medical necessity. Because of this recommendation, Mariah's insurance company agrees to fund the device.

In the school environment, a teacher, SLP, occupational therapy practitioner, and PT work with Mariah's family on developing individualized educational plan (IEP) goals that will help Mariah use her new communication device in all of her environments. They also introduce a computer that allows her to scan the alphabet and select letters with a switch. She now has the ability to take a spelling test and write sentences for a book report.

As the team trains Mariah to use her new equipment, other problems become evident. For instance, her device is heavy and cumbersome and has to be set up for her every time she wants to use it. Some volunteers from the community hear of this difficulty and design and build a lap tray for her that incorporates into the device and attaches easily to the wheelchair.

As Mariah grows and develops the need for more independence, her device, a Dynavox, is programmed to control the television and videocassette recorder. In the future, she will also be able to use the device to turn lights on or off and control other appliances in her environment.

The team also determines that it is time to investigate powered mobility devices. Based on Mariah's ability to use switches, a set of four switches, each representing a different verbally spoken direction, is incorporated with her AC system. As each switch is activated, a specific direction is spoken by a simple communication device. The occupational therapy practitioner or teacher working with Mariah can steer the wheelchair based on the directions given. This device is used for evaluations as well as practice. Everyone involved, including Mariah, is sure that a similar system could be used to operate her wheelchair, so the new powered chair is ordered.

The team constantly reevaluates Mariah's needs, tries new ideas, and implements new plans based on successes, failures, and feedback from everyone on the team. Much of the planning is by trial and error, but one thing remains constant: the group of people works together with the common goal of helping Mariah become independent using AT.

SUMMARY

AT is a tool that occupational therapy practitioners use in all aspects of treatment and service provision. This tool is especially powerful when used in the pediatric setting. AT fosters function and independence in children with disabilities, and this is the primary goal of occupational therapy. With their skills in activity analysis and adaptation, occupational therapy practitioners are vital members and leaders of AT teams. The importance of a team approach to technology integration, keeping technology simple, and setting achievable goals is seen as a valuable component of successful AT provision.

Many aspects of AT exist, including AC, ECUs, mobility devices, and computer-related technology. The field is constantly growing and changing. For occupational therapy practitioners to include AT as a service provision, they must make an effort to stay up to date and informed on new products and developments in this complex and advancing field.

References

1. Angelo J: *Assistive technology for rehabilitation therapists*, Philadelphia, 1997, FA Davis.
2. Deleted in proofs.
3. Cook AM, Hussey SM: *Assistive technologies: principles and practice*, St Louis, 1995, Mosby.
4. Congressional Report on Public Law 100-407, *The technology-related assistance for individuals with disabilities act (Tech Act) of 1988*, Washington, DC.
5. Hays R: Childhood motor impairments: clinical overview and scope of the problem. In Jaffe KM, editor: *Proceedings of the RESNA first Northwest regional conference*, Washington, DC, 1987, RESNA Press.
6. Lewis RB: *Special education technology; classroom applications*, Pacific Grove, Calif, 1993, Cole.
7. Mathena C, Snyders C: No mode is an island, *Link-Up* 7(1):1, 1996.
8. Schmeler M: Ten tips on documenting the need for assistive technology, *TeamRehab* 9(8):16, 1998.
9. Smith RO: Technology part II: adaptive equipment and technology. In Royeen CB, editor: *AOTA self study series: classroom applications for school–based practice*, Bethesda, Md, 1992, American Occupational Therapy Association.
10. Sylvester L: Functional seating and wheeled mobility for children. In Ratliffe KT, editor: *Clinical pediatric physical therapy*, St Louis, 1998, Mosby.

REVIEW *Questions*

1. Who are the possible members of an AT team?
2. What types of responsibilities might the COTA have on the AT team?
3. How has federal legislation impacted the field of AT?
4. What factors might be considered in deciding which type of a switch should be ordered for a child with cerebral palsy?
5. What are some examples of computer-related adaptations that assist a child with input?
6. How might a young child begin using AC?
7. Explain the concept of DME.
8. Describe the types of children who might benefit from mobility aids.
9. What are three documentation strategies that could be helpful in the search for funding?

SUGGESTED *Activities*

1. Contact your local Tech-Act Center (a federally funded organization in each state), and find out what types of services they provide.
2. Visit an Alliance for Technology Access Center and try out the different types of demonstration equipment they have available.
3. Interview a person who uses AT to find out the selection process, their satisfaction with the item, suggested adaptations, and reimbursement issues.
4. Contact an occupational therapy practitioner in a local school system for ideas on how AT is used there.
5. Visit a dealership that sells or supplies wheelchairs and other types of assistive technology. Make a list of the products available and their cost.
6. Design a light-technology device that would assist a child with a learning disability with copying from a chalkboard.
7. Contact the websites for the AOTA, Rehabilitation Engineering Society of North America (RESNA), or Closing the Gap (see Chapter 16 Appendix) and review information on AT.

CHAPTER 16 APPENDIX A

Resource List of Organizations for Current Information on Assistive Technology

Alliance for Technology Access
2175 East San Francisco Boulevard, Suite L
San Rafael, CA 94901
(415) 455-4575
Website: *http://www.ATAccess.org*

**American Occupational Therapy Association
  (AOTA)**
P.O. Box 31220
4720 Montgomery Lane
Bethesda, MD 20824-1220
(301) 352-2682
Website: *http://aota.org*

Closing the Gap
P.O. Box 68
Henderson, MN 56044
(612) 248-3294
Website: *http://closingthegap.com*

The Council for Exceptional Children
1920 Association Drive
Reston, VA 22091-1589
(800) 845-6232
Website: *http://www.cec.sped.org*

**Rehabilitation Engineering Society
  of North America (RESNA)**
1700 N. Moore Street, Suite 1540
Arlington, VA 22209-1903
(703) 524-6686
Website: *http://www.resna.org*

Trace Research and Development Center
Waisman Center
University of Wisconsin—Madison
1500 Highland Avenue
Madison, WI 53705
(608) 262-6966
Website: *http://www.trace.wisc.edu*

United Cerebral Palsy Association
1660 L Street Northwest, Suite 700
Washington, DC 20036
(800) USA-5UCP
Website: *http://www.assisttech.com*

Positioning and Handling

JOYCE A. WANDEL

CHAPTER *Objectives*

After studying this chapter, the reader will be able to accomplish the following:

- Define and describe therapeutic positioning and handling techniques
- Explain the benefits of using positioning and handling techniques for children with central nervous system movement disorders
- Identify ways of selecting therapeutic positions
- Describe the purposes, advantages, and disadvantages of supine, prone, side-lying, and upright antigravity positions
- Describe the types of sensory inputs used in several handling techniques and explain the purpose of each
- Explain the role of positioning and handling techniques in activity-focused occupational therapy

DEFINITIONS

Positioning and handling techniques are two tools used by occupational therapy practitioners. **Positioning** is a static process that improves a child's ability to maintain postural control while participating in activities. Positioning techniques can be as simple as holding or placing the child in a particular posture or can involve the use of specialized adaptive furniture and equipment. The certified occupational therapy assistant (COTA) may use positioning to assist a diplegic child with achieving a stable posture using the wall and a bench. If the positioning is successful, that child may then proceed to learn lower extremity dressing skills. **Handling** techniques are dynamic and guide a child's movement responses by influencing the state of muscle tone or triggering new, automatic movement responses that result in functional actions. These methods are used with children whose movement disorders stem from damage to the central nervous system, such as children who have cerebral palsy (see Chapter 8) or genetic disorders such as Down syndrome (see Chapter 11). Both methods are adjuncts to therapy and are often used as part of a child's overall daily therapeutic plan for increasing movement skills during occupational performance.

BENEFITS

The occupational therapy practitioner who uses positioning and handling techniques examines the ways these methods can create opportunities for children to interact more effectively and independently with their environment. For example, a fifth-grade student with ataxia who cannot stand independently may need positioning assistance to perform classroom activities on the blackboard. A high-school freshman who cannot balance while sitting and has poorly integrated primitive postural reflexes may need to establish trunk stability while seated so that she can learn computer skills. In each case the practitioner can facilitate improved postural control and skilled movement through positioning and handling; the opportunity for improved function results. The many additional benefits that can be derived from use of these techniques include the following:

Increasing a child's physical comfort and reducing fatigue: Providing various positioning options for the child who has little independent movement control can eliminate risk of pressure sores developing or support a state of mental alertness while the body remains relaxed.

Promoting skeletal alignment: Proper bone and joint **alignment** allows the child the best use of available movements and also minimizes or prevents muscle and connective tissue contractures and bone and joint deformities. A child with hypertonia may choose to use the W-sit position because it provides a wide, stable base of support. However, this position can lead to tightening and contractures in the lower extremity muscle groups, as well as hip, knee, and ankle joint malformations. This child needs a sitting position that keeps the bones and joints aligned and moving in their correct planes.

Providing the child with a wider range of sensory experiences that enhance learning options: If independent movement options are limited to a few repetitive positions and patterns, the child may not gather the sensory input needed from the environment to foster continual development of skills.

Assisting the child with learning voluntary control of movement: Handling techniques can facilitate development of righting reactions and equilibrium reactions or can reduce the strength of primitive reflexes that prevent a child from developing the ability to use both sides of the body in a coordinated manner. Combining handling and positioning establishes a better balance between the pull of spastic muscles so that body parts can work together for better quality of movement during activity.

POSITIONING AS A THERAPEUTIC TOOL

The Shankar family is preparing for a traditional Hindu celebration. All family and friends are expected to partake of a meal while seated on the floor. Six-year-old Sanjay Shankar has spastic diplegic cerebral palsy, which prevents him from using his arms and hands unless he is sitting with assistance and using supports. Because of his increased muscle tone, his legs extend outward, with his toes pointing in and his hips rolling back so that he sits on his sacrum. This sitting position causes his upper body to bend forward. Unless Sanjay uses his arms to brace himself upright, he collapses forward.

The COTA who treats Sanjay during his outpatient therapy sessions makes a home visit to the Shankar household before the celebration. Mrs. Shankar indicates where the meal will be served. She and the COTA identify a place against the wall where Sanjay can sit. The COTA shows Mrs. Shankar how to position Sanjay with his back, shoulders, and hips aligned straight against the wall and his legs folded and crossed in front of him. She suggests placing a low bench or stool in front of Sanjay so that he can easily reach his food without having to hold a plate and can also rest on his arms and elbows to maintain his stable, upright position.

Use of positioning techniques should begin as early as possible for children with neuromotor dysfunction because the techniques are one of the best ways to help children use any movement abilities they have. Positioning affects all activities, from sleeping, going to the bathroom, traveling, and eating, to attending school and playing.[1] No one perfect or ideal position can be used with all children. Chosen positions must enhance the many different kinds of activities in which a child engages. The occupational therapy practitioner should always try to choose positions that most resemble the typical positions in which activities are performed. As a therapeutic modality, positioning can promote normal development; compensate for lack of functional abilities; and prevent, minimize, or delay the onset of contractures and deformities that may result in loss of movement, surgeries, and compromised health.[4]

General Principles for Positioning

- *Provide support.* Carefully observe ways that children use to independently maintain various positions (such as prone, supine, side lying, sitting, kneeling, and standing). Use positioning to support only those parts of the body of which they cannot achieve or maintain **postural stability** independently for the chosen activity. The right amount of positioning support allows the arms, hands, and legs to be available for purposeful activity. Too much support stops children from using the independent movement control they already possess.
- *Position for symmetry and skeletal alignment.* Achieve effective and efficient movement of the extremities by keeping the head, neck, trunk, and pelvis aligned. Proper skeletal alignment allows children to shift weight off their center of gravity, which can trigger the righting and equilibrium reactions needed to regain upright postural control. Proper alignment also maintains joint integrity, which prevents joints from dislocating or partially dislocating, also known as *subluxing*. Positioning **symmetry** can help distribute body weight over bony prominences, thus eliminating the skin breakdown that can develop when a bony area receives constant pressure.
- *Offer variety.* People normally use various positions as they engage in daily activities, regardless of their age. Position variety is particularly important for the development of perception and cognition as a child matures. For example, infants' early feeding interactions occur while they are in reclining postures, whereas those of toddlers occur in upright sitting positions, and older children may eat while lying in front of a television. Each new experience broadens children's perceptual and cognitive understanding of the environment. Children develop positional preferences that facilitate and enhance the activities they perform. They may enjoy being stretched out on

a chaise lounge for recreational reading but find it best to read classwork while seated at a desk. Occupational therapy practitioners should offer children enough positioning variety to establish which ones are the best choices for a particular activity and child. They should also show parents, caregivers, and teachers the positions that work best for the child.
- *Consider safety and comfort.* Many factors must be considered when choosing a particular position. Does the chosen position prepare a child for a new, unfamiliar activity? If so, can the child remain stable and feel secure in the position? Will the child ever be left unattended or with minimal monitoring while in the position? Can the child breathe comfortably in the position? Does the position promote optimal vision and hearing?
- *Select developmentally appropriate positions.* A small infant is fed in a reclining position, which is appropriate for the level of the infant's oral-motor skills. Older children must eventually use upright positions to develop mature swallowing, sucking, and chewing movements and for socializing during meal times.
- *Determine whether handling interventions are needed to achieve proper positioning.* Handling techniques are often needed to balance muscle tone, break up or inhibit asymmetrical, primitive postures, or help a child adjust to an unfamiliar sensory experience that is introduced by a new position. An occupational therapy practitioner may use handling for a few seconds or many minutes to place a child in a desired position. Never force a child's body parts into a position. Rather, use the handling techniques discussed in this chapter to address the neuromotor problems that interfere with proper positioning.

Choosing a Positioning Method

Ward groups positioning methods into the following three approaches[5]:

1. Using the body of the occupational therapy practitioner (or caregiver) for support in activities that involve frequent positional changes and weightshifts (such as dressing) may be most effective.
2. Positioning for activities in which the practitioner's hands need to be free (that is, to work with a child on skills such as handwriting or feeding) can be accomplished with the use of either standard furniture (appropriate for the child's body size) or by selecting specialized adaptive equipment. Many types of reclining, seating, standing, transport, and mobility systems are available from various manufacturers.
3. Positioning equipment may be specifically designed to fit the needs of children with severe or multiple

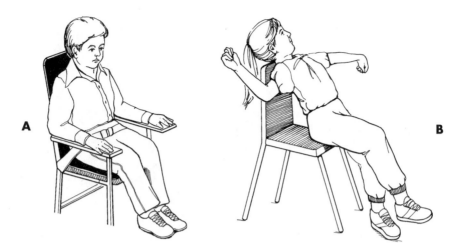

FIGURE 17-1   A, Child positioned in stable sitting posture. **B,** Child extends her neck to look up at her teacher, triggering a strong pattern of extensor spasticity. (From Case-Smith J, Allen AS, Pratt PN: *Occupational therapy for children*, ed 3, St Louis, 1996, Mosby.)

disabilities. Custom approaches are often used when a child has established contractures and deformities, and body parts cannot be properly positioned into or supported by the standard equipment.[5] To create such a customized positioning solution, occupational therapy practitioners can couple their knowledge about movement (and its relationship to occupational pursuits) with their skills in fabricating supportive equipment.

When selecting a positioning method, the occupational therapy practitioner evaluates each child's tolerance for the position, the length of time the child can comfortably maintain the position, the adaptability of the position to the activity it supports, and the age-appropriateness of the position for the particular activity. The occupational therapy practitioner keeps documented records and descriptions of successful positions for each child and notes those positions that pose risks, such as compromised respiration, for the child. Good record keeping enables the occupational therapy practitioner to generate good positioning plans for the child to use at school, at home, or in other environments.

Positioning Choices

Each positioning option offers potential advantages and disadvantages. Infants begin to develop stability and mobility skills in prone, supine, and side-lying postures (see Chapter 6). For very young children and those with severe movement limitations, these three horizontal positions often make the best use of movements they can elicit independently (or with minimal assistance). Positioning choices are also governed by the targeted activity. A therapeutic play activity that requires a child to skillfully reach for and manipulate small objects necessitates a positioning technique that gives the child solid support throughout the pelvis and trunk. Reach and manipulation skills demand isolation of small movements, thus good proximal support optimizes the child's ability to concentrate on these movements. An additional factor to consider is the spatial relationship among the child, activity, and other individuals interacting with the child. The position should allow the child to use vision, hearing, and touch to the child's best advantage. A child with strong extensor spasticity may be positioned in a chair with appropriate degrees of flexion at the ankles, knees, and hips; however, if the child must look upward to make eye contact with the person speaking, that small head movement may easily trigger the spasticity and cause the child to push out of the functional sitting position (Figure 17-1). Always consider whether a child has freedom of movement within a given position. A child who cannot move independently by using weightshifts needs assistance from the occupational therapy practitioner or caregiver. Generally, a child who does not move independently should not stay in any one position for more than 20 to 30 minutes.

Supine positioning

Children may be positioned on a flat or inclined surface using wedges, pillows, rolls, or towels. A key element of supine positioning is that the head be in a midline position and slightly flexed forward (Figure 17-2). Children who exhibit strong extensor muscle tone in this position must also have their hips and knees held in flexed positions. The presence of a strong asymmetrical tonic neck reflex (ATNR) must be counteracted with sym-

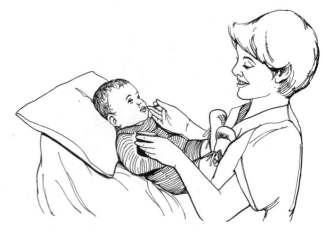

FIGURE 17-2 Supine positioning on a pillow includes maintaining some neck and leg flexion. (From Case-Smith J, Allen AS, Pratt PN: *Occupational therapy for children,* ed 3, St Louis, 1996, Mosby.)

BOX 17-1

Advantages and Disadvantages of Supine Position

ADVANTAGES	DISADVANTAGES
Allows child to see environment (for example, to watch television or play with toys suspended on a mobile)	Is most difficult position from which to raise arms against gravity
Is easiest position for visual fixation and tracking when head is positioned and supported	May increase extensor tone
Allows child to actively work to strengthen neck and abdominal flexor muscles	Places minimal demands on child to develop head control
Provides position of rest and comfort	Encourages shallow abdominal breathing
	Often elicits ATNR

metrical body positioning. Box 17-1 describes the advantages and disadvantages of supine positioning.

CLINICAL *Pearl*

When positioning a child in a supine position, remember the following hints: (1) Support the head in a flexed, forward position. (2) When working with a baby on your lap or an older child on the floor, keep the knees and hips flexed to minimize effects of extensor tone and encourage use of abdominal muscles.

Prone positioning

Placing a firm foam wedge under the child's upper body, with the edge of the wedge just below the axillary area, can place the child in a prone position (Figure 17-3). Determine the correct degree of incline according to the child's ability to independently hold the head up during the selected activity. Keep the neck extension below a 45-degree angle to prevent this head movement from triggering hyperextension throughout the body. If the wedge angle is not high enough, the child's head can drop for-

ward toward the floor and trigger too much flexion. A child with contractures in the hip flexor muscles may require pillows under this body area for comfort (Box 17-2).

CLINICAL *Pearl*

When positioning a child in a prone position, remember the following hints: (1) Put small children or infants in a prone position across your lap for therapeutic dressing and undressing. (2) Make sure wedges and rolls placed under children are not so high that they cause excessive extensor tone or so low that children with very low tone or strength cannot lift their heads.

Side-lying positioning

Most children require external support to maintain alignment in the side-lying position (Figure 17-4). Side lying is a good positioning choice for children whose muscle tone becomes too high or low in prone or supine positions. Side-lying positions also give children a stable, midline head position and keep their hands in their line of vision. Hands remain free to reach for and manipulate objects without having to resist the pull of gravity (Box 17-3).

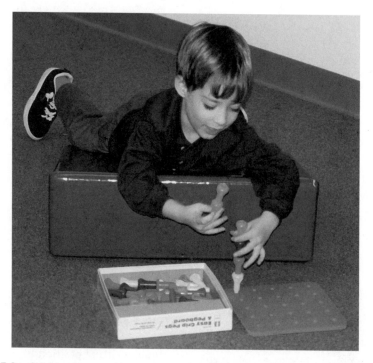

FIGURE 17-3 Child in prone position over a wedge. Note the axillary position, wedge height, and amount of neck extension.

BOX 17-2

Advantages and Disadvantages of Prone Position

ADVANTAGES	DISADVANTAGES
The prone position enables children to practice independent head control. The prone position provides children with an opportunity to stretch hip and knee flexor muscles. The prone position leads to higher-level motor skills such as elbow propping, crawling, and reaching.	Children who are unable to independently turn their heads may have trouble breathing. Children who are unable to lift their heads or prop their bodies on their arms may have difficulty learning to reach, push up, or use vision properly.

BOX 17-3

Advantages and Disadvantages of Side-Lying Position

ADVANTAGES	DISADVANTAGES
Best position to minimize excessive muscle tone; neutral position Easiest position in which to align arms, hands, and head in midline with gravity eliminated Little use of ATNR Good for independent play and development of eye-hand coordination	Difficult to maintain severely affected child in this position without proper equipment. Requires careful positioning of the head to maintain correct cervical spine alignment.

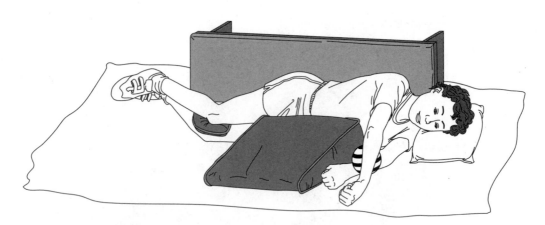

FIGURE 17-4 Side-lying position that provides child with opportunity to bring hands together to play with a toy.

CLINICAL *Pearl*

When positioning a child in a side-lying posture, remember the following hints: (1) Be sure to alternate sides. (2) Use small rolls or pillows to help the child maintain a position, such as using a towel roll in front of a child who tends to push back into extension to allow the child to lean forward and eliminate extensor tone influence. (3) Provide adequate padded surfaces for shoulders and hips to prevent pressure sores and diminished circulation. (4) During play and social interactions, make sure the occupational therapy practitioner or the toys are well below eye level to discourage extension.

Upright antigravity positions
Sitting
Sitting skills emerge in the normal child at about 7 to 9 months of age. Sitting requires the child to maintain postural control of the head, trunk, and extremities against the pull of gravity. Once the child can assume a stable sitting posture without having to brace upright using the arms, the child can then begin to shift weight away from the center of gravity to reach, retrieve, and manipulate objects. Sitting and other upright postures provide important visual and kinesthetic experiences that advance the child's perceptual and cognitive development. Skills such as self-feeding, going to the bathroom, doing school work, and many play activities illustrate the importance of sitting. For children with muscle tone abnormalities, assuming a sitting position often requires the use of handling techniques and positioning devices.

Sitting positions vary greatly. At floor level, children may long sit (sit with their legs straight), ring sit (sit so that their legs form a circle), Indian sit (sit with their legs bent and crossed), or side sit (sit with their legs to one side) (Figure 17-5). Almost all children can obtain a sitting position in a chair, no matter how severe their disability, by choosing the correct type of chair and incorporating as many of the elements of a normal sitting position as possible (Figure 17-6). Some children can maintain a good sitting position in a standard chair with a few modifications, such as a small, low stool placed under the feet or a rolled towel placed behind the shoulders (Box 17-4). The optimal sitting position emphasizes the following:

- The body is positioned as symmetrically as possible, with weight evenly distributed on both sides of the body (on the buttocks, thighs, and feet) and the head aligned with the trunk.
- The head is held in midline and flexed forward slightly.
- The hips, knees, and ankles are flexed 90 degrees or slightly less.
- The feet are supported in a dorsiflexed position, either on the floor or with use of a raised surface.
- The knees are abducted and in good alignment with hips.
- Any table or lapboard used is at elbow height.

CLINICAL *Pearl*

When occupational therapy practitioners use their body to support a child in a sitting position on the floor for active play skills, they should remember to seat the child between their knees and control the child's trunk from the back in an attempt to keep the shoulders and arms forward.

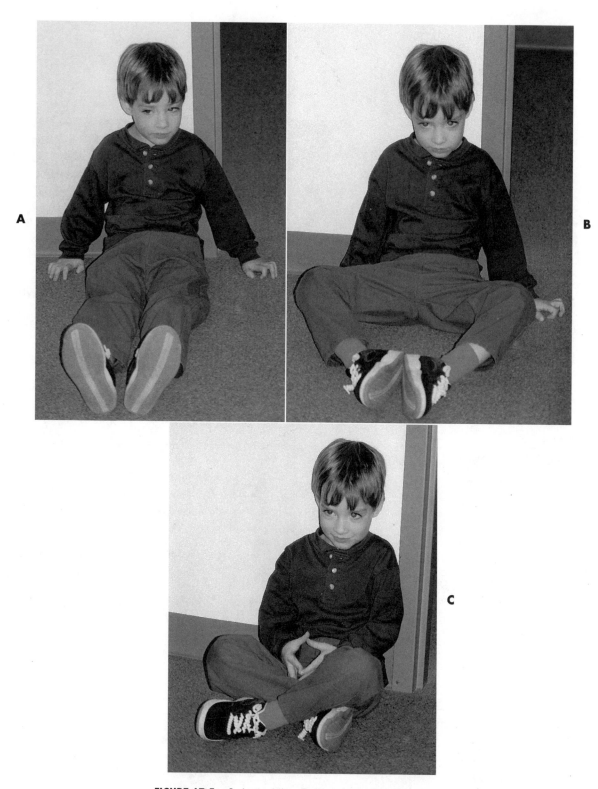

FIGURE 17-5   A, Long sitting. **B,** Ring sitting. **C,** Indian sitting.

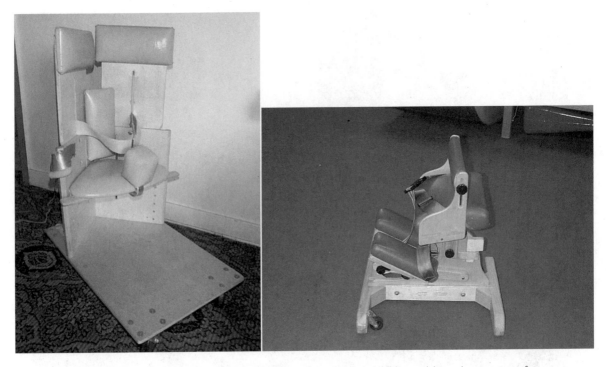

FIGURE 17-6 Two examples of adapted seating systems that help inhibit spasticity and compensate for limited postural control.

BOX 17-4

Advantages and Disadvantages of Sitting Position

ADVANTAGES	DISADVANTAGES
The sitting position allows children to develop head and trunk control and upper body balance reactions.	Children with minimal trunk control may try to compensate by using abnormal postures.
The sitting position provides an expansive perspective of the environment.	Children who cannot voluntarily shift weight to change positions may experience compromised circulation in weightbearing body areas.
The sitting position provides opportunities for midline activities and advanced eye-hand coordination tasks.	The sitting position can cause increased contractures in hip flexor and knee flexor muscles.
The sitting position frees the hands for play, self-care, self-help, and communication activities.	

BOX 17-5

Advantages and Disadvantages of Standing Position

ADVANTAGES	DISADVANTAGES
The standing position allows the child to view the environment from an upright orientation and to interact with others at eye level.	Older and larger children may require the assistance of two people for positioning in standers.
The standing position activates balance receptors in the soles of the feet.	Children with little independent postural control may fatigue rapidly when placed in upright antigravity positions.
The standing position facilitates controlled use of neck and facial muscles used for eating and speaking.	Full weightbearing on the hips and lower extremities may be painful for children with muscle contractures or skeletal deformities in these body areas.

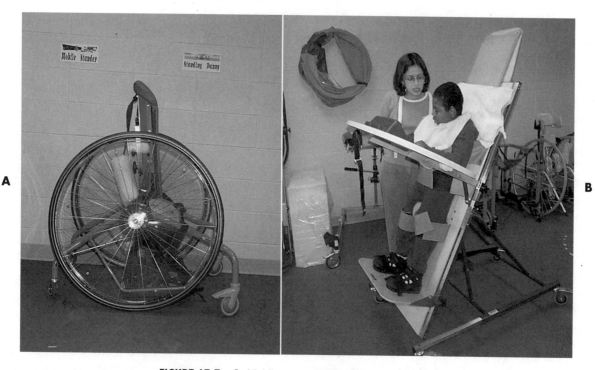

FIGURE 17-7   A, Mobile prone stander. **B,** Supine stander.

Standing

Full weightbearing on the hips and lower extremities fosters healthy bone development, keeps optimal range of movement in muscle tissue, and maintains good circulation. Even children who can stand somewhat independently need positioning assistance to achieve these goals and good postural alignment. Using supine and prone standers (Figure 17-7) helps many children achieve proper upright standing positions. Standers support the body from either the back or front surface and can be secured in a full vertical tilted position. Reclining a stander can be used to adjust to children's muscle tone and keep their joints properly aligned (Box 17-5).

CLINICAL *Pearl*

When positioning children using standing equipment, remember the following hints: (1) Prone standers can be helpful for children with increased extensor tone. Tilt the stander forward just enough to decrease the tone and help the child maintain the head in a midline position. Attach a tray to the front of the stander so that the child's arms and hands can be placed in front, thus giving the child an opportunity to explore objects. (2) Supine standers that support from the lower trunk downward can be helpful for children with diplegia. Using this type of equipment can free the arms and hands. Place two or more children who are using supine standers close to one another so that they can engage in a game of catch or other active game.

HANDLING TECHNIQUES

Two-year-old Lupita Vargas has low muscle tone and overly mobile joints as a result of being born with Down syndrome. Lupita is a very active child. She typically moves around using a "bear walk" (that is, walking on her hands and feet and locking her elbow and knee joints to support her body weight as she moves forward). Lately Lupita has been making attempts to stand upright and reach for toys and other objects. She pulls herself up using furniture but once upright stands with her feet spaced widely apart. She holds her arms bent at the elbows away from her body and turned upward for balance. When Lupita attempts to move out of this stance by taking a step or reaching for her toys, she quickly loses her balance and falls.

David, the COTA who is working with Lupita, has realized that Lupita needs to develop increased stability in the muscles and joints throughout her pelvis and trunk to stand up independently. He knows that the stability would allow Lupita to move her extremities more freely and help her develop the rotational, diagonal movement patterns and balance reactions needed to interact with her surroundings. During her current therapy session, David places his hands over her hips to give Lupita the pelvic stability she needs to bring her feet closer together. Following the cues provided by David's hands, she shifts her body weight side to side, forward, and backward over each leg. As Lupita begins feeling stability in the lower part of her body, she is able to use both of her hands to reach toward her favorite doll, which David has placed on the couch in front of her. David moves the doll to a different place on the couch each time they practice this so that Lupita experiences weightshifting in many directions. Each time she moves, she has to use an equilibrium reaction to bring her body back to an upright stance while holding her doll. David continues to use hand placement on Lupita's hips to give her the sensory experience of stability, which helps to guide her through movement patterns that she will eventually be able to use more independently. David also helps Lupita's mother learn how to foster the development of her daughter's functional motor skills. Mrs. Vargas is pleased because she realizes she can incorporate these handling methods many times throughout Lupita's day, such as when selecting her clothes from the closet rack or reaching for her afternoon snack on a small table.

Whereas the goals of using positioning techniques are to establish stable, functional body postures, handling techniques encompass several active, hands-on interventions. However, just as with positioning, handling is designed to produce an adaptive response from the child so that movement responses are more functional, exploratory, and appropriate for a task.[3] Choosing and applying an appropriate handling technique can be overwhelming to a new or inexperienced COTA. The COTA needs to find opportunities to observe and work alongside an experienced registered occupational therapist (OTR) who can be a mentor for skill development in these methods.

Each handling technique's effectiveness is based on providing specific, graded sensory information to influence the parts of the central nervous system that govern and produce skilled, automatic movements. The most frequently used types of **sensory input** include vestibular, proprioceptive, and tactile input, in addition to the visual input provided by the environment. Therapeutic sensory input is provided at select body locations, which are frequently termed *key points of control*. Key points can be at proximal body areas, such as the shoulder girdle, trunk, or pelvis, or can be distally located on the extremities.[4] Assisting a child with feeling functional or more advanced movement skills helps integrate the sensory feedback of effective movement. With repeated opportunities, patience, and cognitive training, many children continue to learn to use new motor skills.

Handling techniques can either facilitate or inhibit muscle tone, activity level, and levels of alertness (Box 17-6). The occupational therapy practitioner often uses a combination of techniques during a therapeutic intervention. Copeland and Kimmel describe the following five **inhibition** handling techniques[1]:

1. *Neutral warmth:* The occupational therapy practitioner gently wraps the child's body with a soft cotton or thermal blanket for 15 to 20 minutes to re-

---

BOX 17-6

Indicators for Use of Inhibition and Facilitation Techniques

INHIBITION	FACILITATION
Hypertonicity	Hypotonicity
Active primitive reflexes	Inactive primitive reflexes, lack of balance reactions
Excessive activity and motion	Excessive relaxation, semiconscious state
Behavioral excitation	Behavioral nonresponsiveness, flat affect
Excessive sensitivity or reactivity to handling and touch	Decreased reactivity to handling and touch

---

duce extreme hypertonicity. Neutral warmth of 96° F to 98° F can relax muscles, thereby reducing muscle tone. The practitioner monitors the child's level of alertness, attempting to create a relaxed physical state while not causing the child to go to sleep. The child should be able to breathe freely and be in a comfortable position, such as supine or side lying.

2. *Slow stroking:* Using an open palm and the pads of the fingertips only, the practitioner applies a firm but light pressure and stroking motion down the child's back, moving in a cephalocaudal direction. To stroke, the practitioner uses alternate hands to touch each side of the child's spine, beginning at the base of the skull. Just before lifting one hand from the base of the spine, the practitioner uses the other hand to begin stroking. Stroking is done rhythmically, and hands never move against the direction of body hair. Typical positions used when applying stroking are prone, side lying, or between the occupational therapy practitioner's legs in a relaxed, sitting position on the floor. Three to five minutes of stroking a safe time frame. Slow stroking can also improve abnormal muscle tone in the arms or legs (Figure 17-8).

3. *Gentle shaking or rocking:* Shaking is a good technique to reduce tone in an extremity. First, choose a position for the child that is appropriate for the planned activity. Using the flat pads of the fingertips, the practitioner grasps the top portion of a child's body part, such as the arm. The body part is gently and rhythmically shaken while the practitioner's hand moves downward on it. Slow rocking is rhythmical and can include al-

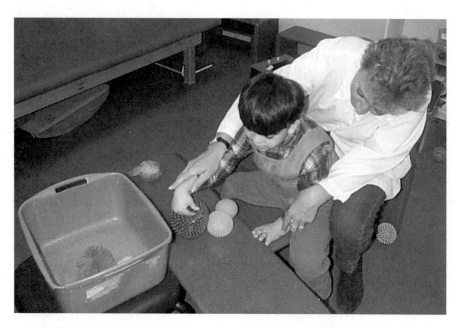

FIGURE 17-8   Slow stroking motions are applied using the whole surface of the palm.

ternating rotational movements with the practitioner's hands placed at proximal key points such as the shoulders.

4. *Trunk and hip rotation:* The practitioner can easily manipulate the trunk and hips using handling techniques while assisting the child with transitioning from one body position to another. The practitioner maintains stability on one body side with one hand. With the other hand, the practitioner assists the child with making movements in diagonal planes. Using proximal key points of the trunk and pelvis reduces hypertonicity by inhibiting patterns of total flexion or extension, particularly those elicited by primitive reflex activity (Figure 17-9).

5. *Slow rolling:* Slow rolling involves handling primarily the trunk and pelvis. The practitioner places the child in a supine position and from one of the key points slowly rolls the child from a supine to a side-lying position and then back to a supine position. The practitioner repeats this pattern in the opposite direction and continues alternating the pattern slowly and rhythmically until the child's muscles relax.

Although practitioners use inhibitory handling techniques more often than facilitation techniques, facilitation methods are sometimes needed to increase low muscle tone, increase levels of alertness, or strengthen the intensity of sensory input to elicit a response. **Facilita-**

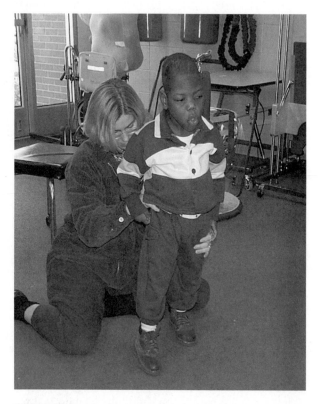

FIGURE 17-9   Handling at key points can facilitate movement.

tion handling techniques include bouncing, swinging, or rocking in an anterior-posterior movement plane and moving the child into upright antigravity positions. Occupational therapy practitioners can use a vast array of equipment, such as therapy balls or vestibular boards, in their facilitation techniques; they can also use themselves as the source of the movements. Occupational therapy practitioners should take care to protect the hypermobile joints of children with particularly low muscle tone from potential dislocation. Whether using inhibition or facilitation techniques, occupational therapy practitioners must carefully monitor each child's response to the sensory input. Many children with motor system impairments have delayed responses to sensory stimulation or may be experiencing the sensation for the first time. Until occupational therapy practitioners become familiar with each child's individual responses, they must proceed slowly. After a minute or so of using a particular facilitation technique, the practitioner should stop and wait a few seconds to assess the way the child responds physically and emotionally. When occupational therapy practitioners couple their knowledge of positioning and handling methods with sensory integration, they can refine the appropriate type and amount of sensory stimulation needed (see Chapter 15). Each child's potential response is intertwined with the child's cognitive and perceptual competencies. By working with the OTR, the caregivers, and teachers, the COTA can obtain the data needed to integrate good positioning and handling interventions into the child's various daily activities and environments.

INTEGRATING POSITIONING AND HANDLING INTO ACTIVITY-FOCUSED TREATMENT

Although mastery of positioning and handling techniques are important therapeutic tools for the occupational therapy practitioner, they are only used as part of the process of increasing a child's repertoire of occupational behaviors. Using principles from the neurodevelopmental treatment approach, Erhardt outlined three phases, or components, of the treatment process that are used with children who need to develop improved movement skills.[2] Neurodevelopmental principles are included in each phase.

- *Preparation:* Use positioning and handling techniques to normalize muscle tone and inhibit abnormal re-

flex activity. Identify the optimal amount of support needed for children to use movement abilities available to them. Use comfortable postures for teaching children new skills.
- *Facilitation:* Strengthen existing skills and very gradually decrease supports as children acquire new skills. Grade activity demands so that children can pay attention to the task itself rather than the way the task is done. Allowing children to problem solve during tasks helps produce automatic, spontaneous movements.
- *Adaptation:* Gradually alter positioning and handling. Vary positions and change sensory cues to increase children's abilities to use skills in a various situations.

In the previous scenario about Lupita Vargas, the COTA (David) helps Lupita achieve stability in a standing position by placing his hands on her hips and then follows this by facilitating weight shifting. David uses facilitation methods to help Lupita repeatedly reach for her doll, which he places in a different location each time. In the facilitation phase of the session, David attempts to grade and strengthen Lupita's new reaching skills and balance reactions. When David and Mrs. Vargas explore other ways Lupita can use her new abilities, they apply the adaptation phase of the treatment process and continue to strengthen Lupita's repertoire of available motor skills.

SUMMARY

Positioning and handling techniques are valuable therapeutic tools used to assist children who have central nervous system damage. Positioning techniques provide the child with stable postural options that can increase interaction with the environment, facilitate the child's ability to engage in meaningful activities, and prevent development of health problems caused by the child's motor disorder. The COTA can recommend positioning approaches and specialized equipment to fit the individual needs of each child. Handling techniques also help the child actively engage in activities using the most functional movement possible. By understanding the types of sensory inputs influencing the nervous system and learning to select and grade them appropriately, the COTA can support a child's acquisition of independent play, work, and self-care skills. Used together, positioning and handling techniques are powerful tools in activity-focused treatment.

References

1. Copeland M, Kimmel J: *Evaluation and management of infants and young children with developmental disabilities*, Baltimore, 1989, Brookes.
2. Erhardt RP: *Developmental hand dysfunction: theory, assessment and treatment*, ed 2, San Antonio, 1994, Therapy Skill Builders.
3. Porter R: Sensory considerations in handling techniques. In Connolly B, Montgomery P, editors: *Therapeutic exercise in developmental disabilities*, Chattanooga, 1987, Chattanooga Corporation.
4. Schoen S, Anderson J: Neurodevelopmental treatment frame of reference. In Kramer P, Hinojosa J, editors: *Frames of reference for pediatric occupational therapy*, Baltimore, 1993, Williams & Wilkins.
5. Ward D: *Positioning the handicapped child for function*, ed 2, St Louis, 1984, Phoenix Press.

Recommended Reading

Alexander R, Boehme R, Cupps B: *Normal development of functional motor skills: the first year of life*, San Antonio, 1993, Therapy Skill Builders.

Bly L: *Motor skills acquisition in the first year of life*, San Antonio, 1994, Therapy Skill Builders.

Boehme R: *Improving upper body control*, Tucson, 1988, Therapy Skill Builders.

Campbell P: *Introduction to neurodevelopmental treatment: application with infants and children with posture and movement disorders*, ed 3, Tallmadge, Oh, 1990, Children's Hospital Medical Center of Akron.

Dunn Klein M: *Pre-dressing skills*, San Antonio, 1983, Therapy Skill Builders.

Finnie N: *Handling the young cerebral palsied child at home*, New York, 1975, EP Dutton.

Jaeger L, Gertz, J: *Home program instruction sheets for infants and children*, San Antonio, 1999, Therapy Skill Builders.

Levitt S: *Treatment of cerebral palsy and motor delay*, London, 1977, Blackwell Scientific Publications.

Logigian M, Ward J, editors: *Pediatric rehabilitation: a team approach for therapists*, Boston, 1989, Little Brown.

Parham L, Fazio L, editors: *Play in occupational therapy for children*, St Louis, 1997, Mosby.

Scherzer A, Tscharnuter I: *Early diagnosis and treatment in cerebral palsy*, ed 2, New York, 1990, Marcel Dekker.

Sheda C, Small C: *Developmental motor activities for therapy: instruction sheets for children*, San Antonio, 1990, Therapy Skill Builders.

Short-DeGraff M: *Human development for occupational and physical therapists*, Baltimore, 1988, Williams & Wilkins.

Trefler E et al: *Seating and mobility for persons with physical disabilities*, San Antonio, 1993, Academic Press.

REVIEW *Questions*

1. Describe the differences between positioning and handling techniques. What is the primary focus of each?
2. Review each of the benefits that can be achieved through positioning and handling techniques. In what ways do they match up with performance components from the "Uniform Terminology for Occupational Therapy Practice?"
3. What are the principles used by the occupational therapy practitioner when selecting helpful positions for a child?
4. Why is it important for the COTA to identify more than just one or two positions for a child who has very little independent movement?
5. What are some of signs the COTA might observe that suggest a position poses risks to a child?
6. Therapeutic handling involves using a combination of facilitation and inhibition techniques. What are the indicators for each handling approach?

SUGGESTED *Activities*

1. Choose two or three daily living activities such as eating, dressing, or performing oral hygiene tasks. Try performing each activity in three different positions; choose both horizontal and upright positions. In what ways does the position affect your ability to perform each task? What makes a position comfortable or uncomfortable? With each position, do you notice any changes in the types of sensory input that indicate how to perform the task?
2. Observe normal children of different ages playing. How often do they change or adapt positions? Which positions provide the most stable postures? What do you notice about the ways children transition from one position to another? Note the qualities of normal movement patterns and think about the way these relate to the application of handling techniques.
3. You are a COTA who has been asked to develop a positioning plan for a 5-year-old boy who has spastic diplegia and is entering kindergarten. Suggest positions that would help him participate in activities such as sitting in a reading circle, participating in sand play at floor level, and putting on his jacket to go home. Refer to an adaptive equipment catalog to determine which types of equipment you might recommend for use in his classroom.
4. Find a partner and practice several of the handling techniques described in this chapter. Execute your movements based on the sensory cueing you experience while your partner is handling you. Provide verbal feedback about the way their handling feels.
5. Look at Figure 17-5. In what ways might you use positioning and handling to improve this child's ability to perform the activity?

Glossary

abduction Movement away from the midline of the body or body part identified as the middle point of reference (for example, spreading the fingers apart or moving the arm away from the side of the body)

abnormal movement patterns Ways of moving the body that reflect pathological conditions in the areas of the central nervous system that are related to movement control

achievement behavior Actions that emphasize performance standards (winning) and competition with others; Reilly's third hierarchical stage of play behavior in which the child or adolescent is driven by competition, and play involves extrinsic motivation characterized by planning and risk taking

acknowledgment Providing feedback to individuals that assures them they have been "heard"

acquired condition; acquired disorder An illness or state of health that is not inherited and interferes with an individual's ability to be functionally independent

acquired immunodeficiency syndrome (AIDS) A severe immunological disorder caused by the retrovirus HIV that is characterized by increased susceptibility to infections and certain rare cancers; transmitted primarily through body

active range of motion (AROM) Movement that occurs as a result of muscles contracting

activities of daily living (ADLs) Self-maintenance activities such as dressing and feeding

activity Specified pursuit in which an individual participates

activity analysis A tool that helps occupational therapy practitioners prioritize, plan, and implement effective treatment; involves identifying every characteristic of a task and examining each performance component, performance area, and performance context

activity configuration The process of selecting specific activities to use during an intervention

activity synthesis Modifying, grading, or changing the structure or steps of an activity into a whole; includes adapting, grading, and reconfiguring activities

acute care Health services provided to an individual whose illness has had a sudden onset and short but severe course

adapting activities Modifying a task or using adaptive equipment to make a task easier

adaptive Tending toward or suitable for

adaptive equipment Commercially available or custom-designed devices used to assist an individual with performing tasks successfully

adaptive response A successful response to an environmental challenge

addiction An intense psychological and physiological craving

adduction Movement toward the midline of the body or body part that has been identified as the middle point of reference (for example, moving the fingers together or moving the arm toward the side of the body)

adolescence The period of time that begins with puberty (age 12 years for females and age 14 years for males) and ends with adulthood

adulthood The period of time that begins after an individual matures or becomes the legal age

agonist A contracting muscle that is resisted or counteracted by another muscle (the antagonist); the prime mover that creates movement at a joint

align To move toward a straight line; posturally, to keep body segment bones and joints correctly oriented toward each other, particularly in the proximal areas of the head, neck, trunk, and pelvis

amputation   The loss of a body part (often part of an arm or leg)

anaphylactic shock   An often severe and sometimes fatal systemic reaction caused by an allergic response to an insect bite or exposure to an allergen; includes symptoms such as hives, itching, respiratory distress or cessation, and fainting

anhedonia   A loss of interest in previously enjoyed activities

ankle-foot orthosis (AFO)   A splint that helps to stabilize or align the ankle with the foot

anorexia nervosa   A mental disorder in which the individual has an intense fear of gaining weight or becoming fat, even in cases in which the individual is below the normal weight for age and height

anoxia   A condition characterized by a lack of oxygen resulting from an inadequate supply of oxygen to the respiratory system or the blood's inability to carry oxygen

antagonist   A muscle that counteracts the action of another muscle; the muscle that relaxes and lengthens as agonist contracts

antisocial personality disorder   An enduring pattern of behavior characterized by a disregard of the rights of others; begins in childhood or early adolescence and continues into adulthood

anxiety   A state of uneasiness, apprehension, uncertainty, and fear resulting from the anticipation of a threatening event or situation

anxiety disorder   A mental disorder characterized by a state of uneasiness, apprehension, uncertainty, and fear resulting from the anticipation and avoidance of a threatening event or situation

apnea   Temporary absence or cessation of breathing

arthrogryposis   A congenital disorder marked by generalized stiffness of joints; often accompanied by nerve and muscle degeneration, resulting in impaired mobility

assessment   The use of skilled observation and the interpretation of tests and measurements to determine the need for occupational therapy services; the act of appraising; a test or evaluation

assisted performance   Performance requiring some type of outside help (for example, verbal or physical cueing or prompting)

assistive technology (AT)   A concept that encompasses the process by which an individual with disabilities acquires or sustains independence by using assistive technology devices

assistive technology device (AT device)   Any item, piece of equipment, or product system that is used to maintain, increase, or improve the functional capabilities of an individual with disabilities

assistive technology service (AT service)   Any service that directly assists an individual with disabilities in the selection, acquisition, or use of an assistive technology device

assistive technology team (AT team)   A group of professionals who make recommendations and carry out training of an individual with a disability using an assistive technology device

asymmetry   Lack of balance or symmetry

ataxia   Abnormal fluctuation of muscle from normal to hypertonic (increased muscle tone); loss of the ability to coordinate muscular movement

athetosis   A type of cerebral palsy characterized by involuntary writhing movements, particularly of the hands and feet

attachment   The development of affection or emotional ties on the part of the infant for the mother

attention span   The length of time during which an individual can concentrate or focus attention on a particular object, idea, or activity without being diverted

attitudes   States of mind, feelings

auditory system   The sensory system related to hearing; the organs of hearing and the sense of hearing

augmentative communication (AC)   A set of approaches used to improve the communication skills of individuals who do not speak or whose speech is unintelligible

automatic movement   Movements performed without volition or conscious effort that align body parts, restore balance, or maintain balance

automatic reflexes; automatic reactions   Responses that are automatic (for example, protective extension, righting, and equilibrium responses); evolve as the primitive reflexes are being integrated during the first 2 years of life

backward chaining   A way to grade an activity in which an individual learns the last step first; begins with the individual completing the last step after watching the occupational therapy practitioner perform the first few steps and progresses to the individual learning the second to the last step (and so on) until the whole sequence is independently performed

balance   Maintaining postural stability against gravity

bilateral coordination   Both sides of the body working together during an activity

binge   Consumption of a significantly larger than normal amount of food; common in individuals with eating disorders, especially bulimia nervosa

biomechanical practice model   A frame of reference that focuses on range of motion, strength, endurance, and preventing contractures and deformities; used primarily with orthopedic disorders

bladder control   The ability to anticipate the need to urinate and wait until an appropriate time to relieve the bladder

bolster   A round, cylindrical piece of equipment that is used during positioning and therapeutic exercises and activities

bolster chair   A specialized chair that has a bolster as the seat

bonding   The development of affection between the mother and infant; the formation of close, specialized human relationships; the emotional attachment process

bony deformity   A permanent change in the shape of a bone, usually at or near a joint, that limits ranges of movement and function

bowel control   The ability to anticipate the need to defecate and wait until an appropriate time to relieve the bowel

bulimia nervosa   A mental disorder characterized by episodes of binge eating followed by episodes of self-induced vomiting

catheter   A tube used to drain fluid from the body

central nervous system (CNS)   The portion of the nervous system consisting of the brain and spinal cord

cerebral palsy (CP)   A motor function disorder caused by a permanent, nonprogressive brain defect or lesion; characterized by disruption in volitional control of posture and movement; produces atypical muscle tone and unusual ways of moving

chromosomes   Threadlike linear strands of DNA that carry genes and play a primary role in the transmission of hereditary information

chronological age (CA)   The number of years, months, and days an individual has lived; used as a standard or reference point to compare developmental status of children with special needs to other children

coactivation   The process of muscle groups (agonists and antagonists) working together simultaneously to produce smooth, coordinated movements

cocontraction   The simultaneous contraction of agonist and antagonist muscles to stabilize a joint and hold a position

cognitive integration and cognitive components   Performance components referring to an individual's ability to use higher brain functions; include level of arousal, orientation, recognition, attention span, initiation of activity, termination of activity, memory, sequencing, categorization, concept formation, spatial operations, problem solving, learning, and generalization

competency behavior   Actions or behaviors that are novel and challenging; play that involves practice or repetition in pursuit of mastery of skill; Reilly's second hierarchical stage of play behavior in which the child is motivated by effectiveness during the play activity

computer access   The methods or means by which an individual interacts with a computer

conduct disorder   A mental disorder characterized by behaviors that violate the rights of others or the rules of society, such as physical aggression toward others, criminal acts (such as mugging, burglary, and shoplifting), truancy, and running away from home

congenital disorder   A condition that is acquired during fetal development or birth as a result of hereditary or atypical circumstances

constructive play   Play that involves building or putting objects together to create a structure

consultation   The act or process of providing advice or information

continuing education (inservice)   Educational programs that practitioners attend to learn new skills

contract development   Developing an agreed-on goal for therapy in conjunction with the family

contracture   A permanent shortening of muscle tissue that results in limited range of movement at the involved joint

convergence   Simultaneous turning of the eyes inward

coprolalia   A vocal tic in individuals with Tourette's syndrome that is characterized by the blurting out of obscene words

corner chair   A specialized chair with a back that is similar to the corner of a room; helps bring the shoulders forward

cotreatment   A means of establishing service competency between an registered occupational therapist and certified occupational therapy assistant; two or more disciplines providing services to the same individual simultaneously

crawl   Reciprocal movement of arms and legs in which the stomach contacts the supporting surface

creep   Reciprocal movement of arms and legs in which the stomach does not contact the supporting surface

curriculum   A group of related courses, often in a special field of study

deformity   A permanent change in the shape of a bone, usually at or near a joint, that limits movement and function

delusion   A strongly held belief that is incompatible with reality (that is, evidence shows that the belief does not exist)

dependent performance   Performance that is contingent on another individual; relying on or requiring the aid of another individual to perform an activity or task

development   The act or process of growth or maturation

developmental age (DA)   The age at which a child or adolescent is functioning developmentally with regard to skill acquisition in specific occupational performance areas or components

developmental disability The result of any condition that interrupts or delays the sequence and rate of normal childhood maturation

developmental dyspraxia Difficulty motor planning that is a result of sensory processing problems

dexterity Skill and grace in physical movement, especially in the hands

diplegia A term describing the distribution of affected muscles in individuals with cerebral palsy in which the musculature in the lower extremities is more affected than the musculature of the upper extremities

discharge planning Preparation for the discontinuation of occupational therapy services

discontinuation Cessation of occupational therapy services

discrete trial A method of teaching a specific skill that is based on repetition, prompting, and reinforcement to strengthen the response and its lasting effects

dislocation Displacement of the normal relationship of bones at a joint

disruptive behavior disorder A mental disorder characterized by socially disruptive behavior that is typically more distressing to others than to the individual with the disorder

divergence The turning of both eyes outward from a common point

documentation The process of recording information in writing or electronically that is pertinent to the occupational therapy process for legal and reimbursement purposes

Down syndrome A genetic disorder caused by the presence of an extra 21st chromosome, which results in mental and motor delays

downward comparison Identifying a situation that is worse than your own

dual diagnosis A situation in which an individual has two disorders or diagnoses (determining nature and cause of disease; opinion derived from an evaluation)

Duchenne muscular dystrophy The most common form of muscular dystrophy; characterized by pseudohypertrophy, especially of calf muscles; seen in males

due process Parents' ability to take legal action against a school if their child's educational rights are violated; derived from the words *due*—owed or owing as a natural or moral right—and *process*—to proceed against by law

durable medical equipment (DME) As defined by third party reimbursement, typically includes wheelchairs and prone and supine standers; to be purchased, must be documented as a medical necessity by the practitioner

dysphoric mood An unpleasant mood defined by feelings of sadness, anxiety, or irritability; common in individuals with mood disorders

dyspraxia Difficulty starting, stopping, or performing purposeful voluntary movements; deficits with motor planning

early childhood Period of time beginning with the end of infancy (approximately 18 months of age) and lasting through 5 years of age; includes toddlers and preschoolers

eating Consuming food

eating disorder A mental disorder characterized by a disturbance in eating behaviors

echolalia A vocal tic seen in individual's with Tourette's syndrome that is characterized by the repetition of others' word

educational activities Those tasks that promote learning, especially in academic areas such as reading, writing, and math

educational system A system of formal preschools and schools that are mandated by federal laws

elevated mood An overly pleasant mood defined by exaggerated feelings of well being

encephalitis Inflammation of the brain

endurance Tolerance level

environment The surroundings; the whole range of factors that influence an individual, including physical surroundings and psychological systems

environmental control unit (ECU) A system that allows an individual with limited motor control to operate electrical devices such as telephones, room lights, and televisions

environmentally induced disorder An atypical condition that is environmentally induced, (for example, resulting from an environmental toxin such as lead)

equifinality The inability to predict how a given situation or event in the present will develop in the future

equilibrium reactions; equilibrium responses Automatic, reflexive, compensatory movements of body parts that restore and maintain the center of gravity over the base of support when either the center of gravity or the supporting surface is displaced; complex postural reactions that involve righting reactions with rotation and diagonal patterns and are essential for volitional movement and mobility; responses that begin at 6 months and persist throughout the lifetime

evaluation The process of using formal and informal measures to quantify an individual's occupational performance in the areas of gross motor, fine motor, cognitive, sensory, and activities of daily living function

exacerbation Worsening of illness symptoms; flare ups

exceptional educational need (EEN) The determination that a disability or handicapping condition exists and interferes with the child or adolescent's ability to participate in an educational program

exploratory behavior   Behavior that is intrinsically motivating and is engaged in for its own sake; Reilly's first hierarchical stage of play that involves pleasurable sensory experiences

extension   Straightening a joint or increasing the angle of a joint

facilitation   Planned, graded physical guidance techniques used to improve movement coordination by increasing inadequate muscle tone, altering sensory responsiveness, or altering behavioral states (for example, hands-on facilitation techniques that are targeted at key postural points such as the shoulders, trunk, and hips)

fading assistance   A method of grading an activity by gradually reducing the level of assistance given until the individual performs a task independently

family adaptation   The reactions and responses of families to new events or crises; family adjustment

family boundaries   The set of behaviors, emotions, and topics of discussion permissible within a given subsystem; family limits

family hierarchies   The categorization of family members according to status; establishes which family members have power and authority

family life cycle   Developmental phases of the family from beginning to end

family resources   The physical, social, or financial support available to a family

family rules   The spoken or unspoken patterns that define order in the family

family subsystem   System of subunits within the family that consists of different individuals with distinct functions and relationships

family system   Interactive system that involves a group of two or more people who provide the child's primary nurturing environment

feeding   Supplying nourishment; giving food to

fetal alcohol syndrome   A disorder that occurs as a result of excess alcohol consumption by the mother during pregnancy; includes birth defects such as cardiac, cranial, facial, and neural abnormalities with associated delays in physical and mental growth

fine motor skill   The ability to use the small muscles of the body, especially the hand muscles, to perform tasks

fixing   Holding an area of the body tightly; used by individuals with limited strength or low muscle tone to aid stability; can result in movement restrictions

flexion   Bending; decreasing the angle of a joint

flight into health   A voluntary suppression of symptoms that resembles a sudden recovery from a disorder

flow of play   Refers to the ease of play; feeling totally absorbed in play and therefore being unaware of the passing of time; continuity of play

fluctuating tone   Irregular changes in muscle tone from one degree of muscle tension to another (for example, from hypotonic to hypertonic)

forward chaining   A way to grade an activity in which an individual learns each step from the beginning; begins with the individual starting the sequence and ends with the occupational therapy practitioner finishing what the individual has not yet learned

framing   The giving and receiving of social cues that mark a given situation as playful; formulates the basic structure of play and provides others with the message, "this is play"

free appropriate public education (FAPE)   Free public education that is mandated for all children and adolescents who have disabilities and are between 3 and 21 years of age

freedom from rules   The capacity to exercise choice or free will; usual course of action or behavior; during play, refers to spontaneity and absence or flexibility of rules in play

freedom stander   A stander that provides minimal support at the trunk, hips, and knees to allow an individual to develop balance and equilibrium

freedom to suspend reality   The ability to participate in "make-believe" or pretend activities; the ability to create new play situations and interact with materials, space, and people in ways that are fluid, flexible, and not bound to the constraints of real life

functional independence   The ability to perform activities of daily living and instrumental activities of daily living, work and productive activities, and play and leisure activities without assistance from other people

fussy baby syndrome   Condition in which the infant is easily upset and given to bouts of ill temper; associated with infants who have sensory regulatory disorders

games with rules   Play activities that require the players or participants to engage in explicit types of conduct, actions, or procedures

gene   A segment on a chromosome that transmits hereditary characteristics

general sensory disorganization   Disorders in which sensory systems are providing inaccurate information; may be associated with impairments in the tactile, vestibular, or auditory systems; associated with infants who are characterized as "fussy babies"

generalization   The ability to perform specific tasks in various environments

genetic conditions   Disorders that occur as a result of abnormal or absent genes

gestation   The period of time from conception to birth during which the fetus develops in the mother's uterus; pregnancy

glenohumeral tightness Excessive tautness or tightness between the glenoid area of the shoulder blade and the humerus of the upper arm; occurs when the shoulder blade is not free to move separately from the upper arm because of fixing or high muscle tone

goniometer A tool for measuring range of motion or movement at a particular joint

goniometry The study or measurement of joint motion

grading activities Changing one or more aspects of a task (usually by increasing or decreasing demands) to make it easier or harder to perform; modifying activities

gravity A physical force that draws all matter toward the earth's center; in varying degrees, a force that is resisted by all humans' upward motions

gross motor skills Activities that require the use of the larger body muscles (shoulder, hips, and knees)

growth Development; increase in size

gustatory The sense of taste; a powerful sense that produces an immediate recall effect

habilitation The act of helping an individual learn new skills

half kneel position Positioned with one leg in a kneeling position (with the hip in neutral) and the other in a front kneeling position (with the hip in 90 degrees of flexion)

hallucination A sensory (that is, auditory, visual, tactile, gustatory, or olfactory) perception that is incompatible with reality (that is, no evidence of the presence of external stimuli supports the perception)

handling techniques Methods of providing specific sensory input to individuals with atypical muscle tone, posture, and movement

head-eye dissociation Also known as *separation of head and eye movements*; the ability to move the eyes independently without moving the head

hearing impairment A disorder in the auditory system that may be a sensorineural or a conductive disorder; are relationships among hearing impairments and the vestibular system, balance, and chronic otitis

hemiplegia A term describing the distribution of affected muscles in individuals with cerebral palsy in which only the musculature on one side of the body is affected

high-technology devices Devices that are expensive and not readily available, such as computers, environmental control units, and powered wheelchairs

home care agency An agency that contracts with nurses and practitioners to provide home-based services

huffing Inhaling toxic substances by breathing them through the nose; seen in substance-related disorders

hydrocephalus Increased accumulation of cerebrospinal fluid within the ventricles of the brain

hypersensitivity Increased awareness of sensory input; may be an aversive response

hypertonicity Abnormally increased muscle tone associated with atypical postural alignment and decreased range of motion at joints; also known as *high tone* or *spasticity*

hypotonicity Abnormally decreased muscle tone associated with atypical postural alignment and excessive range of motion at joints; also known as *low tone* or *flaccidity*

hypoxia A deficiency of oxygen in the body tissues

idiopathic Of unknown cause

iliotibial band (ITB) The very long, tendinous portion of the tensor fascia latae muscle

inclusion The act of including; used in inclusion models, which are based on the premise that students with special needs should be educated in a regular classroom (instead of a self-contained classroom) with support personnel or services provided in that classroom (instead of pull-out services)

Indian sitting A means of sitting in which the legs are bent and crossed over each other

individual educational program (IEP) The written educational plan developed by the IEP team that includes the students' strengths and weaknesses as well as annual goals with short-term objectives

individual family's service plan (IFSP) The written intervention plan that is developed by the IFSP team with a focus on family priorities and resources

infancy The period of life beginning with birth and lasting through 18 months of age; babyhood

infection control Compliance with Occupational Safety and Health Administration (OSHA) guidelines, which include proper hand washing and use of personal protective equipment and clothing, to prevent the spread of infectious diseases

in-hand manipulation Moving objects in the hand

inhibition Planned, graded physical guidance techniques used to reduce excessive muscle tone, calm overly excited behavioral states, and decrease sensory hypersensitivity

inservice training *See* continuing education

intelligence quotient (IQ) A ratio of tested mental age to chronological age that is usually expressed as a quotient (that is, the result of dividing one number by another) and multiplied by 100; determined by using a standardized test that measures an individual's ability to form concepts, solve problems, acquire information, reason, and learn

interdisciplinary team A team consisting of two or more disciplines or professions that are considered distinct

interest Curiosity or concern about something; attention to something

internal control The extent to which individuals are in charge of their own actions and the outcome of an activity

intrinsic motivation A prompt to action that comes from within the individual; drive to action that is rewarded by doing the activity itself rather than some external reward

itinerant teacher; itinerant practitioner A teacher or practitioner who travels

just right challenge Therapy that challenges an individual to achieve by using activities that are not too hard or too easy

juvenile rheumatoid arthritis A chronic disorder that begins in childhood and is characterized by stiffness and inflammation of the joints, weakness, loss of mobility, and deformity

kinesthesia The internal awareness of the excursion (amount) and direction of joint movement provided by receptors in the muscles and joints

kneel position A posture in which both knees are bent and the hips are in neutral

knowledge The acquisition of information or facts about reality

kyphosis Excessive backward spinal curve of the trunk; humpback

learned helplessness A situation in which individuals become needy or dependent as a direct result of having all their tasks performed by their caregiver, who does not encourage or expect independence

least restrictive environment (LRE) A classroom setting with minimal limitations; associated with the premise that children with disabilities have the right to be with nondisabled children

legitimate tools Instruments that are in accordance with established and accepted standards for a profession or discipline

leisure Freedom from the demands of work; engaging in a nonobligatory activity that is intrinsically motivating during free time

level of arousal The amount of alertness and attention needed for an activity; must be at the optimum level for learning to take place

level of severity The relative degree of involvement or disability

level of support The relative degree of assistance required by an individual who is disabled

life cycle events The events that typically occur during an individual's life

life signs Changes in key indicators (for example, color, respiration, body temperature, extremity movements) that can be noted by a practitioner's visual, auditory, and tactile systems

light-technology (low-technology) devices Devices that are inexpensive, easy to obtain, and simple to make

long sitting A sitting position in which the hips are bent and the knees are straight with the legs in front of the body

long-term care Care that is provided in a residential facility when a family or primary caregiver is unable meet an individual's medical needs; includes the goals of providing appropriate medical care and therapeutic intervention

long-term goal The expected outcome of the occupational therapy process

lordosis An excessive forward curve of the lower spine

mainstreaming Derived from the word *mainstream*—the prevailing current or direction of influence; the practice of having students with special needs spend part of their school day in a regular classroom with nondisabled peers

major depressive disorder A mental disorder characterized by feelings of sadness or irritability, anhedonia, significant weight change, change in sleep patterns, restlessness or feeling phasically "slowed down," feelings of worthlessness, difficulty concentrating, fatigue, and thoughts of suicide

mandate An authoritative command; a formal command from a superior court or official to an inferior one

manual muscle testing Method of assessing the strength of muscles based on their specific actions

medical system A group of interacting, interrelated, and interdependent services provided under the direction of a physician

meningitis An inflammation of the membranes of the spinal cord or brain

mental disorder A disorder that manifests in psychological or behavioral symptoms and functional impairments

mental retardation Below-normal intellectual functioning that develops before birth or in the first year of life; results in impaired learning, social adjustments, and atypical development

microencephaly An abnormally small brain associated with disorders such as fetal alcohol syndrome

middle childhood The period of development that extends from approximately 6 years of age to puberty (that is, 12 to 14 years of age)

mild mental retardation A category of mental retardation in which the individuals have a subaverage intelligence quotient (ranging from 55 to 69) and typically require intermittent support; generally allows individuals to master academic skills ranging from third to seventh grade (although more slowly than other individuals)

mobility device Equipment that enables individuals with disabilities to move independently from one location to another

modeling Demonstrating behaviors to another person

moderate mental retardation   A category of mental retardation in which the individuals have a subaverage IQ (ranging from 40 to 54) and typically require some level of support as adults; generally allows individuals to master academic skills at the second-grade level (although significantly more slowly than other individuals)

mood   The persistent, sustained emotion that affects the perception of the world

mood disorder   A mental disorder characterized by a disturbance in mood

morphogenesis   The theory that systems tend to evolve and adapt to the larger environment

morphostatis   The theory that systems tend to maintain the status quo, or stay the same

motor control   The unconscious ability to make continuous postural adjustments and regulate movement; controlled by complex neurological systems working together; associated with two major models: (1) reflex or hierarchical models and (2) systems models, which attempt to explain motor control development and recovery

motor planning (praxis)   Conceiving and planning a novel motor act in response to an environmental demand; depends on adequate processing of tactile, proprioceptive, and vestibular sensory input

movement patterns   The organization of muscle activity components needed to produce various movements; can cause a change in position of the body as a whole or of a particular part (such as an extremity)

multicultural   Of, relating to, or including several cultures

multidisciplinary   Relating to multiple fields of study involved in the care of clients; suggests that although the various disciplines are working in collaboration, they are working in parallel, with each distinct discipline being accountable and responsible for its tasks and functions regarding client care

munching   An immature chewing motion that incorporates an up and down, vertical jaw movement

muscle grades   A relatively subjective means of assessing muscle strength

muscle strength   The ability of a muscle to contract against gravity and resistance

muscle tone   The degree of tension in muscle fibers while a muscle is at rest; the degree of elasticity and contractility in the muscle tissue; the resting state of a muscle in response to gravity and emotion

narrative progress note   A written note that factually states what occurred in a point-by-point manner

neonatal intensive care unit (NICU)   A unit that is specifically designed to address the acute medical needs of newborn infants; characterized by high-technology equipment

neonate   Newborn

neurodevelopmental treatment (NDT)   A treatment approach used with individuals who have central nervous system disorders; an approach developed by the Bobaths in the 1940s with the goal of promoting functional skill development by improving an individual's control and quality of movement

neurological conditions   Congenital or acquired disorders, such as spina bifida and Erb's palsy, that affect the central or peripheral nervous system

neurophysiological treatment approach   A treatment approach used with individuals who have central nervous system disorders; an approach developed by Margaret Rood in the 1940s with the goal of improving an individual's motor control through the application of specific sensory stimulation

nonverbal cues   Facial or bodily signs (such as smiling or frowning) that indicate thoughts, desires, or needs to another person (for example, a girl playing with a ball who smiles at her mother to indicate that she's happy playing with the ball)

normal   Occurring naturally; not deviating from the standard

normative versus nonnormative life cycle events   The usual and expected life events (such as birth, starting school, or adolescence) versus the unanticipated life events (such as frequent hospitalization of a young child or premature death of child or parent)

occupational performance model   A theoretical framework that occupational therapy practitioners use to develop priorities, plan treatment, and implement treatment; based on the premise that all individuals, including children, have the role or occupation of developing competence in the performance areas of activities of daily living, work and productive activities, and play and leisure activities

oculomotor skills   Multiple coordinated eye movements produced by eye muscles; also known as *ocular control* or *ocular motor skills*

olfactory   Pertaining to the sense of smell

oppositional defiant disorder   A mental disorder characterized by negative, hostile, defiant behaviors that exceed normal developmental behaviors

oral motor development   Maturation of the oral motor structures

orientation   Identifying person, place, time, and situation

orthopedic condition   A disorder that involves the skeletal system and associated muscles (that is, joints and ligaments)

orthotic device   A bracing system designed to control, correct, or compensate for bony deformities or muscle imbalance

palmar grasp   A means of holding an object in the palm of the hand; used by infants in ulnar orientation before radial orientation

parallel play   Play during which young children are in close proximity to each other and engaging in similar activities but not interacting with one another

passive appraisal   Ignoring a situation in hopes it will go away

passive range of motion (PROM)   Movement created at a joint by an external force

pectus excavation   A depression in the chest area

pediatric intensive care unit (PICU)   A unit that is specifically designed for infants and children who require highly skilled medical care

perception   The recognition and proper interpretation of stimuli received in the brain from the senses

perceptual coping strategies   Defining events, situations, and crises in ways that promote adaptation

performance areas   Functional abilities that are necessary to perform activities of daily living, work and productive activities, and play or leisure activities; a broad category of human activities that are typically a part of daily life

performance components   Sensorimotor, cognitive, psychosocial, or psychological elements

performance contexts   Situations or factors that impact an individual's ability to engage in daily living activities, work and productive activities, and play or leisure activities

periods of development   Specific developmental stages categorized by age; include infancy, early childhood, middle childhood, adolescence, and adulthood

peripheral nervous system (PNS)   The portion of the nervous system outside the central nervous system (for example, the brachial plexus that innervates the arms)

pincer grasp   A type of pinch in which the thumb opposes the index finger; used to pick up small objects

play   Any spontaneous activity or organized activity that provides enjoyment, entertainment, amusement, or diversion; an experience that involves intrinsic motivation, with emphasis on the process rather than product and internal rather than external control; a pretend experience that takes place in a safe, nonthreatening environment

play goals   Outcomes of play during the occupational therapy process

play modifications; play adaptations   Changes in materials or activities to promote successful play for children who have disabilities

playfulness   Adjective for *play*; a behavioral or personality trait characterized by flexibility, manifest joy, and spontaneity

positioning   Specific ways of placing an individual to maintain postural alignment, provide postural stability, facilitate normal patterns of movement, and increase the individual's interaction with the environment; can include the use of adaptive equipment

postural alignment   A symmetrical position of body parts or the body

postural control   The ability to regulate body position

postural stability   The ability to maintain equilibrium and balance or return to the original position after displacement from the position

posture   The position of the body with respect to the surrounding space; determined and maintained by activation of righting and equilibrium reactions, proprioception, and coordination of the various muscles that move body parts

powered mobility equipment   Battery-operated equipment that allows an individual with a disability to move from one location to another

practice model   A frame of reference that is used to direct the occupational therapy process; helps the occupational therapy practitioner identify problems and develop solutions

praxis   The ability to conceptualize, organize, and execute nonhabitual, novel motor tasks

prematurity   The state of an infant born any time before completion of the 37th week of gestation

preservice training   Instruction that prepares an individual to provide a specific service

pretend play   Play that involves symbolic games, imagination, and suspension of reality

prevocational evaluation   Testing of activities of daily living, learning abilities, and physical capacities needed to begin job training to earn a living

primitive reflexes   A group of reflexive movement patterns that begin emerging at birth and continue until approximately 4 to 6 months; reflexes that are controlled primarily by the lower brain centers; reflexes that enable the body to respond to influences such as head or body position mechanically and automatically with a change in muscle tone; reflexes that provide the developing infant with numerous consistent posture and movement patterns for early interaction with the environment

principles   Fundamental truths; rules; foundations

profound mental retardation   A category of mental retardation in which individuals have a subaverage IQ (that is, below 25) and require pervasive support throughout life and extensive assistance for activities of daily living; generally results in physical disorders in addition to cognitive limitations

progress note   Written or electronically recorded documentation of an individual's change in status or advancement toward goals

pronation Movement of the forearm so that the palm of the hand faces the floor

prone Position in which the individual is lying on the stomach

prone board; prone stander A standing device that promotes lower extremity weightbearing and proper alignment while standing, with the majority of the individual's weight being supported by the anterior surface of the trunk

prone on elbows A position in which the individual lies on the stomach while propped on the elbows

prone on extended arms A position in which the individual lies on the stomach with the elbows straight and the weight on open hands

prone extension A posture in which the individual lies on the stomach in a face-down (prone) position with the head, arms, hips, and legs straight (extended) upward against gravity and the trunk arched so that the arms and legs are above the supporting surface; position that is similar to the superhero Superman's posture while he is flying

proprioception A sensory system that has receptors in the muscles, joints, and other internal tissues that provide internal awareness about the position of body parts

prosthesis An artificial replacement for a lost body part such as an arm, a leg, or an eye

protective extension responses Postural reactions that are used to stop a fall or prevent injury when equilibrium reactions cannot do so; responses that involve straightening of the arms or legs toward a supporting surface

psychiatrist A medical doctor who specialized in the diagnosis, treatment, and prevention of mental disorders

psychosocial skills and psychological components Performance components that refer to an individual's ability to interact in society and process emotions; include psychological, social, and self-management skills

puberty The stage of adolescence characterized by physical and hormonal changes during which an individual becomes physiologically capable of sexual reproduction

pull-out service model Provision of special services outside of a child's classroom

purging Eliminating food through self-induced vomiting; seen in eating disorders

purposeful activities Tasks that have meaning or anticipated outcomes

quadriplegia A term describing the distribution of affected muscles in individuals with cerebral palsy in which the musculature in all four extremities is affected; may also affect musculature of the neck and facial areas

quadruped position A weightbearing position on hands and knees

radial-ulnar dissociation Also known as *separation of skill and stability sides of the hand*; separate, independent control of movements on each side of the hand in which the thumb (radial) side is used for skilled finger manipulations and the little finger (ulnar) side is used for strength and stability

range of motion (ROM) The amount of movement available at a specified joint; measured by occupational therapy practitioners with a goniometer

readiness skills Those abilities in the performance components and areas that are necessary for engaging in educational, home management, care of others, and vocational activities

reading the child in context A moment-to-moment observation and analysis of a child's relationship to social and physical environments and the child's responses to the therapeutic process; a tool that helps occupational therapy practitioners plan and implement treatment

reevaluation Retest; a means of determining whether occupational therapy intervention is effective and should continue

referral A request for a screening or evaluation to determine whether an individual would benefit from occupational therapy services

referral network Derived from *refer*—to send or direct for treatment, aid, information, or decision—and *network*—an interconnected or interrelated chain, group, or system; any individual, organization, or agency that has concerns regarding a child's development

reflex An involuntary posture or movement that occurs in response to a specific stimulus not under conscious control

reflex, or hierarchical, model One of two major models used to understand motor control; suggests that purposeful movement is initiated only when the individual experiences a need to move and proposes that motor learning occurs best when an individual engages in repetition of the same task during frequent and regular practice

reframing Redefining an event or situation so that it is manageable and controllable

rehabilitative practice model A frame of reference that focuses on returning an individual to the highest level of functional independence after an injury or disease and teaching compensatory methods for performing activities; a practice model that is appropriate for many disorders encountered by the pediatric occupational therapy practitioner

related services Special services that may be required for a child to benefit from the special education program; include occupational therapy, physical therapy, social work, school health services, parent counseling and training, speech, assistive technology, transportation, and psychological services

remediation   A remedy; correction of a fault or problem

remission   Lessening of symptoms of an illness

resource classroom   A small classroom in which a child with a disability may spend part of the school day obtaining additional help or support in areas of academic weakness

retinopathy   A pathological disorder of the retina, which is the delicate, multilayered, light-sensitive membrane that lines the inner eyeball

righting reactions   Postural reactions that occur in response to a change in the position of the head and body in space; reactions that bring the head and trunk back into an upright position in space; involve extension, flexion, abduction, adduction, and lateral flexion reactions; begin to emerge between 6 and 9 months of age and persist throughout life

ring sitting   A sitting position in which the legs form a circle with the soles of the feet approximating each other

rotary chewing   A mature pattern of mastication or chewing solids in preparation for swallowing; chewing movement in which the mandible moves in a rotary pattern to grind the solids and mix the bolus with saliva

rotation   Movement around a central axis (with motions in diagonal planes commonly being incorporated by most mature movements); type of movement pattern that greatly increases movement options

rote learning   The acquisition of behaviors that become routine (although not always fully understood or carried out with sincerity); learning that usually occurs through memorization or repetition

rough housing   Physical gross motor play; play that is characterized by gentle wrestling

scapular winging   A term for a shoulder blade that does not rest against the posterior rib cage, with the vertebral border flaring away from the trunk

scoliosis   An abnormal lateral curvature of the spine

screening   An informal or formal measure that determines an individual's need for occupational therapy evaluation and intervention

seizure disorder   A condition in which an individual has sudden attacks, spasms, or convulsions (as occurs in individuals with epilepsy)

self-contained classroom   A specially designated classroom in which students spend the majority of their school day; primarily used with students who have significant cognitive or behavioral disabilities that limit their ability to participate in regular classroom activities

self-esteem   Pride in oneself; self-respect

self-mutilating behavior   Deliberate self-injury

sensorimotor components   Performance components that refer to a child's ability to receive input, process information, and produce output; include sensory, motor, and neuromusculoskeletal skills

sensorimotor play   Play that focuses on movement and sensations and does not involve the elements of make believe or socially shared rules

sensorimotor practice model   A frame of reference that focuses on using sensory input to change muscle tone or movement patterns; a practice model used with children and adolescents who have central nervous system disorders

sensory integration (SI)   Organization of sensory information for use; a theory and intervention originally developed by Dr. A. Jean Ayres; classical use involves suspension equipment

sensory regulatory treatment approach   An approach that expands the original work of Dr. A. Jean Ayres in the area of sensory integration; a treatment approach with the primary goal of promoting sensory regulation (an individual's ability to accurately respond to sensory input from many experiences) and sensory modulation (an individual's ability to accurately perceive sensory input and adjust motor responses accordingly) in children and adolescents

separation anxiety disorder   A mental disorder characterized by extreme anxiety that develops when a child or adolescent anticipates separation or is separated from home or those individuals to whom the child or adolescent is most attached

service competency   The process that ensures two individual occupational therapy practitioners will obtain equivalent results when administering a specific assessment or providing intervention

session objectives   The desired outcomes of a specific treatment session; mini goals or objectives that are steps or building blocks toward short-term objectives

severe mental retardation   A category of mental retardation in which individuals have a subaverage IQ (ranging from 25 to 39) and typically require extensive support throughout life; generally allows individuals to learn basic self-care skills, although they are unable to live independently as adults

shaken baby syndrome   A syndrome resulting from an infant being jerked violently back and forth

short-term objectives   Interim steps or building blocks that are used to reach long-term goals; statements describing skills that should be mastered in a relatively short period

side-lyer   A piece of adaptive equipment used to position a child on the side, which promotes eye-hand regard and brings hands together at midline

side sitting   A sitting position in which the knees point in the opposite direction of the feet and the majority of the body weight is on the knee side

skill   A learned action or behavior

sniffing   Taking in toxic substances by inhaling them through the nose

SOAP note   A method of documentation that contains the following subject areas: *s*ubjective (includes thoughts, feelings, verbalizations), *o*bjective (includes session goal and what occurred), *a*ssessment (includes summary of objectives), and *p*lan (includes future objectives and session goals)

solitary play   A type of play in which the infant or young child is distanced from peers and does not interact with them while playing

spasticity   Increased muscle tone; hypertonicity; often occurs when a stretch reflex is activated in a muscle

spica cast   A cast that is placed on a patient's lower body after certain surgeries or injuries

spina bifida   Split spine (a common disorder seen by the occupational therapy practitioner); comprises three types: occulta, meningocele, and myelomeningocele; common to treat children with myelomeningocele-type spina bifida because of its associated sensory and motor deficits

splinter skill   A specific, often complex task mastered by a child who lacks the underlying developmental capabilities to perform the task; usually attained through compensatory methods and practice rather than by remediating the underlying developmental components

spontaneity   Acting without effort or premeditation; driven by internal forces

states   Classified in six categories for the newborn by Brazelton: deep sleep, light sleep, drowsy or semidozing, alert or active awake, fussy, and crying

subacute care   Level of care that is in between the stages of acute and long-term care and is based on the provision of rehabilitation services; appropriate care for an individual who no longer needs acute care but is still progressing and is not ready for long-term care placement

substance abuse   A pattern of behavior in which the use of substances has adverse consequences

substance dependence   A pattern of behavior in which substances continue to be used despite serious cognitive, behavioral, and physiological symptoms

substance-related disorder   A mental disorder resulting from inappropriate use of drugs, toxins, or medications

suck   To draw (usually liquids) into the mouth by movements of the tongue and lips, creating a suction or a partial vacuum

suckle   To draw liquids into the mouth by a forward and backward movement of the tongue as is done during breastfeeding

suck-swallow-breathe (s-s-b) synchrony   A skill used continuously throughout life that allows an individual to breathe while simultaneously and unconsciously sucking in and swallowing food, drink, or saliva; a skill whose disruption can interfere profoundly with development

supervision   The process of directing and overseeing the performance of others

supination   Movement of the forearm so that the palm of the hand faces toward the ceiling

supine   A position in which the individual is lying on the back

supine flexion   A posture in which the individual lies on the back in a face-up (supine) position with the head, arms, and legs bent (flexed) upward against gravity

supine stander   A piece of standing equipment that is used to promote lower extremity weightbearing and development of flexor control in the neck and trunk; a piece of equipment in which an individual is positioned while lying on the back and after being secured is pulled into a more upright position with a crank

suspension (from school)   Restriction from attending school for a specific period; typically results from violation of school rules

suspension equipment   Equipment that hangs to allow free movement; used during sensory integration therapy and includes bolster swings, platform swings, ladders, and hammocks

switch   A device used to break or open an electric circuit; an item that connects, disconnects, or diverts an electric current; used with children who have disabilities to promote successful interactions with computers, battery-operated toys, and powered mobility systems

symbolic play   Playing that has an imaginative component, involving make-believe or pretend activities; a type of play that depends on the child's ability to create mental representations of objects that are not present

symmetry   Alignment of the body such that the head is in midline, the trunk is straight, and weight is distributed equally on both sides of the body

systems model   One of the two major models used to understand motor control that involves the concepts of feed forward, or anticipatory postural activity; a model suggesting that posture and movement must be flexible and adaptable for an individual to perform a wide range of daily activities

tactile system   Pertaining to the sense of touch obtained through skin receptors

tandem walking   A pattern of walking during which the heel of one foot approximates the toes of the other foot

template (jig)   A guide for accuracy, usually made of plastic, metal, or wood

teratogen   Anything that causes the development of abnormal structures in an embryo and results in a severely deformed fetus

therapeutic use of self   The practitioner's conscious or unconscious use of personality traits and interactions as a tool to facilitate an individual's engagement in therapeutic activities

tic disorder A mental disorder characterized by tics

tics Involuntary and recurrent motor movements or vocalizations

tolerance A state that causes an individual to need to use larger amounts of a substance to obtain the desired results

tongue thrust A movement in which the tongue extends outside the lips, interferes with swallowing, and causes food to be pushed outside the mouth; often seen in individuals with cerebral palsy or Down syndrome

Tourette's syndrome A genetic condition characterized by vocal and motor tics

toxin A poisonous substance of animal or plant origin

transition The passage from one state, stage, or place to another; change

transitional movements Movements that are used to change positions; movements that typically developing infants use (but often very limited in atypically developing infants)

truancy Absence from school without permission; often seen in children with conduct disorder

typical Exhibiting qualities, traits, or characteristics that identify a group; not deviating from the standard or norm

universal design A concept associated with creating accessible environments

values Principles, standards, or qualities considered worthwhile or desirable

vaulting position Arching part of the body (often the back)

vestibular system A sensory system with inner ear receptors that is sensitive to changes of head position in space; affects level of arousal and muscle tone

vision Eyesight; faculty of sight

visual field The entire area that can be seen while the eye is fixing or gazing steadily at a target in the direct line of vision; involves holding the head steady or stable to support the eye control needed to locate, look at, and visually track objects

visual impairment A condition of decreased visual acuity or impaired processing of visual input

visual-motor skills Coordination of the eyes with the hands (or other body parts) such that the eyes guide precise controlled movements; also referred to as *visual-motor integration skills* and *eye-hand* or *eye-foot skills*

visual perception The ability to interpret and use what is being seen

visual tracking Following targets with smooth eye movements

vocational evaluation Testing of all areas of development (physical, psychological, social, and environmental) to determine an individual's ability to be employed

voluntary movement Consciously controlled movements

web space The area between the thumb and index finger that needs to be wide open in a drawing or writing grasp for the fingertips to use sensory feedback to gauge pressure accurately

wedge A piece of positioning equipment that is thick at one end and tapered at the opposite end; used most often to position an individual with motor control problems in a prone position on extended arms

weightbearing Loading part or all of the body onto the arms or legs or distributing the body weight through all extremities (for example, the quadruped position); occurs on the legs and feet in the standing position and on the knees in a kneeling position

weightshifting Movement away from the body's upright center of gravity; used to elicit righting and equilibrium reactions that restore or maintain upright postures

within functional limits (WFL) A term used to indicate that an individual has the necessary muscle strength, muscle tone, and range of motion to perform daily living activities, play activities, and work and productive activities independently

within normal limits (WNL) A term used to designate that performance in the performance components is normal for an individual

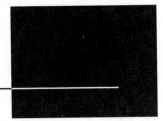

Index

A

AAMR Adaptive Behavior Scales
  (ABS-RC:2; ABS-S:2), 151*t*
ABC School Supply, Inc., 288
Ablenet, 311
AccuCorp, Inc., 286
Achievement, in play development, 101
Achievement Products, 288
Acquired conditions
  AIDS, 184, 185
  latex allergies, 185
Acquired immunodeficiency syndrome
  (AIDS), 184, 185
Active range of motion (AROM), 5, 136
  in Erb's palsy, 174
  in JRA, 164*b*
  play activities for, 301
Activities
  age-appropriate, 5, 60
  purposeful, 198
Activities of daily living (ADLs), 5
  in atypical development, 59
  in cerebral palsy, 122-123
  definition of, 91
  dressing skills, 96-98, 229-240
  examples of, 91*b*
  feeding and eating skills, 91-96, 220-229
  functional communication, 254-268
  functional mobility, 268-270
  grading, 215-216
  grooming and hygiene, 99, 240-245,
    245-248
  health maintenance, 248-252
  living skills checklist, 248, 249
  in mental retardation, 136-137
  in occupational performance model, 213
  in OT evaluation, 33*b*

Activities of daily living (ADLs)—cont'd
  rationale for, 91
  safety skills, 271-272
  sexual expression, 272
  socialization, 252-254
Activity analysis, 106
  child- and family-focused, 198, 200
  process of, 198
  task-focused, 198, 199
  in treatment planning, 214-215
Activity synthesis, 200-201
Adaptation
  activity, 201
  family, 19
  play, 307
Adapting activities, in treatment
    planning, 216
Adaptive functioning skills
  defined, 129
  in intervention plan, 208
  in PDD, 207
ADD. *see* Attention deficit disorder
Addiction, 146
ADHD. *see* Attention deficit hyperactivity
    disorder
ADLs. *see* Activities of daily living
Adolescence
  cerebral palsy in, 122
  cognitive integration in, 85
  emotional development during, 81*t*
  language in, 85
  normal development during, 61
  physiological adaptation in, 85
  play skills in, 103
  psychosocial skills in, 85-86
  readiness skills for, 106
  sensorimotor skills in, 85
Adolescents
  major depressive disorder in, 152*b*
  mental disorders in, 141
  mental retardation in, 133, 135

Adolescents—cont'd
  prevocational activities of, 278
  self-esteem assessment of, 150, 151*t*
  sexual expression by, 272
  social skills at work of, 279
Adrian's Closet, 285
Age-appropriate activities, 5, 60
Agenesis of the Corpus Callosum (ACC)
    Network, 190
Aggressiveness, and mental retardation,
    135
AIDS (acquired immunodeficiency
    syndrome), 184, 185
AIDS-related complex (ARC), 184
Ainsworth, M., 79
Akinetic (drop) seizures, 176*t*
Alberta Infant Motor Scale (AIMS), 189
Alcohol consumption, during pregnancy,
    184
Alert Program for Regulation of Arousal,
    274
Allen Cognitive Level Test (ACL), 151*t*
Allergies
  chemical, 185-186
  food, 185-186, 250
  latex, 185
  susceptibility to, 186*b*
All the Write News Dixon Ticonderoga
    Co., 288
Amelia, transverse, 161*t*
American Association on Mental
    Retardation (AAMR), 131
American Foundation for the Blind, 190
American Occupational Therapy
    Association (AOTA), 5, 15, 291
American Psychiatric Association, 141
American sign language (ASL), 182
  catching, 179
  software for, 336
Americans with Disabilities Act
    (ADA;1990), 41*b*, 43, 331

Page numbers in italics indicate illustrations; *t* indicates tables; *b* indicates boxes.